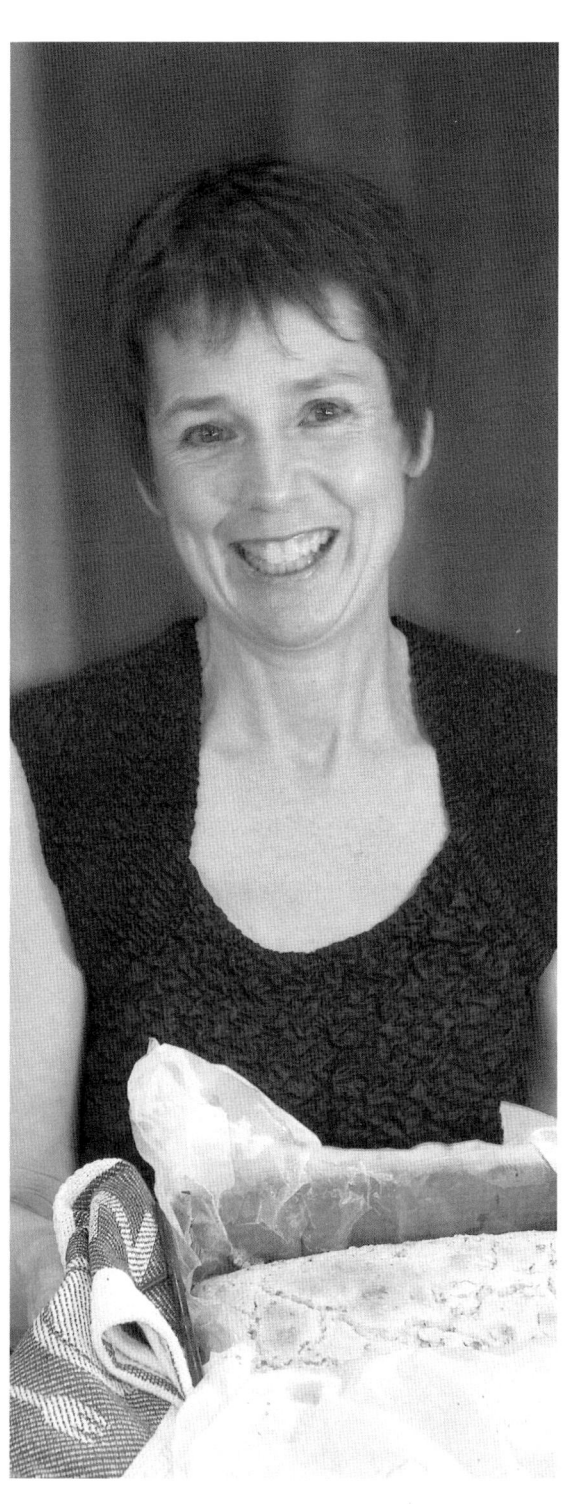

## Kathryn Ale)

D.Th.D., Adv. Dip.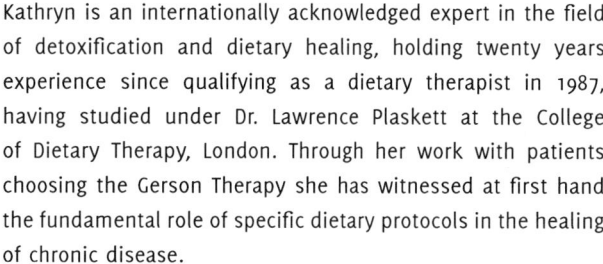

Kathryn is an internationally acknowledged expert in the field of detoxification and dietary healing, holding twenty years experience since qualifying as a dietary therapist in 1987, having studied under Dr. Lawrence Plaskett at the College of Dietary Therapy, London. Through her work with patients choosing the Gerson Therapy she has witnessed at first hand the fundamental role of specific dietary protocols in the healing of chronic disease.

Over the last ten years Kathryn has lectured widely in the UK, USA and Australia, developed training packages for both professionals and members of the public, and is the author of *Get a Life, the Detoxification Diet Made Easy!* - the forerunner to this revised edition. In 1999 Kathryn joined the board of directors of the Gerson Institute with responsibilities for research and development and practitioner training. She developed the training curriculum for the Gerson Therapy™ and produced *Nutritional Healing: a Patient Management Handbook,* described by Charlotte Gerson as "the 'bible' of the nutritional healer of the future."

Kathryn is also a recognised thought leader in the growing trend of the expert patient, where governments around the world are setting the trend toward the patient self-managing their chronic condition. As a consequence, a consumer-centric model of healthcare is now evolving in which patients seek to form partner-relationships with their primary health-care workers. This assists them in best practice management strategies that more closely reflect their own criteria for a best clinical outcome. Invariably strategies involve the combining of complementary and medical treatments, and medical professionals are increasingly required to have a working awareness of complementary protocols in treatment.

Kathryn is now based in Australia where her self-management courses have been well received by both professional and public sectors, with positive feedback from participants who are now equipped to either self-manage their own healing program and make informed decisions in treatment, or to case-manage those of their patients.

# DIETARY HEALING

*the complete detox program*

Kathryn Alexander

...lexander 2007
...xander.com.au

All rights reserved. No part of this publication may be reproduced, stored in or introduced into a retrieval system, or transmitted in any form or by any means (electronic, mechanical, photocopying, recording or otherwise) without the prior written permission of both the copyright owner and the publisher of this book.

Reprinted 2013

Editor:   Michael Berry
Book design:  Adrian Anderson & Kathryn Alexander
Cover design:  Penny Riddoch
Photography:  Penny Riddoch   www.digitalphotodesigns.com
Layout:  Steve Cook

National Library of Australia
Cataloguing-in-Publication data:

Alexander, Kathryn, 1954- .
Dietary healing : the complete detox program.

Rev. ed.
Includes index.
ISBN 9780980376289 (pbk.).

1. Diet therapy.  I. Title.

615.854

Disclaimer
*Dietary Healing, the complete detox program* does not constitute medical advice. If you require advice on any medical or related matter, the author and publishers of *Dietary Healing, the complete detox program* suggest you seek that advice from a qualified professional. As far as the law allows, all people connected with the writing, editing and publishing of this book disclaim all liability arising from the negligence of writer and publisher of *Dietary Healing, the complete detox program*.

# Contents

Foreword — vii
Author's preface — x
My story — xiii

**Part One — Why does it work?**
1. Why detox? — 21
2. Salt and dairy – the de-vitalisers — 29
3. The acid/alkaline balance — 53

**Part Two — How will it work for me?**
4. Vitality & healing — 71
5. Liver cleansing — 93
6. Regeneration and blood sugar control — 157
7. Nutritional supplements – do we need them? — 173

**Part Three — The diet**
8. The diet – not for the faint-hearted — 191
9. The nitty-gritty – shopping & menu planning — 203

**Part Four — The recipes** — 215

Glossary — 268
Index — 274

# Foreword

**by Dr. Lawrence Plaskett**  BA (Cantab), PhD (London), CChem, FRIC

It is with much pleasure that I write to tell you, Kathryn's readers, a little about the background, about Kathryn and about the book itself.

Kathryn has taken the material of naturopathic nutrition and made it come alive and real to anyone who wants to avail him or herself of this unique approach to health. In my view, this edition is a very considerable step forward over the previous edition in the depth and comprehensiveness of its presentation and I congratulate her upon the work. One can only achieve this level of writing in the subject through assiduous learning and through long-term dedication to the practice of the art.

I first met Kathryn in the 1980s when she joined a class in my college in London to study nutritional medicine. She soon became one of the most enthusiastic and accomplished students in the group. It seemed clear to me that she would go far. I did not know then how far that would be.

The work that Kathryn teaches and practices is naturopathic. She does not use all the modalities of treatment that are available to naturopaths – there are so many of these that no one could do that. What stands out in her work is the fullest use of, and adherence to, naturopathic principles while working mainly within the nutritional aspects of the subject.

Today, the American Association of Naturopathic Physicians defines naturopathic medicine as "a distinct system of primary health care - an art, science, philosophy and practice of diagnosis, treatment and prevention of illness". Further, they say, "Naturopathic physicians are primary health care practitioners, whose diverse techniques include modern and traditional, scientific and empirical methods". They see illness as "a series of events that can be changed, or redirected toward order and balance".

Within naturopathy there is strong emphasis upon this regaining of "balance", upon healing being a natural process that only needs to be helped in order to restore health; there is talk of an "inner wisdom that guides internal physical processes" and of the "healing power of nature". These ideas led most of the early naturopaths to speak of the "Life Force" as being a subtle force within the body. The use of the term "Life Force", when it is conceived as an esoteric energy, may well be controversial today, but it can be equated with that "inner wisdom" and with an "inherent self-organising and healing process of living systems".

Naturopathy itself has a long history as there have been essentially detoxifying and revitalising therapies of some sort in most of the ancient civilisations and in most countries of the world. The term 'naturopathy' was not coined, however, until 1895 and it has its origins as a medical system within the hydrotherapy and spa movement of the nineteenth century, most particularly in Britain, Germany and the United States. This was the work of such great names as Louis Kuhne, Vincenz Priessnitz, Father Sebastian Kniepp, David Urquhart, Johann Schroth, Russell Trall, John Harvey Kellogg, Benedict Lust, Henry Lindlahr and Bernarr Macfadden. It was these men and more, who established the ground rules of the subject as it has been passed on to the present day.

Naturopathic concepts and naturopaths have had a hard job living alongside the orthodox medicine of the second half of the twentieth century, which has often been actively hostile. However, modern medical researchers, in particular modern medical biochemists, have long been generating peer-reviewed scientific research that is very fully supportive of naturopathic principles. Perhaps the researchers themselves do not see it that way, so it is a matter of interpretation. However, today we are aware of and can identify and quantify the enzyme systems of the body that carry out detoxification. We know what minerals, vitamins and other cofactors are needed for their optimal function. The literature of this, and related topics that impinge upon naturopathic nutrition is vast, running to tens of thousands, if not hundreds of thousands of published papers. This is just one way in which naturopathy and science are beginning to join hands in the fight against chronic illness. The future, in my view, lies in naturopathy as a fully scientific branch of medicine.

What Kathryn has done here is to describe and explain clearly what anybody who wishes can do to support their health by these methods. I think that with this edition she has retained the appeal of the book to people without scientific knowledge whilst giving a greatly deepened account of how it all works within the body. I see the Law of Cure and several other important naturopathic laws running through the pages of the book alongside the now scientifically established mechanisms by which all of this happens. Therein there lies a very special value in this book.

Kathryn does not quote you all the research papers that support this work from all the medical and biochemical journals all over the world. She concentrates upon clear explanation. The sources of literature proof that are available are voluminous and convincing but quoting them all would make this work unreadable. She is known and will, I feel sure, become even better known, for a clear uncomplicated exposition that transmits these concepts to others and enables people to work with them. Today nutritional medicine has become a university subject in which one may work for an honours degree. For that you must know the literature and be able to quote it. What I most like about Kathryn's writing is that it focuses upon communicating the truly thrilling concepts of healing through naturopathic nutrition. These can fire people with an excitement about making oneself and other people well again and can enthuse people with the sheer discovery that one's body is not just a mechanical material entity, but, rather, is much more. All today's students of nutritional medicine should enjoy that aspect.

These days, I suppose, I have become a kind of "senior statesman" for nutritional medicine. But if I go back many years to when I was simply a scientist exploring this field that was new to me in "Alternative Medicine" I visited an acupuncturist, partly as a personal experiment. He treated two points on my legs that control the 'wood element' and which govern the liver and the gall bladder. It so happened that I arrived for the treatment with reddened and slightly bleary eyes after driving rather too many hundreds of miles. The treatment restored my eyes to normal liveliness and normal clarity within minutes. As an explorer in the field I was very impressed. I tell you of that experience and invite you to correlate it with Kathryn's large and detailed chapter on "Liver Cleansing".

With that I pass you on to Kathryn, now my very capable, gifted and experienced former student, to learn what you will of this marvellous subject and what you may be able to do for yourself and others.

Lawrence Plaskett
Bude, Cornwall, England
29th April 2007


Dr. Lawrence Plaskett graduated from Cambridge University, UK, with a first class degree in Natural Sciences in 1956, specialising in biochemistry, and obtained his doctorate in 1960 from the University of London for his medical research on thyroid hormones, before taking a post as a Lecturer in Biochemistry at Edinburgh University Medical School (1960-65). He was appointed Research Director of the Brooke Bond Liebig Group (1965-74) and subsequently established his own Biotechnology Consultancy Company (1975-82) serving the food and energy industries. From the early 1970s he developed his interest in unorthodox approaches to clinical nutrition and Chinese medicine and he established a multi-disciplined alternative medicine clinic.

In 1982 Lawrence established his own college for nutritional practitioners where he was among the first to teach a wholistic approach to nutrition whereby his life-long experience, working in the borderlands between nutrition and medicine, enabled him to offer a synthesis between many fields that are not often brought together: nutrition, pathology, biochemistry, toxicology, pharmacology, cell biology, naturopathy and homoeopathy. His college continues to operate to this day with Lawrence as principal. Now known as The Plaskett International College (www.plaskett-international.com), it operates in 37 countries. Since 2004, Lawrence has been a visiting fellow and consultant to the Thames Valley University, UK, where his nutritional training course has been adopted as a university course leading to an honours degree.

Between 2002 and 2004 Lawrence was elected to different offices of The Nutritional Therapy Council, the UK's nascent regulatory body for the profession. He was at different times vice chair, acting chair and also chair of the educational sub-committee. He has also contributed to the work of the Expert Committee of the ANH (Alliance for Natural Health), a UK-based, not-for-profit campaign organisation, which works to promote and protect natural health care.

He has in all some 80 publications consisting of research papers, UK and US patent applications and scientific reports on his consulting assignments. He has written several books, many articles and newsletters on nutritional issues, and sections of his work have been translated into French, Spanish, Greek and Mandarin Chinese. His forthcoming book on Nutritional Cancer Therapy is soon to be published.

# Author's preface

Since the publication of *Get a Life: the Detoxification Diet Made Easy!* I have received many letters from people around the world whose lives have been changed, their health problems reversed and their physical and mental wellbeing restored through adopting my dietary approach to healing. It's not always easy changing life-style patterns on a long-term basis, but my readers unanimously praised the book for its simple explanations of how dietary healing works on a biochemical level and, more importantly, how to interpret their own case histories in order to plan their own program. As one reader says, "I sat and read your book from cover to cover last night. I don't have any background knowledge about biology, so I was pleasantly surprised to see how user friendly it was and pleased that I was able to understand a lot of the information and so begin to understand how my body works. It's only taken me this long! I will certainly recommend it to others."

So you can imagine that many readers have been eagerly awaiting a new updated version of that book. However, although I have expanded the text in a few areas to lend greater clarity, the principles governing detoxification and healing follow the natural laws of cure and do not change. Dietary healing programs follow the core principle of restoring the natural healing potential through the two-fold process of cellular detoxification and replenishment of nutrients. Symptoms of disease invariably arise as a consequence of cell adaptation to local conditions; so by changing the internal environment, symptoms may be reversed.

In today's climate, this simplistic approach falls short of the demand for scientifically proven methods of healing. Scientifically proven simply means that we know how and why a specific method or product produces specific effects. It does not automatically mean that it is good for you. However, clinically proven indicates that a method "works", where the overall outcome is beneficial and we see the reversal or improvement of symptoms, even if we don't scientifically understand how or why it has worked.

The following analogy will remind us of the importance of common sense and trusting what we see. Imagine a toxic, polluted lake where all the fish are sick or dying. Would you save the fish by feeding them supplements or high nutrient foods? Or would you clean the lake? Too often, we end up treating the symptoms of internal pollution, rather than removing the pollution itself. Dietary programs that treat both toxicity and nutrient deficiency have powerful and lasting effects on the individual. It's very simple really; once the toxic burden is released, the internal cellular environment is restored and a natural healing process occurs. The body knows how to heal itself; all you have to do is provide the right conditions.

Providing the right conditions at cellular level requires a wholistic approach to detoxification. We are not simply looking at liver and colon cleansing but the loosening and discharging of toxins from all the cells into the circulation. The clearance of toxins from the circulation via the liver and colon then occurs as a consequence of cellular cleansing.

Detoxification occurs at cell level when three basic dietary principles are rigorously applied:

- Salt-free diet (no added salt or condiments containing salt);
- High potassium and alkaline-forming foods (fruits and vegetables); and
- Protein-restriction (but not protein-deficient)

The combination of these dietary principles stimulates the cell to eliminate excess sodium and acidity along with its toxic load in exchange for potassium and a more favourable alkaline environment which supports oxygenation and hence cell vitality. The conditions are then laid for healing to occur. The body cannot heal when the environment is toxic or nutrient and oxygen-deprived.

You can begin to understand that these programs are not about modifying your existing diet but understanding the degree of dietary change that is required in order to secure a detoxification and healing, and that such programs are a long-term commitment. Depending upon your existing condition and the rigor of the dietary protocol you choose, you may also expect healing reactions on the program that will require appropriate management. Once you have achieved your outcome you will then assess whether you really want to return to the old habits that initially caused your problems.

Although the basic principles of dietary healing do not change, our understanding of how and why these programs work has grown with the emergence of new scientific discoveries and explanations. Since the discovery of NMRI (nuclear magnetic resonance imaging) we can now read tissue chemistry electronically and interpret the electrical fields within the cell. The old naturopaths would refer to this as the "dynamic energy", whereas modern-day scientists refer to it as biophysics. We now know that when a cell is damaged or under-functioning, it not only accepts sodium and water but its electrical potential changes. As a consequence it no longer uses oxygen efficiently and the cell may drop into fermentation. These conditions precede the onset of disease. However, the situation can be reversed, provided that the cells are not too damaged, on a high potassium, alkaline-forming, salt-free diet. The high potassium environment sets up a flushing action where the cells take up potassium and eliminate sodium, excess water and toxins. This results in a purification of the cell, a restoration of the electrical potential and good oxygenation.

Similarly, we have better understanding of the liver's detoxification pathways and how their capacity for detoxification impacts on long-term health. Why is it that some people are predisposed to chemical sensitivities, food intolerances or allergies, heavy metal accumulation and hormonal imbalances, while others, with the same environmental exposure and similar dietary habits have no major health issues? It is due to genetic variance which simply means that some people are better detoxifiers than others. The human liver has six major detoxification pathways that, in a toxin-free environment, can more than adequately cope with the end products of normal metabolism. Genetic variance determines the capacity of each pathway, but even if one pathway is "slower" than the others, any comparative deficit can usually be compensated for by the other pathways.

Problems arise when the liver is over-taxed on a regular basis by toxins from foods (additives, preservatives, colourings, amines) and from the environment (chemicals, fumes, dioxins, heavy metals, pesticides). The pathways become overloaded, and in some cases the liver passes the toxins back into the body which gives rise to inflammatory conditions (headache, eczema, asthma, arthritis, auto-immunity) and multiple chemical sensitivities, which may include drowsiness and even stupor. In other cases the liver continues to struggle until eventually we see chronic health problems arising from the accumulation of chemicals (infertility, cancer, thyroid problems, auto-immune disease, immune dysfunction), heavy metals (brain and nerve disorders), carcinogenic by-products (cancer) and poor hormone clearance (infertility, oestrogen-related problems, cancer and insulin resistance).

The liver may then show impairment in its other functions. Take "Syndrome X", or insulin resistance, for example. This represents a build-up of sugar, insulin and cholesterol in the circulation, all of which are risk factors for diabetes, heart disease and obesity. However, an optimally functioning liver will clear excess insulin and glucose. And once these levels fall, so too does cholesterol. A careful study of the case will reveal signs of liver impairment long before Syndrome X makes its appearance.

Too often we start by trying to address the problem without addressing the cause. We may look to conventional medicine to correct the problem by introducing another chemical to fix the symptoms of a chemical poisoning. In fact we look to the same industry that caused the problem to correct it. The results however, speak for themselves. In industrialised countries it is estimated that one-third of the population (across all age-groups) currently suffer some form of chronic degenerative disease (chronic means that the disease will not go away), and this figure is rising.

Similarly, on the complementary front, we add natural products, such as nutritional supplements and herbal remedies, to try and fix the problem. If the cause of the problem is a nutritional deficiency, then this may correct the problem; but if the problem is due to other causes, then the answer lies in removing the cause, reducing the burden, changing the cellular environment and allowing the body to heal itself.

So the advice and the message within this book remain the same; what grows is our understanding of why what we know is good for us, is good for us. This gives us the confidence to stick with a dietary program for the period of time required to allow healing to occur. The body is a biological clock, you cannot turn the clock back, but neither can you hurry it forward. When the body heals, it heals everything; so be consistent and patient. It takes a full seven years to replace every cell of your body. Just remember, what you eat today, becomes your cells of tomorrow.

Kathryn Alexander 2007

# My story

June 1997…………………..

It all started 11 yrs ago when my life came crashing down. I was sick of being a non-person in a non-marriage, and although I was the one who wanted to end it, I think that if I'd known at the outset how difficult the next five years were going to be I might have thought twice. I did make the right decision and it has made me what I am today - a whole person in a whole marriage with a whole family. My lawyer, who was a leading women's advocate in divorce, said at the time that it was one of the worst divorce cases he had ever fought and that whatever I was doing I should put it in a jar and patent it - because it would make me a fortune. I haven't put it in a jar, I've put it in a book for everyone to read, especially for those who sincerely wish to regain their health and experience the strength and fortitude this brings to all aspects of life.

My story really begins when I had just turned twenty. I was studying the piano and harp at the Royal Academy of Music, London when I met and married a budding opera singer who subsequently became an international star. I had a wonderful life with great opportunities to travel and we had two beautiful children. However, as time went by and the travelling increased we grew further apart. Eventually the painful truth, that the career was more important than the family, had to be faced. And so began five years of hell.

I started at a disadvantage with a telephone call from my husband's agent. She gasped down the 'phone, "I'm so terribly sorry, darling, to hear of your news but I know just the right lawyer for you who will have the whole thing wrapped up in no time." It wasn't until a few months into the proceedings that I realised I was being stitched up. The clinching line from my lawyer came when he was trying to convince me to accept a small property with a 90% mortgage in my name assuring me that my husband would meet the payments for the next twenty-five years or so. When I queried the wisdom of this, as there were adequate funds to purchase a house, he said that it was better this way and that I should accept and be grateful as most women who come through divorce end up with far less than this. I sacked him on the spot. I found that my husband's agent had arranged the best firm of divorce lawyers to represent him while I was with a firm that specialised in commercial law.

I chose my own lawyer and the battle began which raged over the next five years. I'm not sure the exact point when reality turned into soap opera but all I knew that on this particular stage I found myself with a script, written by my husband, that was so utterly convincing that court officials, welfare workers, teachers, doctors and the police were all drawn into a web of illusion. Fortunately, some of us didn't play our parts - myself, the children, a very few close friends and my lawyer.

Everything conceivable happened during those next five years. Our mutual friends dropped away from me as though I had leprosy. I was completely snubbed. Some primitive tribal instinct made the wives draw together to make a unified statement to their husbands that they would never dream of behaving in such a way. The bank manager and the accountant suddenly changed into aloof beings, no longer accepting my calls and demanding that I cut my spending. Being as I didn't have any money even during the marriage, or credit facilities, this was a little difficult. We got an interim maintenance order to meet the basics - my first allowance in thirteen years!

One Saturday afternoon my bank card was gobbled up by the machine. I was with my son - we had no money and no food for the weekend. I started to cry and he put his arms around me and said I could share his crisps. I changed my bank and reached an arrangement based on our joint capital assets.

Things got messy. My son's school fees were not paid so I went out and sold the family silver. The following week I had an order served on me not to dispose of any other goods. But the worst moment came when I arrived home with the children from school to find the police and a social worker on my doorstep. They had come to take the children away and to convince me that "under the circumstances the children would be better off with their father." What circumstances? They looked at me stone-faced and said that they weren't at liberty to say, so I said without a court order they weren't at liberty to take the children.

All doors closed; no one would speak to me. Eventually it transpired that serious doubts had been cast upon my suitability as a mother, that I practised alternative therapies akin to witchcraft and that the children were starving from vegetarian food. In addition, I was dating an unsavoury character who had links with cults, terrorist activities and drugs. That was the only time I thought I would break. Through all the years of litigation, the constant weekly stream of affidavits, the demands and the accusations - nothing compared to the horror of losing my children and my lover.

There followed two years of visits from the social worker. She would appear from nowhere at meal times to make sure I wasn't starving the children or practising some form of witchcraft on them. She would arrive with presents from their father because he alleged that I prevented the children from receiving them. The situation deteriorated until eventually neither child would see their father.

Right up until the week before the High Court hearing, custody was being contested. My lawyer was anxious at the lack of character witnesses as most of my long-standing friends had deserted to the other side and were giving evidence against me. The case was set to last a whole week. My lawyer said that it would cost me my future home. Then at the eleventh hour my husband wished to reach a settlement. It was over in two days. Our barristers negotiated the deal and suddenly it all seemed to hinge on a set of gardening books - ones that were stored somewhere in the garage. We gave him the books.

Somewhere in the midst of this ordeal I decided that I would either sink or swim. My health was not good and I knew that I would have to reclaim it if I was to survive in one piece. I also had to think about a career. My interest in nutrition led me to check out most of the courses available until I found one that really made sense - a course which had the motto "Let your food be your medicine and your medicine be your food." It was a brilliant and fulfilling course. All the students were recommended to experience the detoxification program, which, I might add, was stricter than the one outlined in this book!

This was when things really started to change on a very deep level. The physical improvements were undeniable but more remarkable were the changes that occurred mentally and emotionally. I began to feel like I did when I was eighteen. I felt strong, more confident, with greater clarity and no longer a victim. That's not to say that I wasn't frightened at times, and I know that without the support of very special friends it might have been a different story. But at the end of the day, no matter how much support I had, it was my problem and I was the one who had to face it alone. I can honestly say that I not only regained my health but also my will. I came through a time, which would have taxed even the strongest constitution and undermined the most resilient character, with my health, my integrity and a new life.

What more can be said? Health exists on many levels, not just the physical. Complete healing through detoxification touched all those levels and over the last nine years I have helped many patients achieve similar results and to fulfil their potential.

I hope you enjoy this book and that it provides a framework for you to understand your own health, and how you may improve it through diet to allow the self-healing process to begin.

Good luck

Kathryn Alexander  1997

## Post script

Now, 10 years on from my first publication, my commitment to my work has matured. Over the years I have watched a shift in patients' thinking where there is now a greater desire to take a more active role in decision-making regarding treatment. I have seen that the biggest problems arise when patients feel pressured by the medical system into either taking a back seat or making decisions while there remain unanswered questions. The main difficulties occur when cure cannot be offered, but in its place an option that could lead the patient down a path of greater drug-dependency. I have helped a great many patients through those difficult choices, and seen many remarkable improvements in health – improvements that, from a medical perspective, could not have been achieved through diet alone.

I have found that by helping patients gain a greater understanding of their cases and of how their bodies heal, we achieve good results. Much of my work involves giving people greater insight into their cases and retracing the steps to show how they arrived at where they are now. Most people are surprised at how simple it is to put all the pieces in place and that they don't have to be a medical expert to understand their case. As the threads are drawn together a tapestry emerges where the steps that need to be taken become obvious. The language the patient now speaks is outcome. At the end of the day both medical experts and patients speak this same language; confusion only arises when the understanding of the case and the options presented are incomplete.

It's not much different to renovating a house. You may not be a trained architect or a builder, but you can see the state of the house and you have an idea of what you wish to achieve. So you draw out a rough sketch and present this to your architect with your budget, and embark on a series of discussions until the final plan is approved. And so it is with health; you need to know exactly what's wrong, why it's gone wrong and what you need to do to rectify things. Then you formulate a strategy along with an expected time-frame for your healing.

Although I have seen many successful cases, I will relate one of the most moving experiences that happened for me. Last year, when I was teaching in Melbourne, I was contacted by a young patient whom I had helped in 2000. I had never met this patient before; we conducted our consultations by telephone and e-mail. She was only 33 years old and was seriously ill, suffering from advanced myasthenia gravis, an autoimmune disease that affects nerve transmission to the muscles. The disease had reached a stage where there was loss of facial muscle control, speech and breathing were impaired and there was extreme weakness of the arms and legs making it difficult to walk and lift her arms. The medications she was taking were having adverse effects and the medical profession could offer no more help. As she was unable to speak clearly our consultations were slow with her trying to spell the words, and me guessing until I got it right. She had already decided to undertake the Gerson Therapy and asked me to help her and monitor her progress. I did not know at the outset what could be achieved, but my client had high expectations – and she had an inner confidence that her body could and would heal. I monitored her over the first year and then I didn't hear from her until that telephone call, six years later. I recognised her voice immediately and I said "You can talk!" She told me that she was almost fully cured – that she could speak, run, swim and lead a normal life. I invited her along to the teaching group where she told her story. There wasn't a dry eye in the room.

The enormity of her task with so little mobility was almost incomprehensible. How she did the juicing and the enemas I will never know, but she followed the therapy to the letter for three years. Her story unfolded through the questions and answers. How long did it take to see an improvement? "Not long," she said, "after a year I could walk properly." What struck the group was that even in the absence of more immediate improvements, the success of the therapy was partly attributable to the confidence this lady maintained by. Had she not been confident, she may have given up at the first hurdle and discontinued the therapy.

This beautiful young lady had a profound and centring effect on myself and the group. She told us how much she enjoyed doing the therapy, and how much she appreciated each day of the therapy; she looked at the vegetables and felt gratitude that they were going to make her well, and she even said that she envied those in the group who were about to start on their own healing journey. She found that the three years she spent on the therapy were her most fulfilling, as during that time she became attuned and focused which led to a deep appreciation of life itself.

This wasn't a miracle but a story of immense courage, determination and will: courage to acknowledge the starting point and the enormity of the task in hand, determination to stick to the program, and the will to physically do it. It takes courage to face reality: denial tends to deprive you of the mental clarity required to make such life-changing decisions and the willpower to heal.

Most of my patients do not need to undertake such a program as the Gerson Therapy, but whatever program you choose to follow still requires the dedication and determination to follow it through. However, once you are settled into your chosen program the results will come, and after a period of time you will find that a subtle merging of your diet and lifestyle occurs.

Kathryn Alexander 2007

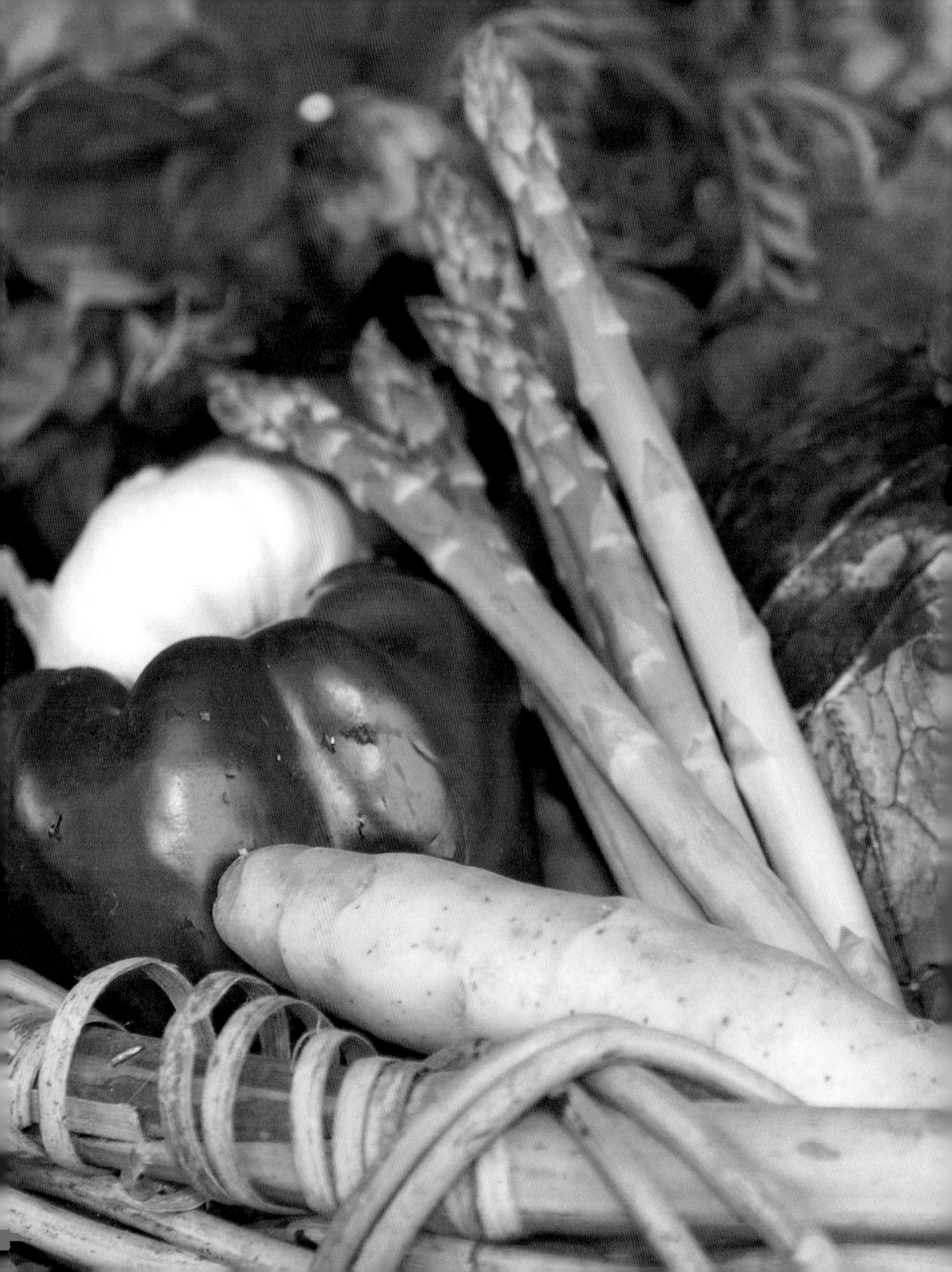

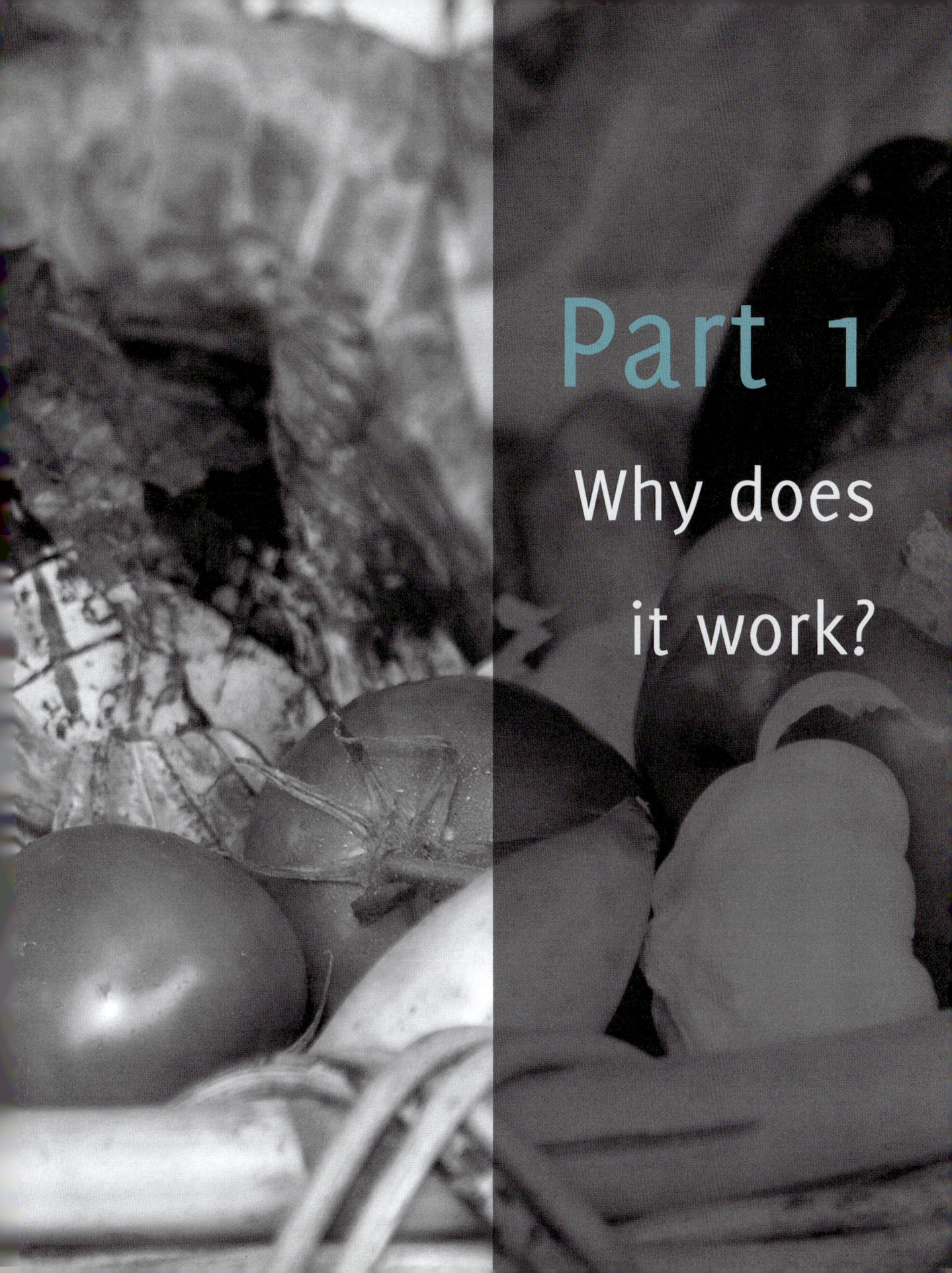

# Part 1

## Why does it work?

I know, through the great number of people I have treated, that it is possible to restore health and the quality of life by making fundamental dietary changes which re-establish the nutrient balance.

If we take a closer look at the word health and remove the "th" we have HEAL, and this to me constitutes health – the body's ability to heal itself or resolve imbalances naturally, without the use of drugs.

# 1

# Why detox?

*1   Why detox?*

**Most people have the common aim** when embarking on any dietary regime to feel good, look good - on the inside and out. We want more energy, better health and a vitality that shines through. Some people will go to extreme lengths to achieve this, whilst others will expect maximum results from minimal efforts! One thing is for certain - maintaining good health involves long-term changes that need to be incorporated into our lifestyle.

So why is detoxification different from other dietary plans? Detoxification means ridding the body of toxins or waste products that have accumulated over the years causing congestion and a clogging of the system. Toxins become tucked away, lodging in the cells, slowly inhibiting vital activities. Eventually, as more and more cells become toxic, tissues and organs start to lose their vitality and the symptoms of disease appear. To maintain efficiency, whether in a mechanical engine or a human body, regular servicing and maintenance is required. As soon as a system becomes overloaded and dirty then mechanical faults or symptoms of ill-health occur.

Detoxification, through the removal of toxins and the release of congestion, raises vitality. This vitality stimulates the body to repair and regenerate itself; disease processes are arrested, followed by the reversal of symptoms. Detoxification promotes and supports self-healing which is the crux of health. So for those of you who wish to regain health, or maintain the health you have, then detoxification will work for you.

# What are the benefits of detoxification?

**Weight loss** is the most immediate benefit as toxins, along with excess salt and water, are driven from the tissues. As the body is 66% water, two-thirds of any weight reduction is due to fluid loss. The body shape changes, particularly for those in their middle years when fluids are beginning to accumulate around the abdomen and thighs, leaving us feeling waterlogged and bloated with tissues that lack tone.

Excess fat is also lost as the body begins to burn this more efficiently. Once congestion starts moving, those fatty deposits that are difficult to shift on ordinary diets will break down. Many toxins are preferentially stored in fat tissue, and it is not until toxicity is lowered generally, and the routes for elimination improved, that fat will be metabolised thereby releasing its toxins. The amount of toxins that can be stored in fat tissue could be lethal in one intravenous dose, therefore it is critical to ensure that the rate of toxin removal does not exceed the capacity for its safe elimination.

*Fat tissue stores toxins. It is important to ensure that its rate of breakdown can be matched by your capacity to eliminate stored toxins.*

**Mental and physical vitality is restored** - not purely from the weight loss but through re-mineralisation of the entire body. This has an effect not only on physical vitality but it also unleashes greater mental clarity and inspiration; new strengths of character can emerge with a greater capacity to fulfil your potential.

**Slowing of the ageing process** occurs as a natural consequence of detoxification. Regeneration of new, healthy tissues occurs at an accelerated rate and increased cell vitality enables the restoration of damaged tissues with a faster turnover of new cells.

**Reversal of symptoms** (including those associated with ageing) occurs once the body starts cleansing; congestion is reduced and symptoms are alleviated. Of the many diseases that detoxification helps a few are listed below:

- Hardening diseases such as **arthritis, hardening of the arteries, heart disease, thrombosis, stroke, gall** and **kidney stones** and the general hardening of organs which compromises their efficiency;
- **Osteoporosis** and other diseases involving accelerated tissue degeneration;
- **Low energy** and **poor blood sugar control**, eating disorders, addictions and cravings;
- Childhood disorders, such as **asthma, eczema** and mental symptoms, such as **hyperactivity (ADHD)**;
- Lowered immune response including **recurrent infection**, poor healing capacity and regeneration;
- Digestive and colon disorders: **ulcers, colitis, irritable bowel syndrome, food allergies**; and
- **Hormonal imbalances, pre-menstrual tension** and **infertility**.

*1   Why detox?*

*In industrialised countries it is estimated that one-third of the population (across all age-groups) currently suffers some form of chronic degenerative disease, and this figure is rising.*

When we read through this list of symptoms we realise just how large a part they play in many people's lives by destroying their quality of life. It is true, that with modern medicine and greater affluence, our life expectancy has increased - but what of its quality? We can't deny that general health seems to be on the decline with an increasing number of people in all age groups affected in one way or another. Heart disease, diabetes and cancer are on the increase, while asthma, eczema, food allergies and hyperactivity have now become common occurrences in younger generations rather than the rare incidence.

Dietary trends over the past 50 years have played a major role in this decline in health, but I know, through the great number of people I have treated, that it is possible to restore health and quality of life by making fundamental changes to diet and restoring the nutrient balance.

## How does it work?
Detoxification stimulates the natural healing process. Once you reduce toxicity and congestion, vitality rises. This is the key to health. A strong vitality constitutes good health.

*Chronic: symptoms that do not go away by themselves.*

What is health? Most people would say that health is the absence of symptoms and a feeling of well-being. But health is a little more than this. If we take a closer look at the word health and remove the "th" we have HEAL, and this to me constitutes health - the ability by the body to heal itself or resolve imbalances naturally, without the use of drugs.

This process may or may not be symptom-free. For example, the body produces symptoms in its healing efforts. Inflammation is a symptom of the body removing harmful substances; fever assists and accelerates this process. Symptoms that resolve naturally indicate a healthy constitution, or strong vitality, but when symptoms fail to resolve and become destructive then health is said to be poor.

So what is vitality? The easiest way to answer this is to imagine a fresh lettuce, with roots, placed in water. You will notice that the lettuce retains its freshness for a couple of days and then gradually starts to wilt. It is losing vitality. As the days go by the lettuce starts to die, becoming slimy and a breeding ground for microbes. There is no vitality left and it is now in a state of decay. From this observation it is obvious that a strong vitality ensures tissue integrity and resistance to pathogens (disease-causing microbes) and disease. Once the vitality declines, cells die and the decaying process begins. Vitality, or the life force, is dependent upon good nourishment.

*Disease is an adaptation to local conditions; by cleansing the internal environment at cell level we restore the conditions required for self-healing.*

How detoxification diets stimulate vitality is the subject of the next two chapters. Our current dietary trends tend to erode vitality by creating nutrient imbalances within the cell. Even if we take nutritional supplements this may not be sufficient to correct the situation. As you will discover, it is only through specific dietary changes that the cells will be induced to flush out their toxins in exchange for nutrients. Nutritional supplements may aid the process but very little will be achieved on a long-term basis when taken in the absence of dietary changes.

## How long will it take?

This depends upon what you wish to achieve. You may achieve your goal in just two months or it may take longer. For those who just wish to lose weight, the time taken is determined by reaching the goal weight. Generally, most people do lose excess weight, particularly in the first few months where losses may average 5 kg in the first two weeks.

I usually recommend between two and six months on the diet. Within the first couple of months most symptoms should disappear. Aches and pains, digestive difficulties, allergies, skin disorders, hormonal symptoms, low energy and mood swings are usually alleviated within this short time-frame and you will experience a greater vitality and sense of well-being.

However, a lack of symptoms does not mean that you are cured. Symptoms are the end-result of a slow devitalising process that has occurred over many years and often results in a named disease. So although you may experience a dramatic remission of symptoms you must remember their absence does not mean that the healing is complete. It takes a lot longer to reverse degenerative effects and it requires a sustained effort. It is not until the body is sufficiently regenerated that a good level of health is achieved.

Take a person who has high cholesterol levels; after a couple of months on the diet the levels may fall to within the normal reference range. I would recommend that this person remain on the diet to allow the liver, which controls the handling of fats and cholesterol, to regenerate. This would also aid the breakdown of fatty accumulations in cells and arteries and improve overall tissue vitality. Hopefully, after a period of time, the diet becomes a way of life where the person has adopted many of the dietary principles on a long-term basis.

As a rule of thumb, the higher your vitality, the quicker the detoxification and regenerative process occurs. You can measure your vitality by how well you resolve illnesses. A person with a high vitality would not need to resort to drugs when they are sick as the body is capable of healing itself. However, many people have chronic conditions that require long-term medication or even experience the sudden onset of a life-threatening illness. Such cases indicate that the vitality has been eroded over the years and the situation will take longer to reverse. Under these circumstances, if you are planning a detoxification, it may be advisable to seek professional guidance so that treatment can proceed at a pace which suits you without causing aggravations. Chapter 4 *Vitality & healing* will lend clarity to this issue and give you greater insight into your own level of vitality.

*Your inherent vitality determines the pace and length of treatment. Those with chronic conditions may need to adopt long-term dietary changes to support their healing.*

## How strict must I be?

Before this can be answered we must look at what the diet entails. It consists of natural (preferably organic), unrefined foods, such as whole grain cereals (brown rice, barley, millet, oats, corn and buckwheat), nuts and legumes (peas, beans and lentils), vegetables and fruits, and fish (if you are not vegetarian). The foods that are omitted are refined and processed foods, salt, sugar, dairy products (for a period of time), wheat, meat, stimulants (such as tea and coffee) and alcohol.

# 1  Why detox?

At first glance you may think that this diet is no different from any other health diet. So what makes it a detoxification diet? The answer lies in the volume of vegetables consumed (often in the form of juices) which actively draws toxins and congestion from the cells. Secondly, through the omission of foods like dairy, animal protein and salt this process is accelerated. With strict adherence to the diet, many people will feel shifts occurring in the body within the first few days. After a few weeks the body starts to gain its own momentum and the detoxifying process kicks in. Most importantly, the diet must be nutritionally balanced to encourage regeneration. Detoxification and regeneration go hand in hand; they are two sides of the same coin.

When a person's vitality is relatively good then I recommend at least a two-month detoxification plan. The diet has very strict guidelines but still allows for plenty of variety. Organisation and preparation are the keys. Finding yourself with "nothing in the refrigerator" is the first step to failure, but if you are well prepared then the diet becomes easy. For this reason I have prepared a shopping list, menu plan and recipes to take you through the first few weeks.

*Detoxification will not occur if you stop and start the program; you need to create a momentum before you experience toxin elimination and healing.*

In order for detoxification to occur it is important that the diet is strictly adhered to. Toxins take many years to accumulate in the tissues and can only be shifted when the body has sufficient vitality. Once this process starts, the movement of toxins occurs in waves as they are released from the cells into the circulation and out through the liver. The momentum that the body gains is critical to this process. If a specific level of vitality is not reached and then maintained, nothing will occur. Just as a car that has to keep stopping and starting at the traffic lights never gains its top speed, likewise within the body – the momentum required for detoxification must be reached before the detoxification and healing process kicks in.

A strong eliminative capacity by the liver is essential for detoxification and therefore we need to ensure that specific dietary items, such as fats and animal proteins, are kept to a minimum while refined carbohydrates (sugars and refined grains), salt and alcohol are excluded totally. These foods increase the burden on the liver, increase congestion and inhibit the elimination of toxins. The congestion in the liver needs to be released in order for the healing process to begin.

*The expression "spring cleaning" is derived from the natural detoxification that should occur in the spring.*

So the actual detoxification plan is very strict; it excludes dairy (except a little yoghurt), eggs, wheat, meat, fish being optional, and there is a high emphasis on vegetables and whole grain cereals, especially brown rice. After the two-month plan other foods are introduced, such as small amounts of chicken and lean red meat, and wheat. Following this modified regime you will still continue to detoxify especially if you have built up a momentum and the liver is eliminating well. This diet serves as a good maintenance plan. At a later stage you may make other dietary changes but hopefully, with the greater insight you have gained through reading this book, you will understand how to balance your foods so that congestion within the tissues does not recur. It is a good idea to give your body a "service" once or twice a year. Spring is a very good time of the year to detoxify because you can maximise on the planetary energy changes occurring at this time.

## How will I feel?

As toxins start shifting from the cells into the circulation you may feel thick-headed, suffer headaches, skin aggravations, aching joints, bad body odour, nervous irritability, experience "taints" in the mouth, and you may feel generally "toxic". Before you become too anxious - this is short-lived, and as your vitality rises you are able to deal with these waves of toxin release more rapidly and effectively.

The body is much like a plumbing system, with nutrients going in and waste products going out. If there is a block in the plumbing system due to congestion, then toxins released into the circulation will be unable to make a safe exit. This is when aggravations occur as the toxins try to make their exit through other routes, such as the skin and mucous membranes.

In order to avoid aggravations it is best to proceed on a detoxification plan where the rate of toxin removal keeps pace with elimination. If removal from the tissues exceeds the rate of their elimination to the outside then aggravations will occur and existing complaints may worsen for a period of time. For these reasons, if you suspect that your vitality may be eroded (you exhibit signs of deep congestion) then it may be advisable to embark on a slower program so that a much gentler elimination is stimulated. At the same time, work can begin on the liver, restoring its function to prepare for a stronger elimination. Eventually the strict detoxification plan can be undertaken without any adverse effects. Chapter 5 *Liver cleansing* will help you understand the liver's function as the body's "main drain" through which toxins are eliminated safely, and outlines the steps entailed in improving liver integrity. As the liver becomes more efficient the effects of toxin removal will be felt less and less.

In most cases a strong elimination can be elicited within the first two months with very few adverse reactions. However, the deeper the disease and the deeper the congestion - the longer it takes. It is important to give sufficient time for regeneration to occur otherwise, for all your hard efforts, the beneficial effects will only be short-lived with symptoms eventually reappearing.

*Ensure that your program does not tax your elimination pathways: the rate of toxin removal must keep pace with elimination from the body.*

*Dietary healing is a two-fold process: detoxification and regeneration. It takes time to regenerate – so factor this into your time-frame.*

When we reinstate potassium within the cells by applying a high vegetable diet, low in added salt, healing occurs.

It is not dietary amounts of calcium that govern our calcium status but rather other nutritional factors that control its absorption and retention.
Of these, magnesium is the most important.

# 2

# Salt & dairy
## – the de-vitalisers

## 2  Salt & dairy - the devitalisers

**Most people don't pay much attention** to the amount of salt in their diet. Salt may not be added to food after cooking but when we take time to read the labels on prepared foods we see that everything from bread, breakfast cereals, cakes and biscuits to canned foods, prepared meals, stocks and sauces has large quantities of added salt. In fact, it has become very difficult to avoid salt. If you add up the daily intake on a normal type of diet, it is easy to consume up to 10g of sodium a day, which is 20 times the amount required by the body!

Most of us are led to believe that there is no long-term health-risk if we consume excess minerals; hence they are liberally added to many products. We are more concerned with not meeting our daily requirements than with the fate of excess nutrients, which we assume will be eliminated if not needed. We are all encouraged to drink milk or take dairy produce daily, and most people are under the impression that dairy is the sole source of our calcium. Marketing tactics, upheld by the medical fraternity, have bred a calcium-neurosis where our society is now consuming vast quantities of dairy produce often at the expense of other foods. Our calcium intake can more than quadruple the recommended daily intake (RDI) with the general assumption that more is better.

This is far from the case; excess salt and excess calcium do damage health; both encourage and accelerate the ageing and hardening process with hardening occuring outside the skeleton in the soft tissues, organs, arteries and joints, while the bones become brittle. High salt and dairy diets disturb the natural mineral balance within the cell and create acidity and congestion resulting in lowered tissue vitality and disease. The subject of this chapter is to discover how the correct mineral balance, as reflected in our natural diet, promotes health and what happens when we deviate from the natural mineral ratios.

Let's take an overview of the minerals found in a natural diet. At this stage we are only concerned with the balance between the four major minerals, sodium (Na), potassium (K), calcium (Ca) and magnesium (Mg) as it is the ratio between these nutrients that governs our cellular activities. If the ratio is maintained through our diet then congestion will not accumulate and our tissues will maintain their vitality.

Table 2.1   Average values for the major minerals: mg/100g

|  | Na | K | Ca | Mg |
|---|---|---|---|---|
| Fruits | 3.2 | 176 | 16 | 9.6 |
| Legumes (dry weight) | 30 | 1,381 | 134 | 179 |
| Root vegetables | 67 | 253 | 53 | 12.6 |
| Leaf vegetables | 23 | 323 | 111 | 17.4 |
| Cereals (dry weight) | 7 | 401 | 41 | 110 |
| Nuts | 5 | 669 | 117 | 223 |
| Meat | 65 | 365 | 6 | 24 |
| Fish | 91 | 443 | 8 | 26 |
| Milk | 50 | 144 | 116 | 12 |
|  |  |  |  |  |
| Total Average | 38 | 462 | 67 | 68 |

Table 2.1 *Average values for the major minerals* gives the average value for the minerals in each food group. You can see that the amounts of naturally occurring sodium are low while those for potassium are quite high. The calcium and magnesium ratio of a diet that incorporates whole grains, nuts and legumes is roughly equivalent. We are not so much concerned with amounts of minerals but the ratio between them. Providing there is more than five times the amount of potassium to sodium in the diet and no more than double the amount of calcium to magnesium (equivalent amounts are preferable) then this is in keeping with a ratio that maintains health. However, let's compare this ratio to a diet that includes 100g of cheese. By adding the values of the major minerals found in cheese we arrive at these new averages.

|  | Na | K | Ca | Mg |
|---|---|---|---|---|
| Cheese 100g | 700 | 82 | 750 | 24 |
|  |  |  |  |  |
| New Total Average | 412 | 424 | 153 | 64 |

Look how the ratio has changed. The sodium/potassium ratio is now equal and calcium far outweighs magnesium. Let's take this one step further and assess the mineral balance on two common diets. Take a moment to review both diet A and diet B (p33).

Assessing diet A, if we add up the mineral values for diet A we conclude:

| Na (Sodium) | K (Potassium) | Ca (Calcium) | Mg (Magnesium) |
|---|---|---|---|
| 6,879mg | 3,404mg | 1,366mg | 236mg |

On this diet the sodium/potassium ratio is reversed where sodium is now in excess of potassium. In addition, the calcium/magnesium ratio is severely damaged. This is partly due to the inclusion of a small amount of cheese, but equally importantly, to the lack of magnesium-rich foods in the diet. In fact, the magnesium does not even meet the RDI at 350mg/day. If the diet also contains tea, coffee or alcohol, then any existing dietary magnesium would be "washed away" resulting in net losses rather than any positive balance.

Now let's look at diet B.

If we add up the mineral values for diet B we conclude:

| Na (Sodium) | K (Potassium) | Ca (Calcium) | Mg (Magnesium) |
|---|---|---|---|
| 1,147mg | 5,348mg | 950mg | 591mg |

*The small amount of salt in seasonings or flavour-enhancers dramatically reduces the sodium/potassium ratio, which erodes our health over the long-term.*

We can immediately see that the sodium/potassium ratio is balanced with approximately five times the amount of potassium to sodium. If meat replaced the legumes the ratios would not alter significantly but beans are marginally higher for both calcium and magnesium than meat. This diet includes very little dairy and yet still maintains a healthy calcium status. The calcium/magnesium ratio is balanced and provided that no tea, coffee or alcohol is taken, will remain so. You will notice that there is more magnesium in the breakfast alone on this diet than in the total daily intake on diet A.

Now let's add a tablespoon of soy sauce to diet B:

|  | Na | K |
|---|---|---|
| 1 tbsp soy sauce | 1,029 | - |
| New total | 2,176 | 5,348 |

The sodium/potassium ratio is now reduced from 5 to 2.5. You can appreciate that small amounts of salt which creep back into the diet can distort the sodium/potassium ratio significantly.

*Dietary ratios between the major minerals*

## DIET A

| Breakfast A | Na | K | Ca | Mg |
|---|---|---|---|---|
| 1 rasher of bacon (50g) | 1,010 | 145 | 6 | 8 |
| 1 sausage | 480 | 135 | 22 | 6 |
| 2 eggs | 122 | 129 | 68 | 15 |
| 2 slices of bread (white) | 432 | 80 | 80 | 20 |
| 1 Tbs of butter (salted) | 116 | 11 | - | - |
| 1 Tbs tomato sauce | 156 | 70 | - | - |
| 1/8 tsp salt | 242 | - | - | - |
| Total | 2,558 | 570 | 176 | 49 |

| Lunch A | Na | K | Ca | Mg |
|---|---|---|---|---|
| Bread (white roll) | 864 | 160 | 160 | 40 |
| Butter (salted) | 232 | 22 | - | - |
| Cheese (100g) | 700 | 82 | 800 | 25 |
| Pickle (1 dsp) | 160 | - | - | - |
| Packet of crisps | 180 | 350 | 11 | 17 |
| Orange | 4 | 280 | 57 | 18 |
| Total | 2,140 | 894 | 1,028 | 100 |

| Dinner A | Na | K | Ca | Mg |
|---|---|---|---|---|
| Meat (200g) | 140 | 700 | 15 | 55 |
| Cook-in-sauce/gravy | 975 | - | - | - |
| Potatoes (200g) | 6 | 660 | 8 | 30 |
| Vegetables (170g) | 76 | 490 | 72 | 26 |
| 1/4 tsp salt | 484 | - | - | - |
| Dessert (flour-based) | 500 | 90 | 67 | 18 |
| Total | 2,181 | 1,940 | 162 | 129 |

Total major mineral values (mg) for Diet A

|  | Na | K | Ca | Mg |
|---|---|---|---|---|
| Total | 6,879 | 3,404 | 1,366 | 236 |

## DIET B

| Breakfast B | Na | K | Ca | Mg |
|---|---|---|---|---|
| Muesli 150g | 107 | 1,004 | 117 | 150 |
| Milk (200mls) | 100 | 288 | 240 | 23 |
| Apple | 1 | 150 | 6 | 7 |
| 2 slices bread (wholemeal) | 432 | 176 | 18 | 74 |
| 1 tbsp butter (unsalted) | - | 11 | - | - |
| Total | 640 | 1,629 | 381 | 254 |

| Lunch B | Na | K | Ca | Mg |
|---|---|---|---|---|
| Baked potato (300g) | 9 | 1,221 | 21 | 62 |
| Butter (unsalted) | - | 11 | - | - |
| Egg mayonnaise (2 eggs, 2 dsp mayonnaise) | 122 | 129 | 68 | 15 |
| Yoghurt (small carton) | 72 | 198 | 270 | 25 |
| Banana | 1 | 420 | 8 | 50 |
| Total | 404 | 1,979 | 367 | 152 |

| Dinner B | Na | K | Ca | Mg |
|---|---|---|---|---|
| Brown rice (50g dry weight) | 4 | 120 | 20 | 50 |
| Vegetables (170g) | 76 | 490 | 72 | 26 |
| Legume dish (50g dry weight) | 15 | 690 | 60 | 84 |
| Fruit salad | 8 | 440 | 50 | 25 |
| Total | 103 | 1,740 | 206 | 185 |
| (+1 Tbsp soy sauce) | 1,029 | | | |
| New total | 1,132 | - | - | - |

Total major mineral values (mg) for Diet B

|  | Na | K | Ca | Mg |
|---|---|---|---|---|
| Total | 1,147 | 5,348 | 950 | 591 |
| (+1 tbsp soy sauce) | 2,176 | 5,328 | 950 | 591 |

*Salt & dairy - the devitalisers*

**I have referred to the major minerals in two separate groups:** sodium/potassium and calcium/magnesium. This is because they are "partners" and it is the ratio between them which influences their availability in the tissues. Once these natural ratios are disturbed, where sodium and calcium levels rise disproportionately, the cell minerals - potassium and magnesium - become vulnerable to erosion. In other words, high sodium diets deplete potassium by promoting potassium losses via the kidneys, and high dairy diets inhibit the uptake of magnesium. The story does not end here, for once the magnesium status is eroded the body cannot absorb or retain calcium, regardless of how much calcium is presented either in the diet or through supplementation, and potassium cannot gain entry into the cell. Consequently many people on high-dairy diets become the most calcium-deficient of all.

It is the interplay and specific ratios between the major minerals that govern health, not their isolated intake. Current dietary trends make us vulnerable to potassium and magnesium deficiencies; these two minerals together control cell vitality. Deficiencies lead to cellular congestion, inefficiency and a loss of vitality with increased vulnerability to disease. Let's look in more detail at these critical balances.

# Sodium/potassium balance

**Man's natural diet contains very little sodium** but large quantities of potassium. The body has evolved in such a way that sodium is recycled resulting in minimal losses. For example, everyday around 23,000mg (23g) of sodium is secreted in the digestive juices and 575,000mg (575g) is filtered by the kidneys. The body, on a salt-free diet, reabsorbs all but 230mg of this total amount which represents the obligatory loss – or the amount required by the body to fulfil its activities. So our total requirements for sodium are very small, a mere 230mg daily.

*Obligatory loss: this value represents the minimum amount of a specific nutrient required by the body on a daily basis.*

**Figure 2.1** The obligatory loss for sodium on a daily basis

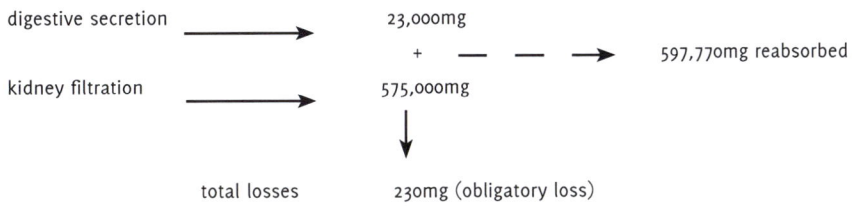

Of the total amount of sodium secreted in the digestive juices and filtered by the kidneys on a daily basis, only 230mg is lost, the rest being recycled by the body. The 230mg lost represents the obligatory loss, or the amount used by the body to fulfil its metabolic requirements.

Our daily requirements for all nutrients are calculated on this basis but the recommended daily intakes are usually set a little higher. These amounts are arbitrary. For example, the RDI for sodium is set at between 1,000mg and 2,000mg/day and yet no symptoms of deficiency are recorded at just 500mg/day. Even in hot climates after a few days of heavy sweating, the glands will start to secrete potassium in exchange for sodium, thereby reducing sodium losses significantly. The old theory about having to take salt tablets if one sweats heavily is not based on fact and does more harm than good in the long-term. Under these circumstances it would be more important to increase your potassium-rich fresh vegetables and fruit juices.

*Our natural diet provides sufficient sodium to meet our requirements.*

However, one can exhibit symptoms of salt deficiency in acute excessive sweating. One patient I was treating had breast cancer and was taking the drug Tamoxifen which hastened the onset of menopause. The hot flushing and sweating were severe and she did exhibit symptoms of salt deficiency. We found that dipping the tip of her tongue into a little salt was sufficient to alleviate these symptoms. The amount of salt required is very small and the body will adjust after a few days. What remains critical is meeting your potassium requirements.

The recycling of sodium is always at the expense of its partner potassium. For example, the kidneys will reabsorb sodium in exchange for potassium, which is then excreted via the urine. On a natural, high-potassium diet this poses no problem. However, as soon as the ratio begins to slip (very easily achieved if you don't eat your fruit and vegetables!) then you will begin to suffer net losses of potassium.

The more sodium you consume, the greater the potassium losses. This is how an excess of one mineral in relation to another can induce deficiencies. So although you may be reaching (and probably exceeding) your recommended daily intake for both sodium (1-2g/day) and potassium (2.5 - 6.0g/day) you may in fact be suffering net losses of potassium leading to potassium deficiency. If you turn to table 2.2 *Sodium values in seasonings and snacks* and table 2.3 *Sodium and potassium values in processed foods* you can see at a glance the values for sodium in many of our common products and how the ratio between sodium and potassium is reversed when foods are processed.

Table 2.2   Sodium values (mg) in seasonings and snacks

| Item | Amount | Sodium (mg) |
|---|---|---|
| Salt | 1 tsp | 1,938 |
| Soya sauce | 1 tbs | 1,029 |
| Baking soda | 1 tsp | 821 |
| MSG | 1 tsp | 492 |
| Baking powder | 1 tsp | 339 |
| Olives | 4 | 323 |
| French dressing | 1 tbs | 253 |
| Worcestershire sauce | 1 tbs | 206 |
| Horseradish sauce | 1 tbs | 198 |
| Tartare sauce | 1 tbs | 182 |
| Mayonnaise | 1 tbs | 150 |
| Tomato Ketchup | 1 tbs | 156 |
| Thousand Island dressing | 1 tbs | 153 |
| Blue cheese dressing | 1 tbs | 153 |
| Margarine | 1 tbs | 140 |
| Butter (salted) | 1 tbs | 116 |
| Pickle | 1 tbs | 240 |
| Stock cube | 1 | 1,030 |
| Salted nuts | 100g | 418 |
| Peanut butter | 28g | 170 |
| Crisps (25g) | 1 pkt | 180 |
| Biscuits | 100g | 365 |
| Crumpet | 1 | 325 |

Table 2.3  Sodium (Na) and Potassium (K) values in processed foods, mg/100g:

|  | Na | K |
|---|---|---|
| Bacon | 2,020 | 290 |
| Corned beef | 950 | 140 |
| Bread | 540 | 100 |
| Butter (salted) | 987 | 23 |
| Margarine | 987 | 23 |
| Cheese: |  |  |
|    Cheddar | 610 | 120 |
|    Cottage | 450 |  |
|    Cream | 300 | 160 |
|    Parmesan | 60 | 150 |
|    Spread | 1,117 | 150 |
|    Processed | 1,136 | 80 |

|  | Na | K |
|---|---|---|
| Fish fingers | 350 | 260 |
| Cornflakes | 1,005 | 120 |
| Kippers | 923 | 485 |
| Baked beans | 500 | 300 |
| Ham | 1,250 | 280 |
| Canned soup | 460 | 40 |
| Canned tuna fish | 400 | 301 |
| Canned sardines | 423 | 590 |
| Canned spaghetti | 350 | - |
| Sausages | 1,300 | 230 |
| Self-raising flour | 1,079 | - |

## Why is potassium so important?

Potassium is so important because it is the key mineral within the body cells and activates many enzyme systems. Potassium is the factory foreman; if he is present within the cell, the enzymes kick into action; but if absent, they go on strike. The enzymes are like factory workers; they receive the raw materials, but in the absence of any tools cannot convert the raw materials into new substances. Our minerals and vitamins represent the tools. Although they are required in minute quantities, compared to the carbohydrates, proteins and fats, without them the body is incapable of converting our food to energy or for tissue maintenance. Taking foods in their natural, unprocessed form ensures that the bulk nutrients (carbohydrates, proteins and fats) come with the array of vitamins and minerals required for their metabolism at cell level.

*Intracellular potassium regulates cell function. When potassium is displaced by sodium, the cell drops into fermentation and we see the onset of disease.*

Potassium, as the general of minerals, governs many systems such as the energy cycle, nerve transmission, and DNA and protein synthesis to name but a few. It ignites the fire of metabolism generating vitality within the cells. If our cells become deficient in potassium they lose their capacity to take up oxygen and will fall into fermentation; eventually activity ceases and the cell dies. This heralds the onset of pathological change leading to chronic degenerative change.

So high salt diets promote potassium losses from within the cells. This occurs gradually over a long period of time. As potassium is lost from the cells, sodium moves in along with water, acting like a wet blanket putting out the fire of metabolism.

## What happens to the excess sodium?

No matter how much salt we eat, our blood sodium concentration is kept constant within a very narrow range. This is achieved in two ways: we get thirsty and retain water which dilutes the sodium concentration to normal, and the kidneys then filter both the excess water and sodium. However, the kidneys only monitor sodium levels in the blood and in the fluid bathing the cells (extracellular fluid). This accounts for just 33% of the total body fluids; 66% is found within the cells and it is here that excess sodium is shunted.

*ICF: intracellular fluids – fluids inside the cell.*

As sodium levels rise in the extracellular fluids a proportion will be removed by the kidneys while any surplus may enter the cells, a situation exacerbated by an intracellular potassium deficiency. Healthy cells are normally low in sodium and therefore a high extracellular sodium would have a tendency to drift down this concentration gradient into the cells. However, the high potassium content within the healthy cell inhibits sodium from entering. If cells become deficient in potassium, then sodium drifts into the cell inhibiting function, heralding the onset of disease.

*ECF: extracellular fluids – fluids outside the cell.*

The cell is geared to maintain a critical ratio between sodium inside and outside the cell rather than a specified amount. This ratio is 13.5 which means that for every one part sodium inside the cell, 13.5 parts exist outside. You can appreciate that sodium concentrations will be raised proportionately within the cell as outside levels rise. This situation becomes even more critical in cases of potassium deficiency where the cell loses its control mechanisms and sodium is free to invade the cell. It is generally accepted that an energy-dependent mechanism operating at the cell membrane, known as the sodium/potassium pump, assists in pumping sodium out of the cell in exchange for potassium.

**Figure 2.2** Exchange of sodium ($Na^+$) and potassium ($K^+$) in health and disease

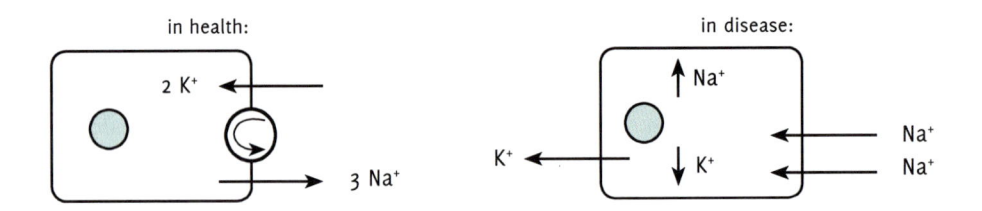

The sodium/potassium pump exchanges two potassium ions for three sodium ions ensuring that sodium is kept out of the cell at all costs. In either potassium deficiency and/or sodium excess, sodium drifts into the cell. The ratio of sodium within and outside the cell is kept constant at 13.5.

Once inside the cell, regulation of sodium by the kidneys becomes a more difficult and slower process. Excess sodium can take up to seven days before it is eventually removed, but the ongoing cumulative effects of excessive salt consumption over a prolonged period of time are deleterious to cell vitality. By removing added salt from the diet and raising the potassium content (vegetables and fruits) you will give the cells an opportunity to start reducing their toxic load.

We owe much of our understanding of the detoxification and healing process to the meticulous work of Dr. Max Gerson during the early to mid 1900s. He proved beyond doubt that by reinstating potassium levels within the cells through the use of vegetable juices, and taking a diet free of added salt, that healing would occur. Much of his later work was done with terminally-ill cancer patients where he achieved a 50% success rate. The diet was very strict and patients would be required to take around

3 litres of various vegetable juices daily along with other natural medications. On his diet, where natural sodium levels would not exceed 500mg/day, patients would eliminate up to 8,000mg daily via the urine over the first couple of weeks with further eliminations occurring over forty-eight hour intervals.

Most medical texts state that under normal conditions daily sodium output can never exceed input, which means that you cannot lose more than you take in. This statement would be true if sodium remained in the extra-cellular fluid as the kidneys would eliminate any excess. However, Dr. Gerson found that on his diet, the opposite was true. So if the blood and extracellular fluid sodium concentration is kept constant, where is the sodium coming from? It is coming from within the cells. The high potassium content of the vegetable juices seems to actively draw out cellular sodium in exchange for potassium.

**Figure 2.3**  High extracellular potassium exchanges with sodium within the cells

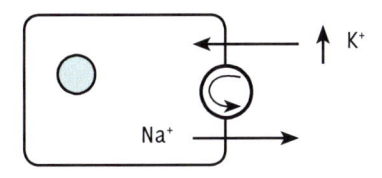

Extra-cellular potassium will be taken up by the cell in exchange for sodium. The cell is purified of excess sodium and toxins and resets its oxidative cycle.

Following the removal of sodium and the reinstatement of potassium, Dr. Gerson found that cell vitality was restored and the body started to heal itself; tumours were reabsorbed by the body and the symptoms of illness declined. However, on the cancer therapy, he noticed that patients needed to maintain the diet for 18 months for complete regeneration to occur. Failure to do this resulted in a return of the symptoms and the cancer. So although patients felt well and had no clinical symptoms, it took a lot longer to change conditions within the body that would not favour the growth of tumours.

*Ensure that you stay with your program after your symptoms have resolved to allow adequate time for regeneration.*

## What does excess sodium mean in terms of health?

As we have seen, excess sodium leads to a general reduction in cell vitality that reflects in the efficiency of the body tissues and organs. Congestion occurs as toxic products from poor cell metabolism accumulate. When vitality is lost, disease sets in which marks a general decline in health. Vitality naturally declines with age and will be accelerated when the cell minerals are lost in favour of sodium.

*Endogenous: made by the body.*

We tend to think of toxins predominantly arising from external pollution in the atmosphere and from the food and water we consume. However, a poorly functioning body will create its own toxins, known as endogenous toxins. When metabolic processes are inhibited as a consequence of potassium deficiency and a lack of other essential nutrients, then intermediate substances are produced called metabolic acids. These are toxic to the cell creating a highly acidic environment that inhibits cell function resulting in cell death. Excess sodium and acidity go hand in hand: an acidic cell will favour the entry of sodium, and the entry of sodium inhibits cells metabolism leading to the accumulation of metabolic acids.

*Exogenous: from a source outside the body.*

**Figure 2.4** The entry of sodium into the cell and accumulation of metabolic acids (toxins)

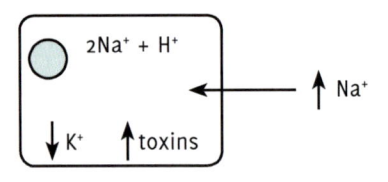

$2Na^+ + H^+$
$\downarrow K^+ \quad \uparrow toxins$
$\uparrow Na^+$

Excess sodium and intracellular potassium deficiencies will directly lead to excess acidity (H⁺) within the cell.

*High Na and acidity (H⁺) go hand in hand. An acidic environment draws calcium from the bones where it precipitates (calcifies) in the soft tissues and joints.*

This has greater implications on health, particularly on calcium. Imagine what happens when you pour milk into a pan of lemon juice; the milk precipitates to form curds while the acidity of the lemon juice is neutralised in the process. A similar fate occurs in the body. An acidic environment causes the precipitation of calcium, causing the formation of salts and crystals which lodge in the joints, arteries and soft tissues. We may feel its consequences in our moveable joints as arthritis, but we remain unaware of the internal hardening until symptoms occur in the organs and arteries many years after the hardening process has begun. Fatty accumulations also occur, and it is of no surprise, given our current dietary habits, that autopsies undertaken on youngsters show hardening of the arteries with fatty change indicating pathological signs well advanced for their years. In short, as our bones become more brittle, our bodies harden, with calcification occurring outside the skeleton - a reversal of what happens in health.

Chronic acidity is also a major trigger for inflammation – a common factor in all degenerative disease. In fact high sodium, high acidity and inflammation form a vicious cycle. When the body reaches its limit of tolerance to toxins (both endogenous and environmental) the inflammatory metabolism kicks in as an effort by the body to either remove or isolate the toxic deposits. In turn, inflammation generates greater acidity and the healthy surrounding tissues are destroyed. Disease tends to manifest in organs and tissues of greatest vulnerability, usually genetically pre-determined.

*Acidic conditions precede inflammation, and inflammation perpetuates acidity. A vicious cycle ensues leading to chronic inflammatory disease.*

As the organs become compromised we may see signs of increased toxicity which include general hardening and inflammatory disease: inflammation of the internal mucous membranes accompanied by mucus discharge; loss of organ vitality, particularly with signs of strain on the heart and kidneys which may lead to elevated blood pressure, fluid retention and weight gain; loss of structural integrity and muscle elasticity leading to hernia, prolapse, incontinence, varicose veins and congestive heart failure; and poor transmission of nerve signals which will have deleterious effects on all organ systems (including the brain). Interestingly, a strong link exists between the sodium/potassium balance and hyperactivity, or ADHD. Although many nutritional factors are involved in this disturbance, a low potassium status predisposes hyperactivity and the constant thirst that frequently accompanies this disorder indicates the kidneys' failure to concentrate urine due to potassium deficiency.

**In short**, a high sodium/low potassium status eventuates in increased cellular toxicity, acidity and congestion, followed by an erosion of vitality that accelerates the ageing process and underpins the development of all chronic degenerative disease.

### Box 2.1 Symptoms of a sodium/potassium imbalance

- Fluid retention, particularly in the lower body, resulting in weight gain;
- Excessive mucus secretions leading to lung congestion, asthma, hay fever, discharges, phlegm;
- Heart and kidney strain resulting in degenerative complaints in these organs;
- Excess acidity collecting in the tissues resulting in osteoporosis and inflammatory conditions such as arthritis, atherosclerosis (heart disease), gout, diverticulitis and colitis;
- General hardening leading to atheroma, arteriosclerosis, fibromyalgia, kidney and gall stone formation;
- Skin disorders such as eczema, psoriasis, dermatitis, boils, acne, abscesses, dandruff, cradle cap (the baby inherits its mineral status from both parents);
- Loss of muscle integrity, elasticity and tone leading to hernia, prolapse, varicose veins, congestive heart failure;
- Impaired nerve impulse transmission leading to heart problems, mental impairment; and
- Congestion with lowered vitality in all tissues.

# Calcium/magnesium balance

## The calcium neurosis

*Absorption and retention of calcium is ultimately governed by magnesium and vitamin D. Deficiencies of these nutrients lead to a low calcium status.*

Calcium enjoys such a high nutritional profile that nothing much is spoken about magnesium. Over the past fifty years our calcium neurosis has increased and yet no one questions as to why we should be calcium-deficient when our dietary calcium often exceeds the recommended daily intake (400mg-1,000mg/day; the higher level being required during growth phases and pregnancy). Advertising campaigns constantly warn us about calcium deficiencies and recommend drinking milk daily.

In fact calcium intakes greater than 1,000mg daily serve no useful purpose. It has been proved that high calcium intake has no effect on bone integrity. In fact there are no known diseases due to a primary calcium deficiency – that is deficiencies arising purely from inadequate dietary calcium intake. Certain tribes living in South America and Africa consume only 200mg-300mg of calcium daily and yet show no deficiency symptoms or skeletal deformities. Rickets (a disease where bones fail to calcify properly) used to be prevalent among poorly nourished children living in dark slum areas, but the condition was found to be due to a lack of vitamin D through inadequate exposure to sunshine rather than a primary calcium deficiency.

*Calcium supplementation inhibits the uptake of magnesium, zinc, iron and iodine, and by default will induce deficiencies of these nutrients.*

If dietary calcium intake was the most important factor in calcium balance, we should not be calcium-deficient on the modern diet. However, it is becoming clear that it is not dietary amounts that govern calcium status but rather factors which control its absorption and retention. Of these, magnesium is the most important. In other words, magnesium deficiency leads to calcium deficiency.

As with the sodium/potassium balance it is the dietary ratio between these two minerals, calcium and magnesium, which determines their overall balance. An adequate magnesium intake will ensure calcium absorption and retention. However, if too much calcium is taken in the diet, it suppresses the absorption of magnesium leading to magnesium deficiencies, ultimately resulting in calcium deficiency. Just as excess sodium causes potassium losses, so excess calcium depletes magnesium.

This ratio is exaggerated on the modern diet which tends to be high in calcium while low in the magnesium-rich foods such as the whole grains, nuts and legumes. Dairy produce is often included in the diet at the expense of these foods, particularly in lacto-vegetarianism where cheese is often preferentially taken as a source of protein over nuts, legumes and whole grains.

If we take another look at the calcium/magnesium balance in natural foods (table 2.4 *Average values of calcium and magnesium*) we can see that adequate amounts of both minerals are found across the food groups, and provided that the diet incorporates sufficient variety, then calcium and magnesium will be consumed in an equal ratio. However, once you start incorporating dairy produce in any significant quantity the ratio favours calcium. It is interesting that many traditional cultures use only small amounts of dairy to complement protein and calcium requirements, and not as the main part of the meal, thereby keeping the mineral ratio.

Table 2.4  Average values of calcium and magnesium, mg/100g

|  | Ca | Mg |
| --- | --- | --- |
| Cereals (dry weight) | 41 | 110 |
| Cheese | 750 | 24 |
| Fish | 8 | 26 |
| Fruits | 16 | 9.6 |
| Leaf veg | 111 | 17.4 |
| Meat | 6 | 24 |
| Milk | 116 | 12 |
| Nuts | 117 | 223 |
| Legumes (dry weight) | 134 | 179 |
| Root veg | 53 | 12.6 |

You can see that on a well-balanced diet, which includes whole grains, nuts and legumes, there are adequate amounts of both calcium and magnesium in a ratio that is beneficial to health.

The refining of grains damages our magnesium status further. Most of the nutrients, including magnesium, are found in the outer coating of the grain which is removed during refining. In addition to this, our staple grain wheat, once refined and the magnesium removed, is then enriched with calcium. The table below gives the values for calcium and magnesium prior to and after refining. You can see that the ratio between these minerals is completely reversed.

### Calcium and magnesium values:  mg/100g

|  | Ca | Mg |
| --- | --- | --- |
| Wheat flour (brown) | 41 | 163 |
| Wheat flour (white) | 150 | 20 |

Excess dairy and the refining of grains are not the only culprits in magnesium deficiency. There are other dietary and lifestyle-related factors which exacerbate magnesium's vulnerability.

*Magnesium is a borderline mineral; soil depletion and the use of nitrate fertilisers further erode the magnesium status of our foods. Additionally, sugar, tea, coffee and alcohol wash away what little dietary magnesium we may ingest.*

## Major culprits in magnesium deficiency

*Dietary factors include:*

- **Tea, coffee** and **alcohol** are diuretics and "wash" magnesium away in the urine. You can end up with net losses of magnesium if you consume large quantities of these items; and
- **High fat** and **refined carbohydrates** (sugar, bread, cakes, pasta) increase the requirement for magnesium. These foods are "empty" of magnesium and other nutrients and yet require it for their metabolism. Therefore they draw on any existing supplies stored in the body and will erode the magnesium status substantially.

*Life-style related factors include:*

- **Emotional** and **mental stress** increase energy requirements and will deplete the body of magnesium - the main mineral involved in energy production.
- **Physical stress** such as **heavy, sustained exercise training**
- **Low blood sugar** (see chapter 6 *Regeneration and blood sugar control*) and erratic eating patterns
- **Stimulants** (tea, coffee, chocolate, other caffeine-containing drinks such as cola, and drugs such as the amphetamines and cocaine).

All in all magnesium fares very badly with current lifestyle trends, the consequences of which undermine our total health picture. As magnesium is the main mineral which governs our energy (along with potassium), detoxification and regeneration cannot occur unless magnesium is reinstated. We shall find out later the critical role magnesium plays in detoxification, the re-establishment of potassium within the cell and in the regeneration of tissues. But before we move on, it is worthwhile exploring just how magnesium controls our calcium status.

### How does magnesium control our calcium balance?

*Blood calcium is maintained within a very narrow range; low levels affect nerve and muscle function and may lead to tetany.*

Parathyroid hormone (PTH) controls calcium concentrations within the blood. The parathyroid glands, situated at the four corners of the thyroid gland, detect any fall in blood calcium. When this occurs they secrete PTH which stimulates the bones to release calcium, the kidneys to reabsorb calcium from the kidney filtrate, and the conversion of vitamin D to its active form which acts as a carrier for the absorption of dietary calcium (figure 2.5 *Mode of action of PTH*). These three modes of action ensure the absorption, retention and subsequent stabilisation of blood calcium. Without these mechanisms we would sustain huge calcium losses; not only would we forfeit all our dietary calcium (due to inadequate conversion of vitamin D to its active form which carries calcium across the intestinal tract), but we would also incur losses from the calcium-rich digestive juices and from the kidney filtrate. To give an idea of the importance of PTH, the kidneys filter around 9,600mg of calcium daily, 9,340mg of which must be reabsorbed. The obligatory loss for calcium is only 240mg, but without PTH these losses would be much greater.

*Health issues relating to the Ca/Mg imbalance*

The secretion and the activity of PTH depend upon magnesium. In magnesium deficiency PTH cannot be secreted; it cannot convert vitamin D to its active form, nor will it stimulate the kidneys to reabsorb calcium. Hence high dairy diets, which are low in magnesium and further depress its absorption, ultimately may lead to calcium deficiency and increased losses from the bones. In order to maintain a good calcium status it is essential to incorporate magnesium-rich foods, such as whole grains, legumes and nuts in the diet. If you turn to table 2.5 *Calcium and magnesium status of foods per average portion* you can see the values for both these minerals in the various food groups.

**Figure 2.5** Mode of action of PTH

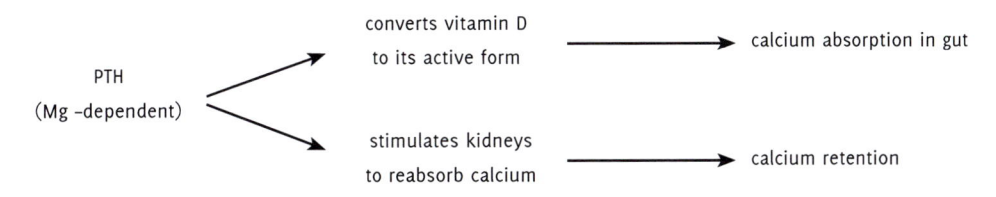

PTH (Mg –dependent) → converts vitamin D to its active form → calcium absorption in gut

PTH (Mg –dependent) → stimulates kidneys to reabsorb calcium → calcium retention

PTH governs the blood calcium status. When blood calcium falls, PTH stimulates the bones to release calcium, the kidneys to reabsorb calcium from the filtrate, and the conversion of vitamin D to its active form which facilitates gastrointestinal absorption of calcium. PTH is dependent upon an adequate magnesium status; therefore magnesium deficiency, by default, causes calcium losses.

## What does a calcium/magnesium imbalance mean?

I mentioned earlier the critical role that magnesium plays in the detoxification process and the reinstatement of potassium within the cell. Magnesium is required for the operation of the sodium/potassium pump at the cell membrane which, if you remember, pumps sodium out in exchange for potassium. Even if you do not take excess salt in the diet, a magnesium deficiency, by default, allows sodium to drift into the cell and results in intracellular potassium losses.

I have treated many people on detoxification programs and supplementation of magnesium can make a great difference in the speed of treatment. This does not mean that you should all rush out and buy magnesium. First you need to assess how strong an elimination your body can cope with (see chapter 4 *Vitality & healing* and chapter 5 *Liver cleansing*). If the pressure is too extreme it can result in a worsening of conditions.

In general, if you suffer high blood pressure, asthma, eczema, kidney disease or other chronic forms of disease, I would recommend starting with the high potassium/low sodium program and introduce magnesium later into the regime. Eczema and asthma, in particular, indicate very deep mineral imbalances with poor calcium handling, but the picture may be too congested to allow safe supplementation with magnesium and instead give rise to exacerbations. Magnesium and potassium-rich foods are introduced into the diet while dairy and salt are removed to correct the imbalance. However, after a period of time magnesium may be safely introduced, if still required by that stage. With high blood pressure, the sudden removal of sodium along with water from

*It is better to incorporate magnesium-rich foods in the diet rather than relying on magnesium supplements as many of these foods are also a rich supply of other nutrients including zinc and iron.*

## 2 Salt & dairy - the devitalisers

**Table 2.5** Calcium and magnesium status of foods per average portion

| Fruits | Ca | Mg |
|---|---|---|
| Banana | 8.4 | 50.4 |
| Blackberries 90g | 56.7 | 27 |
| Blackcurrants 75g | 38 | 12 |
| Grapes, white x 20 | 20.2 | 6.7 |
| Lemon 100g | 110 | 12 |
| Mango 160g | 16 | 28.8 |
| Melon, Cantaloupe | 34 | 36 |
| Honeydew 180g | 25 | 2 |
| Orange | 57.4 | 18.2 |
| Raspberries 75g | 30.7 | 16.5 |
| Rhubarb 150g, cooked* | 139 | 19.5 |
| Strawberries 120g | 26.4 | 14.4 |
| Tangerine | 29.4 | 7.7 |
| Watermelon 180g | 9 | 19.8 |

| Vegetables | Ca | Mg |
|---|---|---|
| Avocado pear (1/2) | 11.2 | 21.7 |
| Broccoli 45g | 34.2 | 5.4 |
| Broad beans 120g | 25.2 | 33.6 |
| Brussels sprout 120g | 30 | 15.6 |
| Carrots, raw 60g | 28.8 | 7.2 |
| Chinese leaves 40g | 61.6 | 64 |
| Leeks 160g | 97.6 | 20.8 |
| Onion 90g raw | 27.9 | 7.2 |
| Okra 60g | 42 | 36 |
| Parsnip 120g | 43.2 | 15.6 |
| Peas 80g | 24.8 | 18.4 |
| Potato (jacket) 260g | 20.8 | 62.4 |
| Spinach 100g* | 600 | 59 |
| Swede 100g | 42 | 7 |
| Sweet corn 100g | 3 | 23 |
| Turnip 100g | 55 | 7 |
| Watercress 20g | 44 | 3.4 |

| Nuts mg/100g dry weight (average serve 40g) | Ca | Mg |
|---|---|---|
| Brazil nuts | 180 | 416 |
| Cashews | 38 | 265 |
| Almonds | 250 | 260 |
| Peanuts | 61 | 180 |
| Walnuts | 60 | 130 |
| Sunflower seeds | 132 | 44 |

| Cereals mg/100g dry weight (average serving 50g) | Ca | Mg |
|---|---|---|
| Barley | 39 | 40 |
| Buckwheat | 38 | 54 |
| Maize | 52 | - |
| Millet | 23 | 184 |
| Oats | 60 | 120 |
| Rice (brown) | 37 | 100 |
| Rye | 40 | 108 |
| Wheat germ | 18 | 319 |
| Wheat flour; brown | 41 | 163 |
| white | 150 | 20 |

| Pulses mg/100g dry weight (average serving 50g) | Ca | Mg |
|---|---|---|
| Chickpeas | 167 | 180 |
| Kidney beans | 157 | 202 |
| Lentils | 44 | 88 |
| Tofu | 504 | 23 |
| Butter Beans | 96 | 185 |
| Haricot | 203 | 203 |

the cells into the circulation may initially elevate the pressure, but this is rarely the case. It is interesting that medical drugs used for reducing the blood volume in cases of hypertension (high blood pressure) cause potassium and magnesium losses - the very minerals you need to reinstate in order to regenerate healthy tissues and a healthy heart.

**Figure 2.6** Magnesium and the sodium/potassium pump

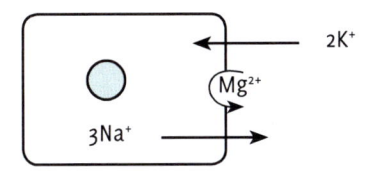

Magnesium helps power the sodium/potassium pump which exchanges sodium for potassium.

**Magnesium and energy** Many people find that no matter how much they eat they feel permanently hungry, never have any energy and suffer cravings for chocolate, sugar and caffeine. This is usually the downfall of any diet - the inability to stick to it due to the cravings! So if your diet is giving you sufficient kilojoules to meet your energy requirements, how is it that you crave more?

*Magnesium deficiency leads to poor blood sugar control and low energy, particularly noticeable during the late afternoon.*

The explanation is quite simple. A magnesium deficiency means that you can neither extract the energy from food nor utilise it. Imagine the domestic fuel scenario. The energy from solid fuel, such as gas, oil or coal is converted to electrical energy which is routed to your home. When you require this energy you plug into it. In a similar manner our food is the fuel that is burned to release its energy. This is converted to chemical energy (ATP) which is available when required. You just have to tap into it. Magnesium is critical in both the conversion of food energy to chemical energy and then to metabolic activity. Think of magnesium as the plug on your electrical gadgets; without these you cannot access your energy supply. In short, magnesium controls your available energy.

**Figure 2.7** The conversion of fuel to energy

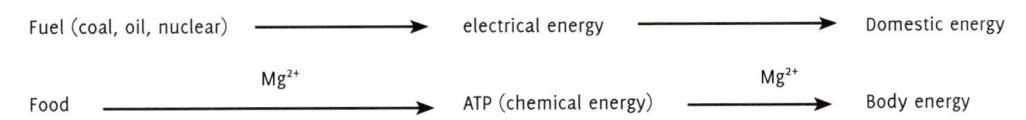

Fuel (coal, oil, nuclear) $\longrightarrow$ electrical energy $\longrightarrow$ Domestic energy

Food $\xrightarrow{Mg^{2+}}$ ATP (chemical energy) $\xrightarrow{Mg^{2+}}$ Body energy

Magnesium is the co-factor required for all energy exchanges within the body; both in the transfer of energy for ATP synthesis and its subsequent transfer to energy-dependent mechanisms.

**Magnesium and our nerves and muscles** Our nerves and muscles are very susceptible to a calcium/magnesium disturbance. The tense, irritable picture where our nerves feel edgy and our muscles cramped and tense, is an indicator of a poor magnesium status. We tend to think of relaxation as being a passive process but it is in fact a very active one. Relaxation requires a magnesium-driven pump to remove calcium from active sites in the muscle fibres which are

*Taking salt to alleviate muscle cramps will exacerbate the problem in the long-term.*

*Nervous irritability and muscle tension are clear indicators of magnesium deficiency.*

responsible for contraction. Painful cramping signifies magnesium (and potassium) deficiencies - hence bananas (which are high in magnesium) are often recommended for muscle cramps.

Similarly with our nerves. In magnesium deficiency, repetitive electrical impulses are sent down the nerve fibres which lead to irritability. Magnesium actively pumps sodium, which is responsible for the nerve impulse, from the nerve fibre so restoring the resting state of the nerve. Many patients who experience anxiety, depression and tension can be helped with magnesium supplementation rather than resorting to anti-depressant drugs.

Heart disease and asthma deserve a special mention here as magnesium deficiencies cause spasms in the coronary arteries, contribute to irregular heart rhythms and constriction of the bronchioles. It is easy to blame environmental pollution for the rise in asthma, but even in areas which are considered to be environmentally "cleaner", asthma is still on the increase. The removal of dairy does much to alleviate the condition in many cases. This will automatically go some way to redress any calcium/magnesium imbalance which, in turn, will positively affect the sodium/potassium balance. Dairy products are low in magnesium, and therefore by default support the accumulation of sodium and acidity in the tissues. This predisposes a catarrhal picture which exacerbates congestion in the lungs.

**Magnesium and regeneration** Finally, magnesium is essential for the regeneration of tissues. As most of our energy-dependent processes require magnesium (hence the analogy with the domestic plug), so tissue renewal and maintenance are no exception. In magnesium deficiency the tissues with the highest turnover (or those replaced more frequently), such as the cells of the immune system, the digestive tract, the liver and even your hair follicles, become compromised and symptoms in these organs will be the first to manifest. Lowered resistance to infection, poor digestion, gastro-intestinal disturbances, ulcers, allergies and hair loss may all form part of the deficiency picture.

**Magnesium and the trace mineral balance** Once magnesium is reinstated then deficiencies of the trace elements such as iron, zinc, manganese and chromium are often resolved without any specific nutritional supplementation. This is because magnesium is integral to many of the energy-dependent mechanisms that are required to carry nutrients across the intestinal tract and also for the manufacture of liver proteins which transport certain minerals, such as iron, to the tissues. In many cases it may be pointless supplementing the trace elements before you have re-established the four major minerals. Once the cells are detoxified then these minerals are retained more efficiently by the cells and taken up by the enzyme systems powering their activity.

**Box 2.2  Symptoms of calcium/magnesium imbalance**

- Acidity and the hardening process is accelerated;
- Lethargy and fatigue;
- Cravings, addictions and mood swings;
- Poor regeneration of body tissues leading to recurrent infection and digestive disorders, hair loss; and
- Irritability in the neuromuscular system: muscle cramping, heart disease, asthma, anxiety and nervous irritability.

# Tips for Restoring the Major Mineral Balance

Unless the major mineral balance is redressed then detoxification will not take place.

- Always make sure that your potassium intake is five times that of your sodium (don't add salt or use products which have salt added);
- Eat plenty of magnesium-rich foods such as legumes, nuts and whole grains. Wheat germ is an excellent source of magnesium. When cooking, use the minimal amount of water required as magnesium, along with other nutrients, is leached into the cooking liquid;
- Omit tea, coffee and alcohol from the diet as these items have a diuretic action and "wash" magnesium from the body via the kidneys;
- Omit sugars, refined carbohydrates and fatty foods. These come without magnesium and draw on existing supplies for their metabolism;
- On detoxification diets dairy is usually omitted initially as it may exacerbate any calcium/magnesium imbalance and encourage the entry of sodium into the cell. On a maintenance plan natural yoghurt may be included.

### Case History 2.1

**Sarah was 40 years old** and going through early menopause. Her menstrual cycle was irregular, she was depressed, felt pre-menstrual all the time and had started having hot flushes. She decided against hormone replacement therapy as there was a tendency to thrombosis.

Sarah's eating habits were erratic and she noticed that she became anxious and shaky if she missed food. These bouts of shakiness inhibited her from going out in case she had an "attack". She also suffered chocolate cravings. Over the last twelve months she had diarrhoea with loose and foamy stools, three to four times daily. Her dentist had noticed bone loss in her jaw.

Sarah suffered recurrent tonsillitis as a child, receiving antibiotic treatment regularly. Her adenoids and tonsils were later removed. During her teens she became anorexic but her weight never dropped critically low. Sarah also regularly suffered from cystitis and thrush.

My main concern was that Sarah might have osteoporosis and I recommended a bone density scan. The results showed that she was "critically osteoporotic" and treatment was advised to start at once. Sarah decided to wait a further eighteen months to see whether she could regenerate bone or at least stabilise the situation. I was not surprised by the result as the onset of early menopause is always a risk factor for osteoporosis. But more indicative was her nutritional state during adolescence and both her pregnancies when requirements for calcium and protein are increased. Failure to meet requirements results in a reduction of bone density from the outset which predisposes osteoporosis in later life. In addition, stress factors, including low blood sugar symptoms (cravings, shaky if misses food), play a major role in bone degeneration. Hormones released under any stress (including low blood sugar) cause the breakdown of bone protein. Finally, calcium and other nutrient losses would have been sustained over the last year due to the diarrhoea.

We had to stabilise Sarah's blood sugar levels (there can be no regeneration while the body is in a constant state of breakdown) and we had to reduce the diarrhoea. Over the next few months following the detoxification diet, Sarah improved dramatically. Although Sarah was both calcium and magnesium deficient, magnesium supplements were not used initially until the cleansing process was well under way. In addition, magnesium can have an aggravating effect on the bowel. Later in treatment magnesium was incorporated into the prescription to ensure retention of dietary calcium. Osteoporosis is not essentially a calcium-deficiency disease, although it can be aggravated by deficiency. It is an abnormal loss of the protein matrix upon which calcium is deposited. Magnesium, zinc and vitamin C are all essential for bone protein synthesis - both magnesium and zinc being inhibited by large doses of calcium!

Sarah tried hard at the diet in the beginning and her health improved dramatically. Her next bone scan showed that the bone density had increased by 3%. She was delighted and although she no longer followed the diet rigidly she had adopted many of the principles. She was more surprised when, three years later, her periods returned.

It is possible to construct a good diet along the principles outlined in this chapter. For many people the detoxification plan may be too rigid or their current lifestyle makes such planning impossible. But there is a great deal that you can achieve just by becoming aware of what you eat and choosing more wisely. However, if you wish to reverse the degenerative process then merely adopting a good eating plan will not be sufficient. For those who wish to achieve a greater potential, then read on. In Part 2 we focus on how you can make the program work for you, within your individual case.

….there is no other way, than through the use of vegetables and fruits, to reduce acidity in the tissues. It does not matter how many nutritional supplements you take or what dietary changes you make, if you do not incorporate appreciable quantities of fruits and vegetables into the diet, then this process will not be stimulated, congestion will not be reduced and the disease process will not be reversed.

# 3

# Acid/alkaline balance

## 3  Acid/alkaline balance

**You will by now be familiar with the term acidity** and what this means to the hardening and degenerative process. The anomaly is that the body constantly produces acids as by-products of normal metabolism. We know that the body needs to maintain its slightly alkaline pH within a very narrow range. At an optimum of pH 7.4 there are 0.0016 mmol of acid in the body. As the body produces 10.4 mmol of acid per minute this represents a staggering 6,500 times the amount held in the body at pH 7.4! This is where breathing comes in. Most of the acid produced is in the form of carbonic acid, which can be converted to carbon dioxide and water. The carbon dioxide is "blown off" via the breath, and the water eliminated by the kidneys. So breathing keeps pace with acid production – the more acid you produce (the faster the metabolism), the faster you breathe. If we stopped breathing for 4 minutes, the body's pH would drop to 3.0, our cells would cease to function and we would die.

However, some acids are not volatile (cannot be breathed off) and as the cells cannot operate in a strongly acidic environment, these acids need to be "buffered" or neutralised. The cell has plenty of neutralising agents (phosphates) but when these phosphates become saturated, or used up, the bones are called upon to buffer the excess acidity. In the process calcium ions are exchanged for hydrogen ions (our measure of acidity), calcium is lost from the skeleton and precipitates in the soft tissues to form insoluble salts and crystals leading to hardening and inflammation: the greater the acidity, the greater the bone calcium losses.

It is the acidity and the consequences of acidity within the tissues that we are attempting to reverse on detoxification programs. Once the cell has its optimal pH for metabolic activity, the cell will take up oxygen, our fuel will burn efficiently, toxins will not be produced and hardening will not occur. We have explored the role of salt in this degenerative process and the necessity of potassium and magnesium-rich foods to facilitate the removal of both sodium and acidity but we can go further than this by identifying groups of foods which either promote acidity or actively remove it. You will then start to gain an insight into why certain foods (and the amounts suggested) are included in the diet and why other foods are omitted entirely in order for detoxification to occur.

## How do we produce acids?

As mentioned, our bodies naturally produce huge amounts of acids daily which are generated as a by-product from the burning of fuel. Our carbohydrates, fats and proteins can all be used as an energy resource but first they are broken down into acids, such as ketogenic and glucogenic acids, before they enter the energy cycle. This cycle is dependent upon adequate oxygen and the presence of specific minerals and vitamins. Remember that vitamins and minerals are like the tools of the workmen, or enzyme systems, which convert food to energy. This cycle creates yet more acids, known as intermediate acids before they are eventually reduced to carbonic acid ($H_2CO_3$) which can safely be eliminated by the lungs and kidneys as carbon dioxide and water (see figure 3.1 *Metabolism of foods in the energy cycle*). If there are nutrient or oxygen deficiencies then our fuel is not fully metabolised and the intermediate acids accumulate resulting in toxicity, congestion and lowered vitality.

*Carbonic acid is a volatile acid and can be exhaled via the lungs.*

We also create greater amounts of acidity if we are stressed, take stimulants such as caffeine-containing drinks, eat chocolate or drink alcohol. In addition, diets high in foods which are stripped of their nutrients (refined foods and fats) predispose congestion of the tissues. For example, in severe B1 deficiency, pyruvic acid accumulates causing oedema of the tissues and subsequent heart failure. While most of us do not suffer from such gross deficiency states, undoubtedly borderline deficiencies do occur which may insidiously erode health over many years.

**Figure 3.1** Metabolism of foods in the energy cycle

$$\left.\begin{array}{l}\text{CHOs}\\ \text{Fats}\\ \text{Proteins}\end{array}\right\} \xrightarrow{B6, B2, Mg} \text{gluco- \& ketogenic acids} \xrightarrow{B1, B2, B3, B5, Mg, K, Mn + O_2} \text{intermediate metabolic acids} \rightarrow H_2CO_3 \begin{array}{l}\nearrow H_2O\text{ (kidneys)}\\ \searrow CO_2\text{ (lungs)}\end{array}$$

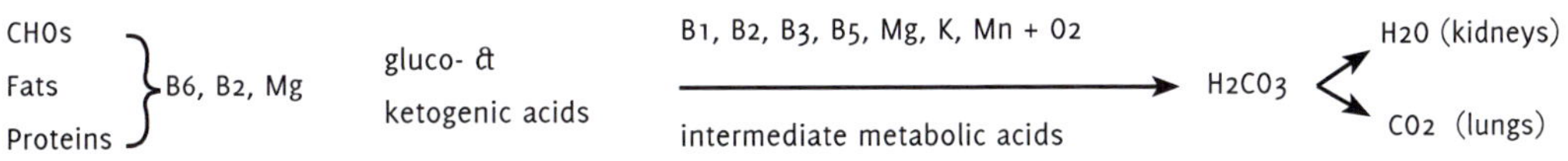

A range of minerals and vitamins are required as co-factors in the conversion of fuel to energy. During the conversion glucogenic and ketogenic acids are formed. Provided that there is an adequate supply of nutrients and oxygen, these acids will eventually be degraded to carbonic acid which is easily eliminated via the lungs and kidneys.

All foods require vitamins B6, B2 and magnesium to enter the energy cycle as acids. From here the breakdown of these acids requires a variety of other nutrients plus oxygen for their ultimate reduction to carbon dioxide and water. Oxygen and nutrient deficiencies lead to the accumulation of intermediate acids in the cells and toxicity. You can see that in spite of the volume of acidity generated by the body that there are fast and effective ways of dealing with it.

*Vitamin and mineral deficiencies are a major cause of acidity.*

However, other types of acids, known as the metabolic acids produced by high fat and high protein diets, take a lot longer to eliminate, eventually being disposed of through the kidneys. The kidneys bear the brunt of acid elimination and on the modern, highly acid-forming diet, the biological age of the kidney may not reflect its chronological age, hence the saying the "ageing Western kidney." Kidney disease is certainly on the increase, these organs having a major influence on the health of the heart and bones. It is interesting that many of the herbal medicines for arthritis, which focus on the removal of excess acidity from the tissues, act by stimulating kidney function and regeneration.

## 3 Acid/alkaline balance

*Metabolic acids, derived from protein and fat metabolism, take seven days to eliminate via the kidneys.*

As the kidneys lose their efficiency the acidic load may become greater than the kidneys can comfortably handle. Like sodium, acidity from metabolic acids takes around seven days to eliminate during which time it is stored in the cells. This delay in elimination creates a cumulative effect increasing the acidic burden within the cells. As the general acidic burden rises, calcium becomes leached from the bones in exchange for the acidity. The acidity is thus buffered, leaving the calcium to precipitate in the soft tissues.

In simple terms, if we return to our analogy of adding lemon juice to milk, buffering is the process that occurs when the the alkaline milk exchanges its calcium for the acidity of the lemon juice. In the process whey is formed (a dilute acid) and curds precipitate.

Sodium may also precipitate to form the salt, sodium urate. This occurs when uric acid concentrations are elevated as seen in gout. These crystals cause intense inflammation and pain particularly in the big toe joint. However, sodium urate crystals are more readily dissolved than the calcium salts.

### What must we do to reduce this acidic load?

Obviously eat less of the acid-forming foods and more of the alkaline-forming foods. If you look at figure 3.2 *Dietary contributions to the acid:alkaline balance* you will see at a glance the three groups of foods: the alkaline-formers, the acid-formers and the neutral foods. The neutral group consists of foods which do not create excess acidity but neither do they actively reduce it.

**Figure 3.2**  Dietary contributions to the acid:alkali balance

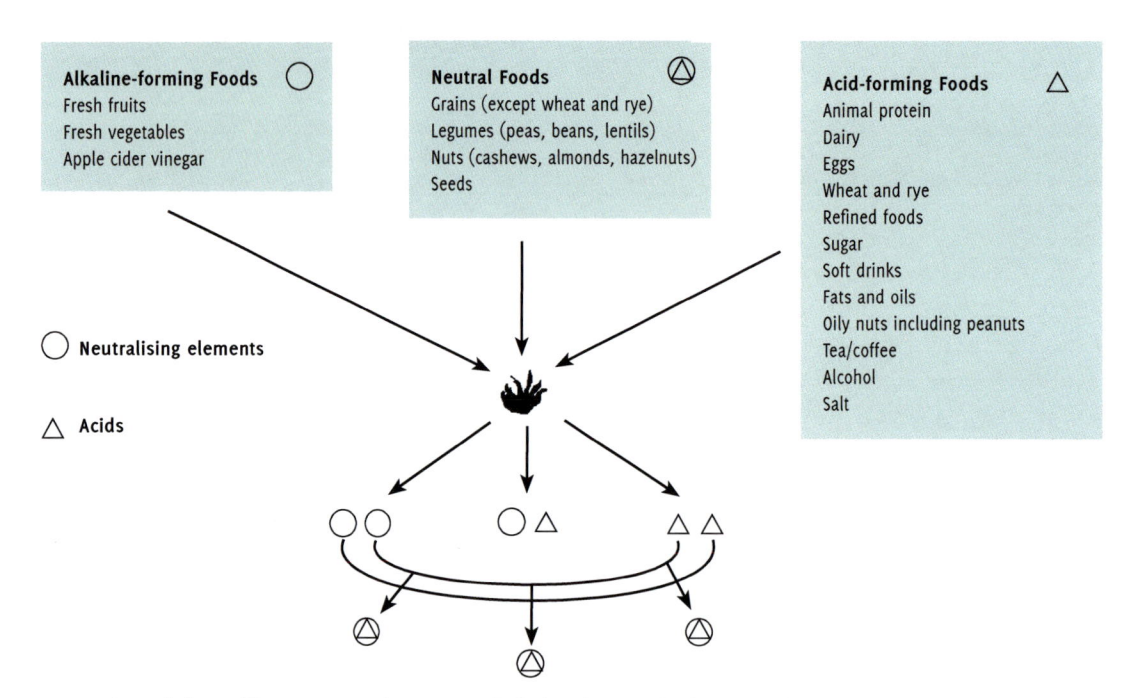

**Alkaline-forming Foods** ○
Fresh fruits
Fresh vegetables
Apple cider vinegar

**Neutral Foods** △
Grains (except wheat and rye)
Legumes (peas, beans, lentils)
Nuts (cashews, almonds, hazelnuts)
Seeds

**Acid-forming Foods** △
Animal protein
Dairy
Eggs
Wheat and rye
Refined foods
Sugar
Soft drinks
Fats and oils
Oily nuts including peanuts
Tea/coffee
Alcohol
Salt

○ Neutralising elements

△ Acids

Balanced diets will ensure a predominance of alkaline-forming foods over acid-forming foods. In this way you will protect your body from the ravages of prolonged acidity and degenerative disease.

# Alkaline-forming foods

**These are the fruits and vegetables.** Do not be confused by their acid taste into thinking that they must create acidity in the tissues. Quite the reverse is true. Their overall effect is to create an alkaline environment within the cells. Vegetables and fruits, once metabolized, leave a high concentration of potassium ($K^+$) and hydroxyl ions ($OH^-$) within the cell. In simple terms, the hydroxyl ions (alkaline) neutralise and mop up the acids or hydrogen ions ($H^+$) to form water ($OH^- + H^+ = H_2O$), while the potassium flushes sodium, excess water and toxins from the cell. By increasing the alkaline reserves within the cell, the cell becomes more negatively charged, the positively charged hydrogen ions having been neutralised. Once the negative potential is restored, oxygen is drawn into the cell and potassium is reinstated. Then a curious sequence of events occurs. As the electrical state is rectified, potassium binds at specific sites which, in turn, generates its own electrical field. This field pulls water molecules into a formation, lining up in tight layers leaving no room for toxins, sodium or excess water, and the cell is naturally purified. In truth, there is no other way, other than through the use of vegetables and fruits, to reduce acidity in the tissues. It does not matter how many nutritional supplements you take or what dietary changes you make, if you do not incorporate appreciable quantities of fruits and vegetables into the diet then this process will not be stimulated, congestion will not be reduced and the disease process will not be reversed.

*pH is the measure of acidity. "H" stands for hydrogen ions: the greater the acidity, the greater the concentration of free hydrogen ions in solution.*

**Figure 3.3** Purification of the cell on a high potassium, high alkaline-forming diet

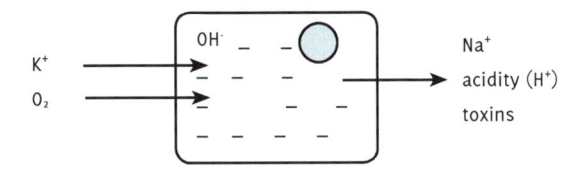

*The electrical state of the cell is governed by the pH. An acidic environment reduces the electrical potential and lowers cell vitality.*

As the cell becomes increasingly alkaline ($OH^-$), due to the high potassium, high alkaline forming diet, its negative potential increases and potassium and oxygen enter the cell. The oxidative cycle is restored, and sodium, acidity ($H^+$) and toxins are driven from the cell.

On a detoxification program between 40%-80% of the diet is met by vegetables and fruits. This is the percentage of the energy value of the diet. So on a diet providing 6,300 kilojoules (1,500 calories), then 40% (2,520 kilojoules) must be met by fruit and vegetables which represents a staggering 2.5 kilograms daily - hence the use of juicing. This detoxification program advises the lower figure of 40%, as diets with the higher content are difficult to sustain over a long period, particularly if working or raising a family. However, for those with serious conditions who can commit to a stronger regime (such as the Gerson Therapy) then higher amounts may be advisable.

*Generally, I would not recommend juicing beetroot as it is too high in sugar. Celery may not be recommended initially as it is high in sodium.*

### Vegetable juices

should be made from organic produce (you don't want a cocktail of chemicals), such as carrots, lettuce, green capsicum, red cabbage, red or green lettuce (not iceberg as it lacks nutrients), and small amounts of dark green leafy vegetables combined with apple. Generally 250g of mixed vegetables to 250g of apple will give 250ml of juice. We usually avoid juicing beetroot as it is high in sugar and can aggravate conditions where there is poor blood sugar control or insulin resistance. Celery may also be omitted from the juices in the initial stages as it contains high amounts of natural sodium which oppose the potassium push that you are trying to achieve. Similarly, some of the darker green leafy vegetables, such as kale, spinach and chard are not only high in sodium but also contain high amounts of oxalic acid that bind calcium making it unavailable. If you follow Dr. Gerson's green juice recipe (below) you will see that the principal green vegetable is lettuce, to which we add small amounts of the dark green leafy vegetables. It is not recommended that you substitute other greens if you can't access all the vegetables, however you should be able to source green capsicum, red cabbage and cos lettuce throughout the year. This combination, along with the apple, makes a more than satisfactory green juice.

**Dr Gerson's Green Juice Recipe**

- 1 small wedge red cabbage
- 1/4 green capsicum
- 1 leaf endive
- 1 leaf chard/silver beet
- 2 leaves beet tops
- 2 sprigs watercress
- large handful of cos, green or red leaf lettuce (not iceberg)
- 1 medium green apple, cored

### Apple cider vinegar

has long been heralded a great reducer of acidity and its use is advocated in hardening diseases such as arthritis and stone formation. It is a concentrate of the apple, so creates a stronger alkalinising effect on tissues. 10mls diluted in a little warm water can be taken half an hour before meals to reduce acidity. The saying "an apple a day keeps the doctor away" is derived from the known beneficial effects of apples. Vegetable juices mixed with apple juice taken over a period of time exert deep cleansing effects on the body tissues.

### Lemon juice

is traditionally known as a great cleanser. It is both sour and an astringent and benefits the liver so may be taken on the program. Conversely, orange juice may aggravate conditions, particularly catarrhal symptoms and arthritis, and is therefore best avoided if you suffer these problems.

# Other cleansing therapies

## The Gerson Cancer Therapy®
requires 13 x 240ml [8 fl oz] freshly made vegetable juices taken on an hourly basis throughout the day: 5 apple and carrot juices, 3 carrot only juices, 5 green juices and 1 orange juice. This amounts to around 3.12 litres of juice, or the equivalent of 3.75kg vegetables, 2.25kg apples, and 2 oranges on a daily basis. Vegetable juicers that grind the vegetables and then press the pulp are recommended over centrifugal juicers which destroy the valuable oxidising enzymes critical for the success of the therapy. In addition, your daily meals include raw fruits and salads, cooked vegetables and fruits (stewed in their own juice), potatoes and oatmeal. Animal protein is not allowed during the first six weeks, and after then only in the form of fat-free, salt-free pot cheese and/or yoghurt from skimmed milk, and buttermilk. This therapy is an 18-month to two year program.

*When choosing a juicer, opt for a machine that either grinds or triturates the vegetable matter. Centrifugal machines are not effective at extracting all the nutrients and tend to destroy the anti-oxidants making the juice more vulnerable to oxidation.*

## Dr. J. Christopher's 3 day cleanse and regenerative diet
advocates the three-day cleanse where the aim is to replace nine litres of toxic lymph with nine litres of alkaline fluid over a three-day period. This is a mono-diet, where the juices are prepared from one fruit or vegetable only; three litres are taken daily, interspersed with distilled water for three consecutive days. Each mouthful should be "chewed" stimulating the digestive juices. On the fourth day the cleanse is broken by adding raw vegetables to the diet. This is a very strong elimination and should not be undertaken unless supervised by a qualified professional. Dr. Christopher does not recommend this plan unless the patient has undergone a preliminary preparation period using diet and cleansing techniques to pave the way for the great elimination that may ensue. I would not recommend "chewing" the juices on a regular basis, as the acid can erode the enamel from the teeth. In fact I always recommend brushing your teeth with water after taking vegetable juices.

Dr. Christopher's dietary principles on his regenerative diet include vegetables and salads as the main part of the diet, fruits, herbs, potatoes, nuts and whole grains (but not milled). These whole grains should be "cooked" by low heating so that technically they could still sprout. Grains like barley and whole wheat can be successfully "cooked" overnight in a wide-necked thermos flask by adding 1½ cup of boiling water to 1 cup of the grain and sealing with the lid - but I doubt that they would still sprout! These cereals are delicious with stewed fruit. The use of all animal protein, dairy products, eggs and milled grains are prohibited. He also recommends three teaspoons of cayenne pepper daily (taken in capsules) to cut mucus and remove catarrh (both caused by toxicity).

This regenerative diet is recommended over an eight week period, often followed by the three day cleanse and a further eight weeks on the diet. However, this type of diet may prove too stringent for most people and often does not lead to long-term dietary changes, which are essential if you are going to maintain health. In addition, depending on your constitution and your current level of toxicity (see chapter 5 *Liver cleansing* to help you determine this) you may feel dreadful and give up at the first hurdle. Others, who suffer from ill health due to long-term nutritional deficiencies, could become even more deficient suffering a further decline in health rather than any regeneration.

## 3   Acid/alkaline balance

*Fasting can be deleterious if you are nutrient-deficient and may lead to a decline in health. Very little detoxification occurs on a total fast.*

**Fasting** on the other hand, is not dangerous (unless you are nutritionally-depleted) but neither is it the best method of detoxifying. In my experience very little detoxification occurs when the body is deprived of nutrition. Detoxification is an active process and the tissues, particularly the liver, require a steady supply of nutrients and glucose to perform the task. Fasting initiates the release of glucocorticosteroid hormones from the adrenal glands and switches the liver metabolism into keto-acid production (ketones). Ketones become the fuel source of the tissues. Not only does this produce enormous acidity within the body, but your general metabolism shuts down and concentrates on the bare essentials only, certainly not on detoxification or tissue regeneration. This is not to say that people will not experience some benefits during their fast. For example, you may see a remission of symptoms with the removal of specific foods known to cause aggravations. So conditions such as arthritis, eczema and asthma may abate. However, unless these improvements can be sustained once you break the fast, then no real healing or reversal has taken place. By using your commonsense and following the guidelines in this book, you should be able to determine how nutritionally deficient you may be and also assess how strong a detoxification plan you can comfortably handle.

# Acid-forming foods

**Obviously, we want to cut down** as much as possible on the acid-forming foods without prejudicing our health. We have talked about salt and its effect on acidity and we know that certain foods, such as the refined carbohydrates (white flour, white rice, sugar etc.) and fats (butter and margarines, refined oils) which come stripped of their nutrients also promote the build-up of acids and toxins in the system. The stimulants (tea, coffee, cola, chocolate) and alcohol are also major culprits. This leads us to animal products – meat, dairy and eggs – which are concentrated forms of protein.

**Protein** is essential for growth and tissue maintenance, the RDI standing at 1g protein/kg of body weight. These are very small amounts. If we look at some average values in foods you will see that it is easy to achieve these amounts, and that many people can exceed them four-fold.

*Protein requirements stand at 1g/kg body weight daily. Animal protein is a concentrated source where just 350g of meat will provide enough protein for a person weighing 70kg.*

### Average protein value of foods  g/100g

| | |
|---|---|
| Meat/poultry | 20g |
| Fish | 17g |
| Cheese | 25g |
| Grains | 12g |
| Legumes | 25g |
| Nuts | 20g |

Taking these food values it is possible to estimate the protein content of certain foods in an average diet:

| | |
|---|---|
| 4 slices of bread | 24g |
| 200g of meat | 40g |
| 100g of cheese | 25g |
| **TOTAL** | **89g** |

This total does not take into account other dietary items that may be eaten during the day, such as breakfast cereals or cooked breakfasts (bacon and eggs), snacks and other grains. Many people have animal protein twice daily and the total protein intake may reach around 200g per day. If you turn to table 3.1 *Percentage of carbohydrates, fats and proteins in foods* you will find a more extensive appraisal of the protein content of foods.

*Acid/alkaline balance*

## 3  Acid/alkaline balance

*High protein diets produce metabolic acids that are only slowly removed via the kidneys. These diets predispose to tissue acidity and degenerative disease.*

Protein is extremely acid-forming because of the amount of sulphuric acid it contains. Wheat and rye are also high in sulphur which is why they join the list of acid-forming foods. Although we need sulphur, the body only maintains a small pool, the excess being discarded. Sulphuric acid is an end-product of protein metabolism and is only slowly removed from the body via the kidneys so people on high protein diets can accumulate acidity within their cells over a period of time.

## Sodium

is inextricably linked to both dietary protein intake and acidity. You can never reduce your sodium levels while your intake of animal protein is high. You may remember that the kidneys recycle sodium and for this reason it can be quite difficult to eliminate excess sodium in the urine as there is a tendency for it to be reabsorbed - especially on high protein diets. This is because the acidity generated by the protein in the form of hydrogen ions ($H^+$), exchanges with sodium ions in the kidney; as H ions are being pumped out into the filtrate for removal to the outside, sodium ions are being reabsorbed and returned to the body. Thus the higher your protein intake, the more sodium you reabsorb. Consequently, you can only reduce sodium and acidity on a low protein/high vegetable diet.

**Figure 3.4** Exchange of sodium ions ($Na^+$) for hydrogen ions ($H^+$) in the kidney

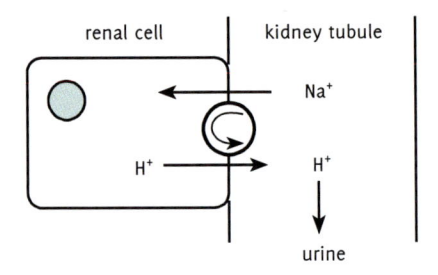

In conditions that predispose high acidity (high protein diets, refined CHOs and fats, stress and stimulants) the kidneys eliminate the acidity in exchange for sodium. Therefore the greater the acidic burden, the more sodium you reabsorb. A vicious cycle ensues as the excess sodium perpetuates acidic conditions within the cells. You can never truly reverse accumulated acidity without addressing all these factors and over a long period of time.

So by reducing animal protein to a minimum we actually accelerate the detoxification process and the removal of acidity and sodium from the cells. Very strict detoxification programs do not allow any animal protein, at least not for the first six weeks and then only in the form of pot cheese or yoghurt. On my diet, for non-vegetarians, I have allowed two meals of fish a week, and on a maintenance plan up to five meals a week may include animal protein, where portions are limited to 100g/serve for females and 150g/serve for males. I have recommended that you keep at least two days of the week vegan (no animal produce, eggs or dairy) so as to keep encouraging elimination.

*Mixing vegetable proteins, such as legumes with cereal grains, will give you a first class protein with a 70% utilisation value.*

If you really wish to speed up your detoxification, it is recommended that protein requirements should be obtained from vegetable sources. You will see from table 3.1 *Percentage of carbohydrates, fats and proteins in foods* that legumes, nuts and cereals all contain significant amounts of protein.

However, it is not a concentrated source as found in animal protein, but forms a percentage of the whole. Although legumes may appear to have as much protein as foods from animal sources, this percentage is derived from its dry weight. As soon as these foods are cooked, their weight increases 3-fold. Therefore, you would need to divide the protein value/100g by 3 to arrive at the total protein you would be receiving. For example, 100g cooked lentils would deliver around 8g protein.

## Complementing vegetable protein

is essential to obtain the correct balance of protein required by the body. Vegetable proteins, such as cereal grains, legumes and nuts are referred to as second-class proteins because when taken in isolation they will not provide all the building blocks (amino acids) for protein synthesis in the body. It's a bit like having an alphabet with half the letters missing - you cannot make all the words you require. Whereas animal protein tends to have all the "letters", vegetable protein will lack some. However, legumes have the letters that cereals and nuts lack and can therefore be used to complement both these foods providing the full alphabet. Nuts and cereals do not complement each other as they have the same amino acids (letters) missing.

**Figure 3.5** Complementary proteins

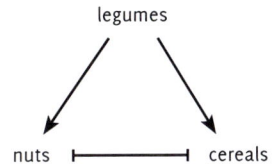

```
         legumes
          /   \
         ↙     ↘
     nuts ⊢——⊣ cereals
```

Legumes will complement both nuts and cereals; but cereals will not complement nuts as they are both deficient in the amino acid lysine.

A word of warning, if you don't complement your vegetable protein then up to half of the protein eaten may be discarded as it can't be used. The body will not wait until the next meal in the hope of finding the additional amino acids. As you can imagine, you can end up losing more protein than you retain. Not only will this place a high acidic burden on the body but the tissues will fail to maintain themselves and body tissue integrity will decline. You will see from the diet sheet that most meals contain complementary protein sources, minimising acidic residue and ensuring that regeneration can occur. Generally speaking, ensure you do not exceed 1g of protein/kg of desired body weight. This will be sufficient to maintain your health on the detoxification plan.

*Vegetables average around 1.5 – 2.0% first-class protein; therefore 1 kg of vegetables will deliver 15-20g of quality protein.*

## Stress

eats into the body. This includes physical, mental and emotional stressors. Physical stress can be caused through skipping meals or inadequate food intake, taking stimulants, excessive physical exercise or physical trauma. Under these conditions the body mobilises both its fats and proteins for energy and you literally start breaking yourself down or "eating yourself away". When this occurs there can be little regeneration, but most importantly, the oxidation of these fuels generates greater acidity. Fats and proteins are regarded as dirty fuels and should not to be used for energy.

*Stress hormones break down body tissues for energy. This is why periods of stress often precede the onset of chronic conditions.*

There is a great danger when people are advised to cut down on dietary unrefined carbohydrate in the treatment of food intolerances, candidiasis or insulin-resistant states, that fats and protein will be used for energy. This creates tremendous acidic waste, robbing the body of its carbohydrate maintenance materials so that the general health of the body may decline paving the way for more chronic symptoms.

# Neutral foods

**This brings me to the third group of foods**, the neutral foods, most of which are rich in carbohydrate. Unrefined carbohydrate is a clean fuel; it comes with its complement of nutrients and therefore can be oxidised safely away leaving no residue in the tissues. Carbohydrate (our source of energy), along with the naturally occurring fats and oils, makes up the rest of the diet.

In this group we have whole grain cereals (except wheat and rye), the legumes (peas, beans and lentils) and the less oily nuts (cashews, almonds and hazelnuts). In addition to providing carbohydrate for energy they supply us with our protein and essential fatty acids. Oils, taken in this natural form, are biologically active and do not pose the problems of saturated fats or refined oils for the body.

Technically speaking, unrefined carbohydrates will produce an amount of acidity by virtue of the protein and fat they contain. However, these foods are not nearly as acid-forming as animal protein, and you are less likely to overdose with protein taken in this form than say eating your way through a large steak several times a week. It is easier to keep to the minimal protein requirement for body maintenance when the diet is predominantly vegetarian, provided that you complement these second-class proteins.

## Tips for supporting your acid/alkaline balance

- 40% of the energy value of the diet should be supplied by vegetables and fruits. Juicing is recommended;
- On average take no more than 45-70g of protein a day (depending on your ideal weight), mainly from vegetable sources;
- Complement your proteins sensibly (legumes combine well with either nuts/seeds or whole grains);
- Unrefined carbohydrates (preferably in the form of brown rice, oats and millet) should supply your energy requirements;
- Reduce fats and oils to a minimum; and
- Keep your fluid intake up (water and juices) taking around 2 litres daily, more if you exercise. This will assist the kidneys in the removal of toxins.

### Case history 3.1

**Rachel was 33 years old** and nine weeks pregnant with her second child when she came to see me. On the advice of her homeopath, she had been following a low carbohydrate diet and not mixing protein with starches for the last eight years. Initially, this regime gave relief from the digestive problems of bloating and the joint pains from which she was suffering. However, her health had suffered a gradual decline and she now found that she was suffering from recurrent infections, thrush, severe pre-menstrual tension and headaches. She had also been recently diagnosed with chronic fatigue syndrome or ME (Myalgic Encephalitis) and felt extremely fatigued. This fatigue had been present before the pregnancy so she did not feel that it was solely due to the pregnancy. Rachel also had catarrh, swollen glands and constipation, and had suffered eczema from birth.

It was obvious that a dramatic decline in health had occurred over the past eight years. We can see an acidic constitution with the inability to handle calcium (eczema) and a low magnesium and zinc picture. As these deficiencies deepen and the congestion rises, tissue regeneration would be compromised often surfacing first in the digestive tract (hence symptoms here) and later in the immune system (lowered resistance to infection).

I felt that Rachel was experiencing allergic reactions to some foods (eczema and joint pains) but the majority of the intestinal symptoms were from food intolerances due to a poor digestive capacity. When food is not completely digested it tends to ferment causing bloating and even the overgrowth of pathogenic organisms like candida, which gives rise to thrush. A toxic colon in turn gives rise to a toxic liver and toxic body, and in order to stimulate the healing process we had to reduce the acidity.

However, embarking on a detoxification during pregnancy is unwise as toxins can flow from the mother to the baby. The baby acts as a receptacle for toxic waste which can compromise the function of an already immature liver. So we set about addressing her current diet. Firstly, we re-introduced the carbohydrates. The omission of these foods was an important factor in the decline of her health. Proteins were being used as an energy resource rather than for tissue maintenance. I also recommended that she no longer rigidly split her proteins from her starches, pointing out that vegetable sources of protein also contain significant amounts of starch. So on a diet with a vegetarian bias the philosophy behind the regime would become difficult to implement. We did remove certain foods known to provoke allergic reactions and intolerances but we followed the basic principles of the maintenance diet - obviously not including vegetable juices.

Rachel also exhibited long-term mineral deficiencies that could not be made good by diet alone. I supplemented magnesium along with calcium so as not to promote a strong detoxification and I also recommended iron and zinc. These two minerals were taken at opposite ends of the day as iron can inhibit the uptake of zinc. Both minerals are equally important for foetal development and zinc deficiencies can occur in women on high iron supplementation. Rachel also took lactobacillus bifidobacterium throughout the pregnancy to establish a good bacterial flora in the colon (essential to reduce colonic toxicity) and to ensure that her breast milk would have the correct bacteria to support the immune system of the baby.

By the fourth month Rachel's energies had stabilised and she had no more headaches. We continued on the program, altering supplementation to suit both mother and baby's needs. She had a little girl. Rachel breastfed her daughter for a few months but her general health seemed poor and the headaches returned. She decided that she would embark properly on a detoxification plan. It was not possible to detoxify while breast-feeding as breast milk is a ten-fold concentrate of the blood. Any toxins passing from mother to baby through the milk would do so at a high concentration. After breast-feeding Rachel went from strength to strength on her detoxification plan. Her energy and digestion remained good, headaches abated and her general resilience improved.

Table 3.1 Percentage of carbohydrates, fats and proteins in foods

| | Protein | CHOs | Fats |
|---|---|---|---|
| **Meat/fish** | | | |
| Beef | 21-24 | 0 | 19-24 |
| Lamb | 18-24 | 0 | 19-35 |
| Chicken | 20 | 0 | 7-12 |
| Cod | 16.5 | 0 | 0.4 |
| Halibut | 18.6 | 0 | 5.2 |
| Herring | 17.3 | 0 | 18.8 |
| Mackerel | 18.7 | 0 | 12 |
| Salmon | 19.9 | 0 | 13.6 |
| Trout | 19.2 | 0 | 2.1 |
| Shell fish | 14-18 | 0-4 | 0.1-3 |
| **Dairy/eggs** | | | |
| Cheese | 18-27 | 1.8-3.4 | 22-30 |
| Milk | 3.2 | 4.6 | 3.7 |
| Eggs (whole) | 12.8 | 0.7 | 11.5 |
| white | 10.8 | 0.8 | 0.2 |
| yolk | 16.3 | 0.7 | 31.9 |
| **Vegetables** | 0.5 - 4.0 | 4-9 | 0.1-0.6 |
| Potatoes | 2.0 | 19.1 | 0.1 |

| | Protein | CHOs | Fats |
|---|---|---|---|
| **Nuts/seeds** | | | |
| Almonds | 18.6 | 19.6 | 54.1 |
| Brazils | 14.4 | 11 | 65.9 |
| Hazelnuts | 12.7 | 18 | 60.9 |
| Peanuts | 26.9 | 23.6 | 44.2 |
| Walnuts | 15.0 | 15.6 | 64.4 |
| **Cereals** | | | |
| Barley | 9 | 76.5 | 1.4 |
| Buckwheat | 11.7 | 70 | 2.7 |
| Oats | 13.8 | 67.6 | 6.6 |
| Rice | 7.6 | 79.4 | 0.3 |
| Wheat (whole) | 12.1 | 71.5 | 2.1 |
| Wheat germ | 25.2 | 49.5 | 10 |
| **Legumes** | | | |
| Kidney beans | 21.3 | 61.6 | 1.6 |
| Lentils | 25 | 59.5 | 1 |
| Soya beans | 34.9 | 34.8 | 18.1 |
| **Fruits** | 0.5 - 3.0 | 9-16 | 0.1-0.4 |

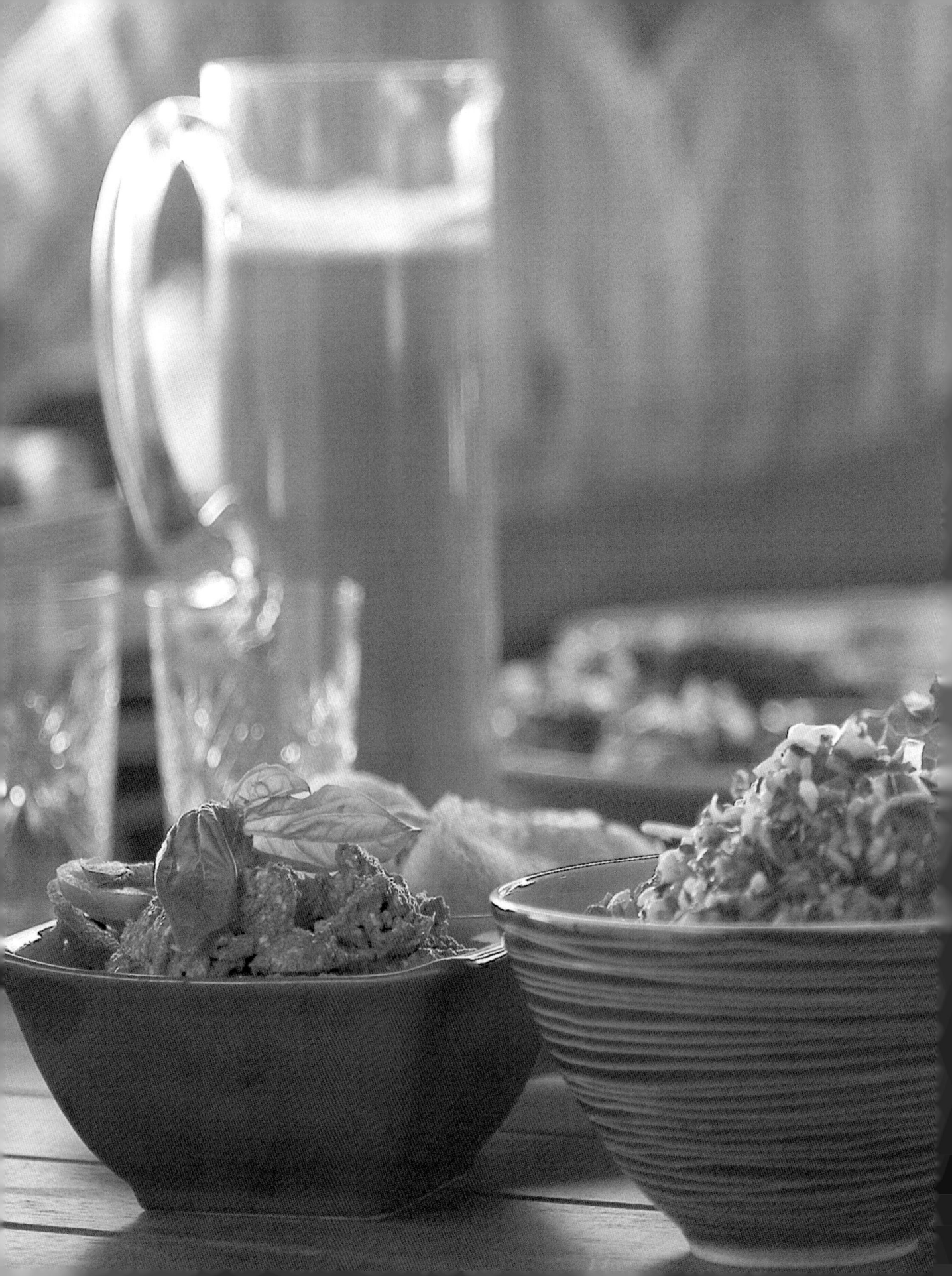

# Part 2

How will it work for me?

Vitality is a measure of your healing energy or how efficiently you can resolve an illness naturally.

Reducing the toxic load raises your inherent vitality; when the vitality is raised healing kicks in. When the body heals, it heals everything.

# 4

# Vitality & healing

# 4 Vitality & healing

**Vitality is the life force** as it manifests physically. A strong vitality gives strength and resilience to the physical body. However, this is a very generalised definition and we need to understand its implications in greater depth before we can begin to measure our own vitality. A correct assessment of vitality is critical for your program as it determines how easily and safely you will be able to eliminate toxins. A poor vitality, where there is deep congestion, usually indicates that detoxification and elimination need to proceed more slowly in order to minimise any adverse reactions that could prove destructive rather than healing in outcome.

So how do we measure vitality? Is it a question of how we feel when we get up in the morning; is it a measure of how long we can sustain heavy exercise, or how early we need to retire to bed? Is it purely a measurement of our fatigue? Some people seem to have loads of energy, never sitting still - do they have high vitality? They may be running on nervous energy which is a far cry from having a strong vital energy, while others, who prefer passive recreations, may in fact have a higher vitality than those with a lot of get up and go.

It is clear that vitality cannot be measured purely on this scale. Vitality is a measurement of our healing energy or, in other words, our capacity to heal ourselves naturally. A person with high vitality will resolve illnesses without having to resort to drugs while those with a lowered vitality will find that they cannot resolve illness without the aid of medical drugs.

To take this one stage further, if you have high vitality you will experience a strong response to illness, the symptoms of which may be inflammation and fever. This response is the body's defence mechanism where invading pathogens are destroyed and removed, and damaged tissue repaired.

**Figure 4.1** Inflammation as a measure of vitality

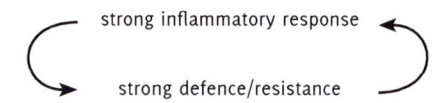

```
     ┌──  strong inflammatory response  ←──┐
     │                                     │
     └──→ strong defence/resistance  ──────┘
```

A strong inflammatory response is an indicator of your inherent vitality and your capacity to resist disease and regenerate healthy tissues.

The inflammatory response is a symptom of healing. If it is suppressed then you delay healing and actually prolong the illness. You may be symptom-free but is the disease lurking in a more chronic form with only acute outbreaks when you are feeling physically low? You can answer this yourself by seeing if you are prone to recurrent infection that surfaces when you are under stress and fails to resolve easily. This may apply, for example, to herpes virus outbreaks.

*Vitality is a measure of how efficiently you can resolve illness naturally, without the use of drugs.*

These marked variances in vitality and resistance between individuals is highlighted when an infectious illness hits a community; some will succumb to the illness, while others will not; some will experience severe disease reactions where vital organs are affected, while others may only suffer mild reactions that resolve easily. Infections can only "seed" if the resistance is low. So the outcome is determined more by the natural resistance of the host than the virulence of the disease itself. Hence, even microbes of very low pathogenicity that would not normally register in a healthy person, can become lethal in a host that has no resistance. This situation can occur following cancer treatment when most of the immune cells are eradicated through drugs or radiotherapy. It can also occur in any condition where the person is immune compromised, such as AIDS, and therefore rendered vulnerable to opportunistic infection.

*It is not the virulence of the disease itself that determines the outcome, but the resistance of the host.*

When general vitality is low, children will succumb to infectious illness even when they have been vaccinated against the disease or at worst, will suffer serious complications from the vaccine itself. If the resistance is such that the child cannot prevent even small amounts of the infectious agent from disseminating to the vital organs, including the brain, then infection seeds in these areas with the resultant complications. This is why I say that the resistance of the host is more important in determining the outcome of disease than the infectious agent itself.

*Vaccination programs do not build natural vitality and resistance, and by default encourage a downward trend in health.*

The treatment of health centres on raising the inherent vitality which automatically improves resistance. The treatment of health is very different from the treatment of disease. You may well be able to rid the body of infection through the use of antibiotics or inhibit the spread of infectious disease through the implementation of mass vaccination programs, but these methods do nothing to improve general vitality. They ignore factors which support vitality, such as diet and lifestyle, and therefore, by default, encourage a downward trend in health. Unless resistance is improved then infectious illness will continue to undermine health; drug and vaccine-resistant strains of microbes will evolve and we will be caught in a never-ending battle between medication and microbes.

**Figure 4.2** The opposing effects on vitality with various therapies

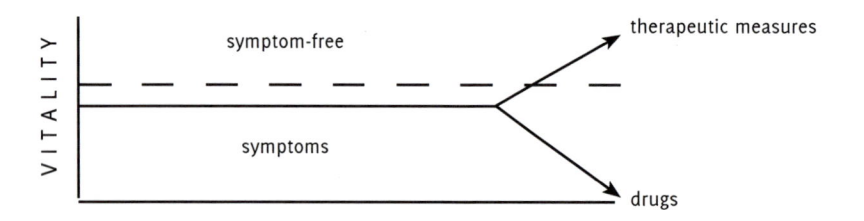

Vitality can move in either direction depending on treatment. Drugs and suppressive treatments lower vitality while therapeutic measures, aimed at improving natural resistance, raise vitality. The aim of treatment is to raise the vitality above the line, so that when stress arises, there is enough vitality in the bank to support and resolve any imbalance.

The treatment of health is not the same as the treatment of disease - try not to confuse the two. Treatments aimed at suppressing the symptoms, or the defence mechanism, ultimately lower resistance and vitality allowing disease to manifest in a more chronic form.

*Acquired weaknesses become inherited weaknesses in the next generation. Inherited weaknesses cannot be changed, but the body can be supported so that these weaknesses do not manifest.*

When vitality is suppressed in this way, body tissues become more inefficient, sluggish and devitalised. Acidity, toxicity and congestion rise and these areas become a breeding ground for pathogens. With increasing congestion the body will start secreting mucus which is a medium for the disposal of toxic waste. The body is now eliminating toxicity through its internal membranes. These areas can soon become infected by pathogens feeding on de-vitalised, decaying matter, and so the congestion deepens. Eventually, with the general lowering of vitality, organic change occurs and the pathological signs of disease will become apparent. The weakest organs (determined by inheritance factors) will be the first to deteriorate, and unless steps are taken to lower the toxic load and initiate regeneration, the acquired weakness may become an inherited weakness in the next generation.

# Vitality & the healing process

**High vitality: the acute phase** is when the body is quick to respond with either fever or inflammation and will resolve the imbalance naturally. If you turn to figure 4.3 *Assessing vitality* you can see a very broad categorisation of the levels of vitality. This type of response is seen in young children who suddenly develop a high fever and yet the next day they are enjoying perfect health. However, if you take medication that suppresses the symptoms rather than taking supportive measures to assist the body's defences, you actually prolong the illness. Fever is an important part of the healing process as it stimulates the cells of the immune system increasing their response for the eradication of pathogens. It is preferable to control fever (before it rises too high), rather than suppressing it, by tepid bathing or cool sponging, while making dietary changes and using herbs or homeopathy to assist the process of ridding the body of pathogens and toxins, leaving the patient with a raised vitality and greater resistance.

*Inflammation and fever are critical defence responses; by suppressing either, you prolong the disease.*

**Moderate vitality: the sub-acute phase** is reached when there is an absence of natural resolution due to a weakened vitality leading to recurrent infection. For example, the odd bout of sinusitis that resolved itself in the past now requires medication. After several years the medication that addressed the complaint no longer seems to work so well and several doses are required just to obtain some relief. At this stage any attempts by the body to alleviate the situation may be unsuccessful. In addition, stress factors (including changes in weather conditions) may increase susceptibility.

*Acute illness may become chronic if suppressed.*

**Low vitality: the chronic phase** is a stage where the condition requires long-term medication. A chronic condition implies that the inherent vitality can no longer rectify the disharmony and the body now adjusts to the new conditions (known as pathological equilibrium) usually at the expense of healthy tissues. At this stage there are underlying inflammatory processes at work as the cells of the immune system attempt to remove debris and toxins at a local level. Local inflammation may arise in places such as the joints (arthritis), arteries (heart disease) and skin (eczema, dermatitis, psoriasis), which then exposes adjacent healthy tissue to free radical damage. In an attempt to repair the injury, growth factors are released from these neighbouring tissues to stimulate the growth of new tissue. However, unless the immune cells can completely remove the irritant, a self-perpetuating inflammatory cycle ensues leading to an overgrowth of scar tissue that creates new problems, such as the occlusion of the arteries, swelling at the joints or the thickening of the skin. (See figure 4.4 *The cycle of inflammation in the healing/disease process*.) Most inflammatory conditions, such as arthritis, gout, asthma, allergy, ulcers and inflammatory bowel disease, fall into the chronic phase.

*Pathological equilibrium: an adjustment by the body to the disease, the symptoms of which are detrimental.*

**Figure 4.3** Assessing vitality

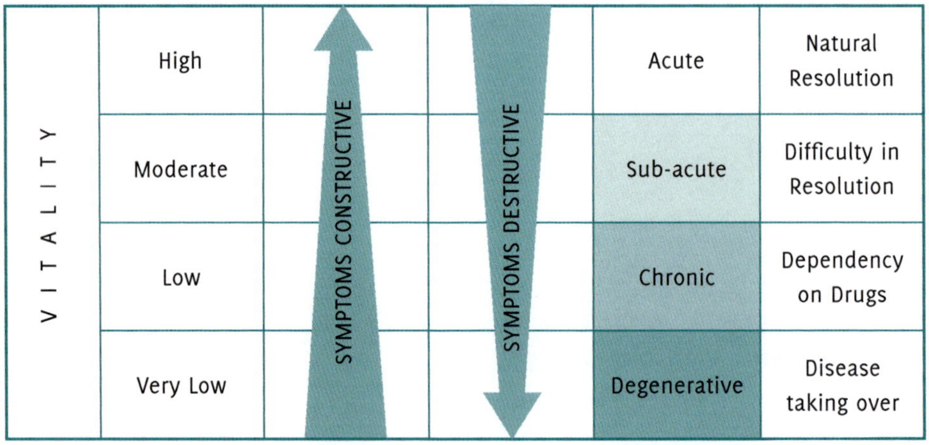

| VITALITY | | SYMPTOMS CONSTRUCTIVE ↑ | SYMPTOMS DESTRUCTIVE ↓ | | |
|---|---|---|---|---|---|
| | High | | | Acute | Natural Resolution |
| | Moderate | | | Sub-acute | Difficulty in Resolution |
| | Low | | | Chronic | Dependency on Drugs |
| | Very Low | | | Degenerative | Disease taking over |

## Very low vitality: the degenerative phase is reached once the disease takes over.

There is insufficient vitality to arouse a healing response and not even medications can halt the spread of disease. Prolonged chronic inflammation leads to the infiltration of abnormal scar tissue into the organs and connective tissue. Scar tissue has no functional activity and will impede circulation, nerve signals and the function of organs. In the brain it gives rise to amyloid plaque (Alzheimer's Disease); in the arteries, atherosclerosis; and in the case of diabetes, where glucose as AGEs (advanced glycosylation end products) embeds in the capillary walls, leads to retinopathy, neuropathy and nephropathy.

In the various autoimmune disorders, where the immune system creates antibodies to its own tissues, we may see organ destruction, such as of the pancreas (insulin dependent diabetes [IDDM]) the thyroid (Graves or Hashimoto's thyroiditis), the digestive tract (Crohn's disease, ulcerative colitis), the joints (rheumatoid arthritis) or the connective tissue (systemic lupus erythematosus [SLE]). Invariably, as one arm of the immune system becomes more irritated, the other arm, which protects against viral infection and cancer, may become under-active.

In order to increase vitality we must stimulate the healing response. This is the key focus of many healing therapies: homeopaths will prescribe remedies that raise the inherent vitality to induce a healing reaction; herbalists will prescribe various herbs to improve the efficiency of body systems in order to reduce toxicity and subsequently raise vitality; and the masseur will stimulate the tissues causing the release of toxins which are removed by the lymphatic system enabling regeneration of tissue. Let's now take a closer look at the actual healing process.

*Inflammatory metabolism*

**Figure 4.4** The cycle of inflammation and the healing/disease process

### a) Normal inflammatory metabolism

```
                inflammatory response to cell injury
                  (toxin, trauma, chemical, pathogen)
                        ↙         ↓         ↘
          free radicals   ←——→   damaged tissue
          anti-oxidants          growth factors
                               ↓
                     scar tissue formation
                            healing
```

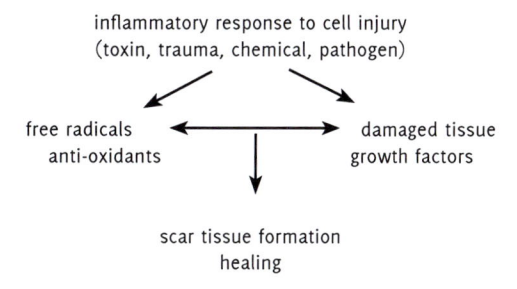

Free radicals generated as a consequence of the inflammatory response should be neutralised by the anti-oxidant enzyme system while growth factors are released from adjacent tissue for the formation of normal scar tissue.

### b) Uncontrolled inflammation

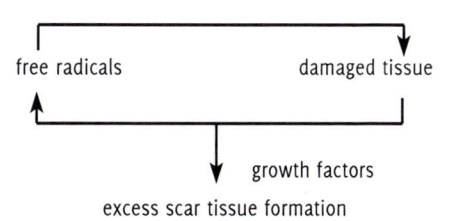

```
          ┌─────────────────────────┐
          ↓                         ↓
     free radicals            damaged tissue
          ↑                         │
          └─────────────────────────┘
                       ↓
                  growth factors
             excess scar tissue formation
```

With anti-oxidant deficiency or a persistent source of inflammation (such as glucose [in diabetes], oxidised cholesterol, heavy metals, toxins, allergens [food and environmental] and antibodies) we see uncontrolled free radical production as a consequence of immune involvement. This perpetuates the cycle of destruction. Growth factors are continuously released leading to the formation of excess scar tissue.

### Case history 4.1

**Theresa was 51** and could barely walk into my office through exhaustion. She was suffering chronic fatigue syndrome for the second time in four years. It took two years to recover from the initial incidence. Currently she was off sick from work but desperate to return for financial reasons.

When I took her case history I began to see patterns of suppression leading to deep congestion, particularly in the liver. From childhood she had been constipated, catarrhal and had both her tonsils and adenoids removed at an early age. During her teens she suffered recurrent sinusitis and received antibiotic treatment. This condition worsened over the years and in spite of two sinus operations the sinusitis was now constant where even antibiotics could not shift the infection.

In her thirties she suffered glandular fever and after a course of antibiotics developed colitis (antibiotics can precede the onset of colitis in certain cases). Later she developed digestive difficulties, had surgery for fibroids, her periods became heavy with associated migraine and she developed a vaginal discharge. Two chest infections had left her very weak and debilitated. She also complained of a painful left breast.

It was clear that no supportive treatment to raise the vitality for natural healing had ever been undertaken. As a consequence, her body had gradually become devitalised and congestion had built up in the tissues leading to deeper disease patterns. Constipation, glandular fever, digestive difficulties, menstrual imbalances along with migraine all point to poor liver function. A toxic lymph system indicates generalised congestion with symptoms manifesting in the lymphatic tissue (tonsils, adenoids, appendix) at an early age.

I recommended that Theresa had a mammogram which gave her the all clear. She started on the diet and was amazed that by the end of the month she was back at work. She stuck with the diet for about six months but I was fairly convinced that she had a long way to go. Unfortunately, the disappearance of symptoms indicated to Theresa that she was cured. However, three years later she telephoned to say that she had just been diagnosed with breast cancer and was devastated because she felt well. She had surgery followed by radiotherapy and went back on the diet. She also had acupuncture and Chinese herbs to assist the process. Theresa now understood that a far longer regeneration period is required to change conditions significantly in the body in order to regain health and that the removal of symptoms does not constitute health.

# Inflammation & the healing process

**We have already established** that by reducing the toxic load the healing response is activated. Detoxification through diet is a very old principle used by the father of medicine, Hippocrates himself. Down through the ages and up until modern times, many eminent physicians have employed these dietary principles in the treatment of disease and there is no doubt of their powerful and effective results. When the vital organs are detoxified sufficiently, the body's acid/alkaline balance re-established and the mineral and enzymes systems are re-instated, then self-healing can occur.

We talk of the healing process as a single response, and yet we have many disease labels. In conventional medicine each disease label has a specific medication suggesting that each disease has a different cause and therefore a different treatment is required. While it is true that each disease may have a unique pathology with a wide range of symptoms, what is also true is that the body's healing response to all illnesses, regardless of the label, is uniform. That response is the inflammatory response. Quite simply, if there is foreign matter in the body, whether it is an infectious agent, a chemical or even your own devitalised tissue, the body's immune cells will remove it along with dead tissue, and this is followed by the regeneration of new healthy cells. This is all part of the inflammatory or healing reaction.

*All diseases, regardless of their label, are dependent on the same healing mechanism: the inflammatory response.*

When inflammation is initiated, there is movement of blood to the area (which accounts for the swelling, redness and heat) and immune cells move from the circulation into the affected area. This mass exodus will marginalise the irritation or infection and prevent further spread. The strength of this resistance determines the outcome. These immune cells also take up malignant or cancerous cells in the early stages of cancer formation. Prevention of cancer from its outset is therefore dependent upon a strong and vital immune response.

Dead tissue, dead organisms and toxins are then taken up by the lymphatic system which acts as an overflow system for the fluids bathing the tissues. The lymphatic vessels are more permeable than the blood capillaries and are able to take up larger particles and waste products. The lymph flows through local lymph nodes where "non-self" tissue is identified and an appropriate immune response is activated which may involve the production of antibodies or the stimulation of specific immune cells, such as natural killer cells. Eventually, the toxic lymph empties into the subclavian vein and is taken directly to the liver to be detoxified and its toxins removed via the bile system. The bile passes to the digestive tract and is removed with the toxins via the colon. Finally, new tissue is regenerated.

*Lymph, carrying toxins, finally empties into the subclavian vein and passes directly to the liver where it is detoxified. Lymph congestion invariably indicates liver congestion.*

*Vitality & healing*

*There may be many areas for regeneration, but you will not be able to dictate what gets healed first! The body will prioritise its own efforts.*

## The healing crisis

is a spontaneous inflammatory response, which may involve fever but is not generated by infection. It usually occurs after a period of detoxification, when sufficient burden has been removed and the vitality restored. Old injuries, either from past trauma or infection, or current injury are revisited with inflammation at the site of the injury which usually resolves within three to five days. This self-limiting inflammatory response is commonly referred to as a flare-up. On a detoxification program, depending on your starting point (or level of vitality) symptoms may flare within the initial two-month period. Invariably, the area of healing is revisited at intervals. We tend to think that when an initial injury has "resolved" then healing is complete. In truth, the body will merely accomplish what it can, given the resources available. If there are insufficient resources, then minimal healing takes place. The higher the resources, the more complete the healing. As we build these resources on this type of dietary program, flare-ups will recur at intervals, reducing in intensity and frequency as the old tissue is replaced with new, healthy tissue. In my practice I have seen old scar tissue inflame and then resolve in this manner until there was no evidence of scar tissue left.

*Survival advantage in cancer is as much dependent upon the healing potential as the disease potential (aggressiveness of the disease). When you increase the healing potential, then chances of recovery are much greater.*

Dr. Max Gerson laid great emphasis on the healing crisis as a measure of the healing potential and capacity for cure. Dr. Gerson knew through clinical experience that if the cancer patient was unable to raise a spontaneous healing inflammation then their chances of cure were slim. Continuous suppression of our healing potential through the use of drugs pushes us deeper into the degenerative stage. Dr. Gerson found that once the body started fighting the disease, the inflammatory response was sufficient to destroy the cancer, which proved that cancer can be eliminated by the patient's own mechanisms. As medical research progresses we are discovering more about the natural chemicals released through immune reactions that cause the destruction of tumours. One such chemical is tumour necrosis factor (TNF), which is released during inflammation and effectively shuts off the circulation to the tumour causing its death. It is also acknowledged that the prognosis of a patient suffering with cancer is better if the immune system can be stimulated. The stronger immune response in children accounts for their higher survival rates as opposed to survival rates for the elderly. Unfortunately, treatments used in cancer tend to eradicate the immune system, and if a patient with low vitality is unable to rebound after treatment then the prognosis is poor.

*Don't confuse the disease crisis with the healing crisis; if you are in the chronic or degenerative phase, then "more of the same" symptoms which fail to resolve are invariably part of the disease process.*

## The disease crisis

occurs when inflammation that is not self-limiting becomes destructive. The body needs to complete the cycle from inflammation to resolution. There are many inflammatory diseases where the irritant remains in the tissues due to an ineffective or poor healing response. A self-perpetuating inflammatory cycle occurs where more and more tissue becomes destroyed giving rise to disease patterns that will not resolve. Sometimes the irritants are due to food allergens, toxic chemicals, surplus cholesterol and glucose or an antibody/toxin complex which becomes lodged in the tissues. However, detoxification can alter the path of such diseases dramatically, enabling inflammation to subside and regeneration to occur.

You can appreciate the importance of interpreting inflammatory reactions correctly. It is all too easy to blame any inflammatory reaction on the healing crisis particularly if you are following a detoxification program. However, it is safe to say that if you are either in the chronic or degenerative phase, then inflammatory reactions are usually symptoms of the disease process, known as a disease crisis, not the healing process. Under these circumstances it may be important to seek additional help in controlling symptoms (herbs and homoeopathy may be useful here) while you are simultaneously building the healing potential through your dietary program. In some cases, the body may be so badly damaged and the disease process so entrenched that reversal is not possible. However, the disease process may be slowed down or even arrested with appropriate application of diet and natural treatments. For some, once the vitality is sufficiently restored, the body is able to instigate a strong healing response that ultimately results in resolution.

Regeneration takes a long time, with damaged organs regaining their function over a 9-18 month period during which time you may see repeated flare-ups. It is therefore necessary to support this process by continuing detoxification until the body is healed. Prematurely ceasing the program, before the body has regained its full capacity, will result in the return of symptoms. Similarly, restoration of tissues depends not only upon detoxification but also the re-mineralisation of the entire body. Those who embark on severe detoxification programs over a prolonged period of time, where they restrict themselves to juicing only, may become more nutrient-deficient and devitalised than they were at the outset. Regeneration will not occur under these circumstances.

By maintaining the program you will naturally gain the momentum critical for the stimulation of the healing response. It is important that the diet is sustainable from your life-style point of view and able to meet your physical demands. Short-term detoxification plans will do nothing to improve your long-term health, will not reverse the disease process, nor instigate any long-term changes in dietary habits.

Remember that the removal of certain food products from a diet, and the associated remission of symptoms supposedly due to these foods, is not synonymous with the healing process. If no steps are undertaken to initiate the healing response then the disease process will not be reversed. It is purely symptomatic treatment and sooner or later the symptoms will return even though those "suspected foods" are still being omitted.

4 *Vitality & healing*

**Figure 4.5** The inflammatory process in healing

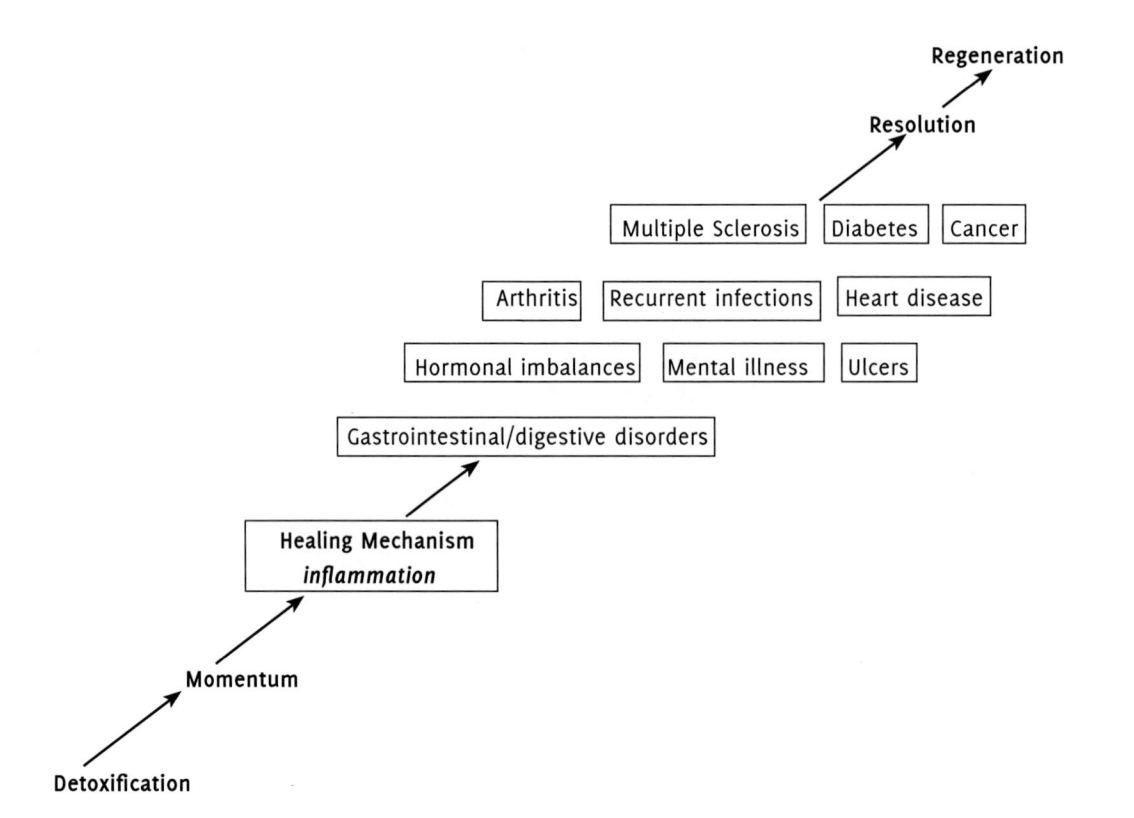

Regeneration
↗
Resolution
↗
Multiple Sclerosis | Diabetes | Cancer

Arthritis | Recurrent infections | Heart disease

Hormonal imbalances | Mental illness | Ulcers

Gastrointestinal/digestive disorders
↗
**Healing Mechanism** *inflammation*
↗
Momentum
↗
**Detoxification**

# Managing reactions

**The healing process**, as we have seen, is a symptom-generating process which may require management from time to time. However, you need to be able to interpret the symptoms within the given case in order to be able to apply the most appropriate methods for supporting the desired outcome. For example, we do not want to suppress the discharge of toxicity nor the healing inflammation, but neither must we let these symptoms run amok if they are part of the disease process or if they are of infectious origin. The problem in management lies in differentiating between the sets of symptoms. This is not as difficult as it sounds – but if you are unsure of how to proceed in a given situation, or if you remain unsure of the origin (for example, an infection) then you should consult a professional.

*Reactions that are self-limiting are usually part of the healing process; those that persist are invariably part of the disease process.*

**Managing the toxic crisis** is achieved by ensuring that the rate of toxin elimination from the tissues does not exceed the liver's capacity to eliminate to the outside. A toxic crisis occurs when the liver is unable to cope with toxin elimination and the consequences are a poisoning of the system with diverse symptoms such as feeling "hung-over" and groggy, headaches, bad breath with taints in the mouth, bad body odour, 'flu-like symptoms with accompanying aches and pains, and even nervous irritability, emotional frustration or anger. The only way to deal with these quickly and effectively is by taking a coffee enema which assists the liver in clearing toxins from the blood (see chapter 5 *Liver cleansing* pp 119-120). If the symptoms resolve with the enema, then you know it was a toxic crisis. Similarly, painful muscle spasms, which may occur following the release of toxic chemicals from the cells into the surrounding fluids, can be alleviated by the use of the warm castor oil pack (p85).

*The coffee enema is the most effective way of relieving the toxic crisis.*

**Managing the detoxification crisis** is achieved by regulating the release of large amounts of toxic bile from the liver into the digestive tract which cause nausea (and even vomiting) or diarrhoea - or both! The coffee enema will not alleviate this crisis, but may intensify it. Although you may wish to assist the liver with the enema, all you will achieve is a greater release of toxins into the digestive tract. The bile is strongly alkaline so by either sipping on gruel (a very thin oat porridge using 1 part oats to 8 parts water, simmered for 1-2 hours, and strained) or peppermint tea throughout the day, you will neutralise the bile. Gruel not only mops up toxins but also soothes inflammation and acidity. Taking gruel both before and after the coffee enema can neutralise toxins as they are released and enable you to continue with the program.

*Taking gruel or peppermint tea helps to alleviate the detoxification crisis.*

*Vitality & healing*

Alternatively, if the coffee enema still provokes too great a release of toxicity, then you may take a chamomile tea enema (p120) which will still help to facilitate the passage of toxins through the digestive tract without provoking a toxic release from the liver. If you have diarrhoea, then taking 1/4 tsp of bentonite clay in a glass of water after each bout of diarrhoea can be extremely helpful. Pectin is a strong astringent, and grated apple that has been left to oxidise (go brown) may help to alleviate diarrhoea.

Occasionally you may experience inflammation at the rectum from the irritating toxins as they are being discharged. I would recommend covering the area with a barrier cream, particularly before you release the enema.

When going through a detoxification crisis you may have difficulty in eating and drinking. You will need to keep your fluid intake up, and for this purpose gruel, sweetened with organic sugar or honey, will settle the digestive tract and provide nourishment. The diet becomes more important than the juices at this stage, as the juices may tend to pass straight through, whereas food slows the transit time and gives more time for nutrients to be absorbed. Take a well-cooked, easily digested diet (porridge, soups, mashed potato, apple sauce etc.) and remove known irritants – particularly raw onions, garlic and tomatoes.

*Lingering infection inhibits the healing process; make sure you deal with this appropriately.*

## Managing the healing crisis is achieved by supporting the inflammatory metabolism.
Invariably, patients may experience toxic and/or detoxification reactions alongside the healing crisis, and if so, then numerous steps may be needed to alleviate the crises. It is very important that you discriminate between infectious illness and the healing crisis. Attempts at healing are undermined when there is a foci of infection, because the combating of infection by the body's immune forces takes precedence over general healing. Low grade or chronic infectious states (including candida) lower the vitality and will need to be resolved before you can expect reversal of chronic complaints.

The main symptoms of the healing crisis are inflammation and pain at the site of old injuries, inflammation at current sites of injury, recurrence of symptoms peculiar to past illnesses, and fever. The management of the crisis by supporting the symptoms is the key to resolution.

## Managing fever without resorting to suppression with drugs, will result in a better outcome.
However, if the fever is prolonged (five hours or more) or rises above 39°C, then bathing in tepid water, using cold compresses, cool water enemas and taking cool drinks may be successful in controlling the temperature. Herbs that are useful for reducing fevers by stimulating sweating include peppermint, yarrow, elderflower and boneset, which may be taken as a tea. These methods for controlling temperature are not the same as suppressive measures. However, it is important to monitor the temperature closely and if it either rises above 40°C, or the burning/shivering stage begins, you may need to resort to an anti-pyretic medication, such as aspirin.

## Managing pain at the site of inflammation can also be a challenge. However, hot and cold packs over the affected area often prove useful.

**The castor oil pack** is a warm pack generally used for releasing mucus congestion of the lungs and bowel, alleviating muscle tension, spasms and cramping, and colicky pain of the internal organs. This warm pack increases circulation to the area which relaxes the muscles, allowing toxicity and congestion to disperse. The castor oil pack can be kept on for as long as required and re-used later.

During the initial stages of detoxification circulating toxins will often lodge in muscle tissue causing contraction, stiffness and pain particularly around the shoulder/neck area. Muscles also contract over local areas of inflammation, including inflammation of the bone. Additionally, colicky pains may be felt in the liver, particularly if you suffer from gall stones or a fatty liver. In all these circumstances, the castor oil pack will prove invaluable for releasing tension and spasm, and may even relieve griping spasms in the digestive and female reproductive tracts when placed over the area.

Castor oil packs can also be used as a gentle stimulant for the lungs, liver and colon. They are particularly useful in any toxic condition where there is a stagnation of mucus, such as lung infection, constipation, diverticulitis, colitis and irritable bowel syndrome. The absorption of the castor oil through the skin lubricates, softens and helps to shift toxic matter and mucus from these areas. A toxic colon pollutes the rest of the body, especially the lymph and the liver.

## *Method and preparation of the castor oil pack*

- Take three flannelette cotton cloths (each about half the size of a tea towel or the size of the area to be covered) and a piece of plastic of the same size (a plastic bag will do). Thoroughly wet one cotton cloth and squeeze dry, placing it flat on the plastic.
- Cover with a second layer of flannelette.
- Spread a generous layer of castor oil over the cloth. Repeat with a third layer.
- Lay this, castor oil side down, over the area keeping the plastic in place, and secure with a wide bandage or towel.
- Place a heated pad (not electric) or a hot water bottle over this. If it is too hot, then you may place an additional towel over the castor oil pack and remove this as the heat pack cools.
- Leave in place for as long as desired, minimum 1½ hours.
- This pack may be re-used. Roll it up for storage (you can store it in the freezer) and apply more castor oil, if required, the next time.

Repeat this procedure for three days and over the next three days massage the area with olive oil. Do nothing on the seventh day and then repeat the entire procedure again for a period of seven weeks.

Of course, this is quite a commitment and I have outlined an entire program. You may choose to do just the odd one now and again, although it is better to try the whole program for long-term benefit. It stimulates a very gentle healing that needs to occur gradually over the weeks.

**The clay pack** is a cold pack that is used on hot, swollen inflammations and may be placed over infected sites. They can be useful for easing pain in hot joint conditions, or reducing oedema where there is tissue injury. Clay adsorbs toxins and excess fluid by drawing it through the skin; it also reduces infection at the site of an open injury.

## Method and preparation for the clay pack

Use a fine montmorillonite or bentonite clay.

- Mix the clay with hot water (200g clay/100ml water) to make a soft paste which should be easily spreadable.
- Spread a thick layer, approximately 0.5cm deep, on a piece of double-thickness muslin/gauze, the size of the affected part.
- Cover with thin gauze (although the pack can be placed directly on unbroken skin) and place over the site, securing it with an elastic bandage.
- The pack should be kept on for up to 3 hours (no longer) or until dried out, and then thrown away. It cannot be re-used. Use twice daily on the affected site until the condition is resolved.

NB: when preparing clay do not let it come into contact with metal; a glass bowl is preferable to plastic. If using a metal spoon do not let it stay in contact for longer than necessary.

Invariably a patient may experience all three crises simultaneously. But all these reactions, the healing, the toxic and the detoxification reaction, are self-limiting which means that they should resolve within a short period of time and you should feel better than you did before the event. Symptoms that fail to resolve are not part of the healing process, but may indicate either a worsening of the disease, or possible reactions against specific food items on the dietary program. In both these instances, it is perhaps advisable to seek further help for clarification and appropriate management.

## Managing the disease crisis
is achieved mainly by balancing detoxification with regeneration. The easiest way to explain this is by using the analogy of an old building that needs to be renovated. There may be much work to be done, but you may find that if you go in too aggressively and remove too much debris that the building starts crumbling. The debris may have been supporting the building! So it is with the human body; we need to ensure a process of removal and simultaneous renovation. Embarking upon a more gentle cleanse will ensure that you do not place undue burdens on an already overtaxed system. Generally, the lower your vitality and the deeper the congestion, the longer it will take.

*Disease moves from the outside in and from the bottom up.*

You will need to determine the direction that your disease is moving to assess whether you are improving (healing crisis) or deteriorating (disease crisis). Generally the disease process moves from the outside in and from the bottom up. For example, disease may start at the superficial level (skin), and if this is suppressed will move inwards to affect the liver and colon; from here to affect the lungs and kidneys, and in the final stage affecting the heart and brain. There is a very old saying that if you look after your liver and kidneys, then the heart and brain will look after themselves.

Nowadays people with skin disorders, such as eczema or psoriasis, are no longer at this superficial stage. There is usually liver, colon, lung and kidney involvement. These links become apparent when inflammation is suppressed at the skin level resulting in a manifestation of the disease at the lung/kidney level as asthma or kidney problems. In Chinese medicine the skin is known as the third lung and the third kidney illustrating its close links with these organs on the disease pathway.

Skin ⟶ Liver/colon ⟶ Lungs/kidneys ⟶ Heart/brain

A further link may be seen in children who suffer with hyperactive disorders. In many cases this is a progression of the allergy/eczema/asthma picture (disease at the liver and lung level) to the brain level. These children have very deep major mineral imbalances due to the modern fast food, high salt and high dairy diet, and iodine deficiency may also be implicated.

It is best to manage the disease crisis under professional guidance as it can be a tricky process of knowing when to pull back, when to push forward and how to deal with inflammatory reactions that are not resolving. It is critically important that non-resolving inflammation is addressed at the outset. Inflammation destroys tissues and generates scar tissue production. Both outcomes have serious consequences.

*Inflammation needs to be resolved at the outset in a disease crisis; delay may worsen the prognosis.*

You may monitor your progress with your chosen professional to ensure that you are going in the right direction. If old symptoms resolve and new symptoms arise in more superficial tissues, then this is a healing reaction. For example, if asthma resolves but gives way to eczema, the skin now carries the toxic burden, but being a less vital organ than the lungs represents a less chronic state. Healing symptoms move from the inside out and from the top down.

*Healing occurs from the inside out and from the top down.*

Ensuring that the rate of toxin removal from the tissues does not exceed your capacity to eliminate toxins to the outside is the subject of the next chapter. The lower the vitality, the more difficult it becomes to remove toxins safely; this is when symptoms may be detrimental. For example, if you suffer arthritis, which reflects a highly acidic constitution, the removal of toxins from the tissues can exacerbate joint pain if they are not taken up by the lymphatic system for delivery to the liver. With high acidity the disease is almost "locked in" and the body has to be gently stimulated to release toxins slowly at a pace that the liver can accommodate so that adverse reactions do not occur.

You will not turn around chronic disease in a couple of months but will need to look at more permanent changes - as perhaps we all should. However, the improvement in health as you progress should make it all worthwhile.

Remember a healthy diet is enough to keep a healthy person healthy but is insufficient in reversing the effects of disease.

Case history 4.2

## Thomas was a hyperactive 3 year old.
His parents had already had to remove him from his preschool group as the teachers could not cope with his behavioural problems and they were now worried about his future education. He was incapable of sitting still and concentrating, he couldn't socialise and was aggressive most of the time. He was even too busy to sit down and eat. When we looked at his diet it consisted mainly of cheese, bread and vegemite, anything salty and anything sweet. He refused all vegetables and fruit except bananas.

He was small as a baby and failed to thrive. The GP suggested growth hormone and consequently his mother never returned to the clinic. He did catch up but remained thin. He also had eczema on his face and arms.

When I enquired about his parents' health it transpired that his father had eczema, asthma and suffered allergic reactions to cats and horses. He admitted that his diet was terrible - he ate lots of cheese, salt and no vegetables.

The pattern of eczema, asthma and hyperactivity is very clear in this case study. It arises from a deep mineral imbalance resulting in an inability to handle calcium due to the high sodium and low magnesium status. It takes a long time to correct this picture but results can be seen within the first two months. We removed dairy and although Thomas did refuse to eat any food for about 3 days he eventually succumbed. The eczema disappeared but the hyperactivity remained. He continued on the diet and through stabilising his blood sugar levels, stimulating regeneration of the liver through the diet his condition gradually improved. It was a trying time for the parents but well worth the effort in the long-term.

# Tips on managing reactions

**Toxic symptoms:** these make you feel "poisoned". They indicate that elimination of toxins from the cells is occurring more rapidly than elimination by the liver. The symptoms include:

- Brain/mental level – headaches, foggy/heavy head, loss of concentration, disorientation;
- Bad taste in mouth, halitosis;
- Mood swings, extreme irritation;
- Nervous irritation as old toxins/drugs are released into the circulation and irritate nerve endings; and
- Joint and muscle aches and pains/inflammation

*To do:* the coffee enema is the only method of effectively releasing this toxicity.

**Detoxification symptoms:** these occur most specifically at gut level and the symptoms are associated with large amounts of toxicity being released from the liver into the duodenum. The strongly toxic and alkaline bile can make you feel extremely nauseous, may cause vomiting of bile and/or diarrhoea. Sometimes an increased efflux of toxicity from the liver follows the coffee enema as it specifically stimulates this release. This is a real tell-tale sign of increased liver activity and detoxification, and is a positive sign.

*To do:*
- If doing coffee enemas, try to maintain them; if they make you feel worse then take at half-strength or try a chamomile tea enema (p120).
- Drinking peppermint tea increases stomach acidity and therefore helps neutralise the bile.
- Taking gruel before and after the enema helps to counteract the effects of the toxic bile. Gruel will "mop up" toxic bile and soothe the digestive tract. Gruel can be added to the vegetable juices to help keep them down.

**Healing symptoms:** these occur when the body is either resolving old injuries/illnesses (bacterial/viral or physical trauma) or discharging toxicity during a healing crisis. During these crises the body resolves scar tissue, heals old fractures and eliminates toxic residue through the skin, mucous membranes, liver, kidney and colon. These reactions are generally accompanied by inflammation, fever and general malaise which is self-limiting. Usually a few days prior to a healing crisis the general energy/vitality rises. The crisis which follows will last from 3 –10 days. You may need to establish that there is no infectious cause as this will determine treatment.

### Managing fever

If the fever rises to 39°C you will need to monitor closely. The following steps may be useful in the control of fever without suppression:

- Bathe in tepid water; use cold cloths/compresses on the forehead and at the nape of the neck (a cloth soaked in witch hazel may assist); take cold drinks or even a cold enema;
- Take herbs such as willow, feverfew, peppermint, yarrow, elderflower and boneset to bring the fever out; or
- Take an aspirin-based medication (or alternative if you suffer stomach ulcers) if your temperature either rises above 40°C, or the burning/shivering stage of fever begins. This will suppress the fever, but is usually advisable if the fever reaches this stage.

### Managing pain

Use the hot and cold packs as appropriate; hot baths and packs can ease muscular pain and tension, while cold packs reduce heat, inflammation and swelling.

#### The castor oil pack (hot pack)

- releases congestion from mucous membranes (respiratory, colon);
- increases elimination via the liver; and
- releases toxic accumulation in muscles (these often show sudden signs of tension when toxins are released).

#### The clay pack (cold pack)

- Reduces swellings from hot inflammations; and
- Adsorbs toxins from the surrounding tissue

Clay accelerates healing of open and internal wounds through these methods of reduction and adsorption. They are used at hot inflammatory sites, infected sites, tumour sites and over swelling/oedemas.

### Herbs and homoeopathics

Herbal remedies and homoeopathics can support the healing crisis. Choose appropriate remedies that will enhance immune function, cleanse the lymph, assist the liver and act as demulcents soothing mucous membranes from the effects of the highly toxic irritants.

Toxic, detoxification and healing
crises all require management.

Supporting the body in its
attempts at discharging toxicity will
ensure you have a smoother ride.

By helping the body to resolve
inflammation in as short a time as possible
will lead to the regeneration
of healthy, new tissue.

Detoxification is about cleansing at cell level; but it is the liver that ensures removal of toxins.

The liver detoxifies and cleans the blood and the lymph of toxins. The entire blood volume passes through the liver every three minutes.

# 5

# Liver cleansing

## 5  Liver cleansing

**If you adhere to some strict detoxification plans** you may find that you start to feel "toxic" or poisoned towards the end of the first or second week. Symptoms may include headache (not to be confused with withdrawal headaches accompanying the cessation of coffee), nausea, bad breath and body odour, coated tongue, mouth ulcers, cold sores, mucus discharge, achy joints and general malaise. These symptoms indicate toxins being drawn from the cells into the circulation and the lymphatic system with no speedy route to the outside. In the event they may end up making their way through the external skin, internal skin (mucous membranes of the respiratory, urogenital and gastro-intestinal tracts) and kidneys. The lymphatic circulation can become over-burdened with toxins which may result in swollen glands as they try to deal with the situation.

However, most people do not wish to go through these rigours and therefore it is important to understand how detoxification works in order to be able to plan the best type of detoxification program to suit you.

Perhaps it is easier if we regard our body as a plumbing system with routes of exit for waste products. In this system the liver is the main drain through which most of our toxins flow to the outside. There are other drains which will excrete poisons, such as the kidneys, the skin, the internal skin and the lungs. However, if their load is increased, because the main drain is not functioning adequately or "blocked", then toxicity and symptoms of congestion will arise in these areas and a backlog is created in the tissues.

**Figure 5.1**  The Pathways of elimination

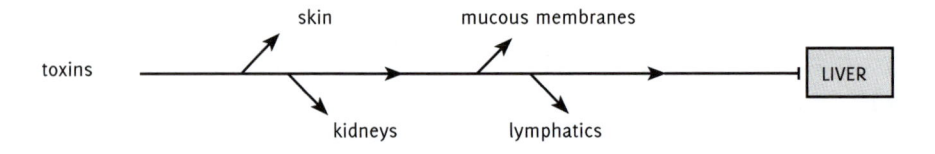

When the liver is congested toxins will start to eliminate through the other channels. It is important that the rate of detoxification at cell level matches the capacity of the liver to eliminate toxins safely.

## Most people will have some reaction to the program within the first month.
The body builds a momentum and then suddenly, you wake up one morning feeling awful. It is very rare, if you are following the diet properly, not to get any reactions. However, in order to limit the toxicity experienced, it is possible to design your own diet so that the pace of detoxification can match your eliminative capacity.

If you turn to chapter 8 *The diet – not for the faint-hearted* you will find a comprehensive section, along with full dietary recommendations, outlining three diet plans ranging from a strong detoxification to a more gentle approach. The strong detoxification plan (Plan A) advocates the use of vegetable juices, raw salads and fruits with no animal protein. However, many people may need to take the process more slowly and this is where Plan B or C would suffice. By reducing the amount of vegetable juices, raw vegetables and fruits (except apples, pears and bananas), and increasing the animal protein, you will immediately reduce the pace of detoxification. If you still feel toxic, make sure that you are eating plenty of brown rice which helps carry toxins out of the system. If you are taking magnesium supplements, then reduce these or omit them from your nutritional prescription. These are all ways that will slow the pace to a more comfortable stride - but you will still continue to detoxify. Most people prefer to get the system moving as efficiently and quickly as possible so that detoxification occurs at a good pace. If this is the case, and you have current health issues, then it may be advisable to seek professional help.

Realistically, it's best to decide on a detoxification plan before you start. How can you tell which one is best for you? We have already seen how to assess the vitality which gives us some indication of how we will cope on the diet. But this, by itself, is not sufficient to make a full assessment. You need to gain more insight into how well your main drain, the liver, will cope with the removal of toxins. Once you have assessed its capacity from your case history, you will be in a position to make a more accurate prediction of how well you will manage.

This chapter explores how we assess the liver's eliminative capacity. There are many symptoms, most of which do not seem to relate directly to the liver, which indicate liver congestion. The term "hypochondriac" illustrates this perfectly. It describes a person who always feels ill and yet shows no clinical signs of illness. It literally translates as - "hypo" meaning under and "chondrium" or ribcage which is the area where the liver resides. The frustration of medical practitioners being unable to clinically diagnose the source of malaise has seemingly justified dismissive attitudes to genuine complaints, earning the patient the derogatory status of a hypochondriac. However, long before clinical tests were available, a person would be diagnosed as "liverish" and given a liver tonic.

*Symptoms of being permanently "under the weather" often indicate poor liver function. In the past a liver tonic would have been prescribed.*

The liver is central to so many activities from balancing our energy and hormones, supporting our digestion, controlling cholesterol levels and assisting in the transport of nutrients. The Chinese call it the "wheel of life" and in our own language, *liver* expresses its vital importance to life itself. The liver is so important that it is the only organ that is not only able to fully regenerate to regain its size, but also carries a 70% functional reserve - which means that clinical tests will only detect abnormalities when we are down to our last 30%! It can be a bit late by this stage to start reversing the process, so it is much better to heed the signs of liver congestion at the outset to prevent its degeneration.

*An optimally functioning liver is central to our health.*

*Liver cleansing*

# Elimination channels

**If you turn to figure 5.2** *Symptoms relating to congestion in the eliminative channels* you will see the five routes for toxin elimination (lymphatic system, internal skin, external skin, kidneys and liver) and the types of illness that arise from congestion in these tissues. Remember, conditions have to prevail within the body before disease sets in. Pathogens do not take hold when the cells are vital; it is only when they become weakened through congestion that infection sets in. Eventually, if vitality is not restored, then organs become inefficient and metabolic disturbances occur giving rise to specific disease patterns.

**The lymphatic system** is an overflow system taking toxins, dead cells, microbes and tissue waste from the cells. It is similar to the circulatory system but has no pumping mechanism, so the movement of lymph relies on exercise. As muscles squeeze, the lymph is pushed forward. This system also has clusters of little nodes (lymph nodes or glands) and patches of lymphatic tissue, which trap foreign substances, food antigens, pollutants, bacteria, virally-infected cells, and abnormal or tumour cells. Lymph nodes and lymphatic tissue are situated at strategic points around the body; the neck and throat (tonsils), the armpits, groin and along the gastro-intestinal tract (Peyer's patches and appendix). It is here that specific cells of the immune system are activated and antibodies formed. It is when they become active that an immune response is elicited and the nodes become swollen and painful.

*Viruses can linger in the body if immune responses are inadequate to eradicate the agent completely.*

This is a healing reaction and if supported the body will eliminate the aggravating factor completely. If suppressed, the pathogen may not be eradicated entirely and if the body is no longer capable of an acute response, the pathogen may remain in a dormant state. If vitality is subsequently lowered due to physical or emotional stress, the pathogen can strike again. This is particularly true of viral infections, such as herpes and shingles. Specific viruses may also be implicated in the onset of certain autoimmune diseases. For example, the Coxsackie B virus is implicated in juvenile diabetes, motor neurone disease and cardiomyopathy.

The eradication of early cancer is also dependent upon a functioning immune system. A specific branch of the immune system recognises tumour cells and will remove them from the body. If the immune system is suppressed by symptomatic treatment or through poor diet, then this can increase the risk of cancer, particularly in later years.

**Figure 5.2** Symptoms relating to congestion in the eliminative channels

**Lymphatic system**
Poor immune response
Recurrent infection
Tonsils/adenoids/appendix
Glandular fever
CFS
Cancer
Fibromyalgia

**Kidneys**
Acidity of tissues
Arthritis/hardening
High blood pressure
Nephritis/nephropathy
Osteoporosis
Fluid retention

**Liver**
Jaundice/Hepatitis
Glandular fever
Irritable bowel syndrome
Haemorrhoids
Digestive disorders
Allergies/food intolerances
Low blood sugar/poor energy
Hormonal imbalances
General congestion

**External skin**
Eczema/psoriasis/dermatitis
Boils, acne
Cradle cap

**Internal Skin**
Infection, ulceration & congestion of the mucous membranes:
*Digestive tract:*
Colitis, diverticulitis, ulcers
*Urogenitary tract:*
Vaginitis, candida, cystitis,
Nephritis, pelvic inflammatory disease
*Respiratory tract:*
Sinusitis, rhinitis, laryngitis
Bronchitis, tracheitis, asthma,
Chronic obstructive airways disease (COAD)

In a healthy body no pathogen, bacterial or viral, should be able to gain access to the interior. Resistance depends on the integrity of the skin and the mucous membranes. If we build this resistance through healthy diet, then the production of antibodies by the immune system is a last ditch attempt at neutralising pathogens when they have breached these defences. A high antibody count to a specific disease is not an indication of higher resistance and vitality but merely shows that the pathogen has survived the initial defences. Antibodies are additional forces that the body has to summon up in order to try and eradicate the disease.

*The immune system is only called to action when the external defences, the skin and the mucous membranes, have been breached.*

When mapping a case history, symptoms of lymphatic congestion (tonsillitis, appendicitis and painful lymph nodes) often appear quite early on. These conditions indicate that the resistance of the external and internal skin is weakened (nowadays mostly due to poor diet rather than living conditions) and that general vitality is lowered with increased congestion within the body. The lymphatic system, which takes tissue wastes from the cells, often becomes so burdened that the tonsils, adenoids and appendix become diseased and may have to be removed.

This does not address the situation; it merely places a greater burden on the remaining lymphatic tissue and nodes. You will find that once you start cleansing the body, even in a young child susceptible to recurrent tonsillitis, the glands subside and regenerate. If you do nothing, then you increase the vulnerability to infections like glandular fever. Glandular fever will only strike when the vitality has reached a low ebb - which explains why some adolescents/adults, particularly when under stress, succumb while others do not. Glandular fever attacks the liver and many people experience a sudden

*Recurrent glandular infections are indicative of a combination of high levels of toxicity with a weakened immune response. Reducing the toxic burden is often sufficient to see resolution of these complaints.*

decline in health dating from that period. Many patients will say that their energies were never the same since having glandular fever. Case histories very rarely show a gradual decline in health but are more often punctuated by illnesses which mark definite water-sheds where health suddenly declines and the "picture" changes to reflect the disease patterns of lowered vitality.

The tonsillitis/glandular fever picture often precedes the onset of arthritis. A congested, overtaxed lymphatic system undermines its capacity to remove tissue waste efficiently. Acidic residues in the form of crystals and salts settle in the joints causing inflammation and pain. Additional symptoms include the sore and swollen glands experienced when people hit a "low". In women this often coincides with the menstrual cycle when vitality naturally dips. This dip is only noticeable when there is no surplus vitality to compensate or buffer the effects.

**Figure 5.3** The threshold of vitality

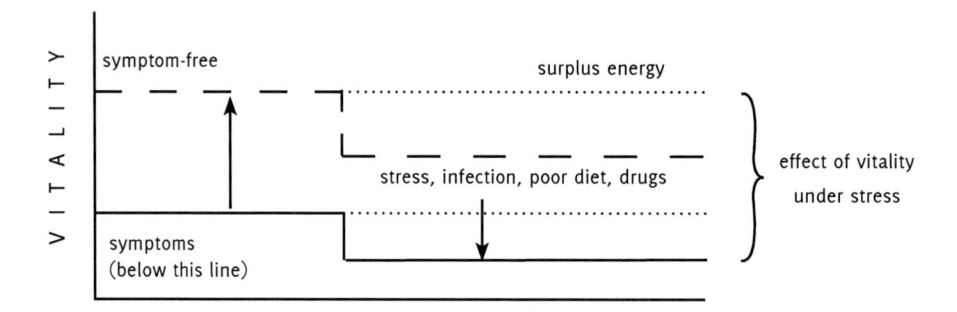

People living on the line have no surplus energy. This is like having no capital in the bank; when the debts come in, there are no reserve funds to pay them. Symptoms that occur as soon as stress arises indicate that there is no buffer. The aim is to get enough surplus energy (vitality) to compensate when under stress so that no symptoms occur.

Once the detoxification process starts there can be an additional strain on the lymphatic system, particularly when the liver is congested (see later), and it may be wise to go more slowly. However, once underway and the vitality raised, it is possible to have an immune response, such as fever, swollen glands and immune reactions, that is constructive rather than an indicator of a lowered vitality. You can tell a healing response by how acute the reaction is and whether it resolves naturally within a short period of time with supportive treatment (rest, sleep, good nutrition, herbs).

As a practitioner, I have witnessed many healing crises (as they are familiarly known). But I would like to relate my own personal experience which occurred during an eight month detoxification plan when I had chickenpox and later, mumps. Neither of these illnesses was circulating at the time, nor had I contracted them when I was a child, even though my sisters had had both infections. It is possible, when your own vitality is low, that you do not mount an immune response to an infection but harbour pathogens without eliciting symptoms. It is the symptoms that tell you that you have the disease. The symptoms are the healing response. As a child my vitality was poor. I suffered with asthma and chest infections and was inclined to be lazy. In truth

**Case History 5.1**

## Sue was 42 years old, working as an infant teacher when she came to see me. Over the past six months various joints had become inflamed. The swelling and inflammation moved from joint to joint, from shoulder, to arm, to wrist, hands and fingers. Her feet were also affected. The joints stiffened and she was prescribed anti-inflammatory drugs. Blood tests were normal and there were no seemingly precipitating factors. Sue was depressed and had given up gardening and crafts. She could no longer drive the car when her hands were painful.

I took her case history and she told me that as a child she had continuous tonsillitis and antibiotics were prescribed. At eight years they were removed which led to a catarrhal picture. At twelve years her sinuses were so badly infected and blocked that she had them scraped. The catarrh worsened over the years giving rise to sinusitis and perennial rhinitis. At seventeen years she suffered glandular fever and was ill for several months. From this time on, Sue felt that her energies were never quite as good. She went on to have three children and up until recently the only health problems suffered were chest colds (put down to infection from the children she taught) which would often last the entire winter and only respond to antibiotic treatment. She also complained of poor energy, constipation and thrush (as a consequence of antibiotic treatment).

Sue's diet included much salty food, especially cheese and ham. She also drank around eight cups of tea or coffee a day and enjoyed sweet snacks.

Liver congestion arose at an early age (constipation and low energy), lowering general vitality and placing a tremendous burden on the lymphatic system. Following the removal of the tonsils, the internal membranes took on the toxic load leading to congestion and infection in the sinuses and upper respiratory tract. Further suppressive treatments continued to compromise the vitality, eventually resulting in glandular fever. Toxicity and acidity continued to rise over the years with congestion moving in deeper to reappear, not in the eliminative channels, but as hardening and inflammation within the joints. Although symptoms were located within the joints this condition reflects a general hardening where disease becomes "locked in". When the eliminative channels are no longer open, local immune responses to the stagnant, toxic waste increase the acidity and the formation of crystal deposits.

Sue went on the detoxification diet, removing all meat, and within the first month the inflammation in the joints disappeared. She hadn't realised how depressed she had become until her energy started rising. Constipation became a complaint of the past and she was amazed that by the third month her nose started to continually run - it was no longer blocked! We did a lot of work on the liver using choline preparations and flaxseed oil and re-established the magnesium levels. She also took apple cider vinegar to help reduce the acidity. Sue remained on the diet for a good six months and then started introducing various foods. We identified a few foods which aggravated the joints, among which were mushrooms, sweet corn, berries and wheat.

I had very little energy. However, as soon as my vitality was raised through detoxification, those childhood diseases "came out" with my body mounting quite a response. Neither illness was severe and with bed rest and proper care I recovered well.

When the healing process begins, symptoms tend to reappear in the reverse order. That is, the symptoms you experienced last are the first to go and the symptoms experienced first are the last to go. It would appear, in my case, that I was able to produce an inflammatory response to the small amounts of pathogen that existed in my body once my vitality was restored, and I noticed that it was towards the end of my cleanse that these symptoms appeared.

## The skin 
is our largest eliminative organ where up to two-thirds of our tissue waste may be eliminated. When the lymphatic system is congested our skin may take the burden, but if this is suppressed then the congestion moves in and affects our internal membranes (mucous membranes) leading to toxicity and infection at these surfaces. Although spots, boils and acne are the bane of many an adolescent's life, if you desire a cure then you start cleansing on the inside by shifting toxins through the lymph and out through the liver. Then the burden will be relieved from the skin and symptoms will disappear.

*Antibiotics damage the natural balance of micro-organisms in the gut. This has a profoundly negative effect on general immunity and the integrity of the colonic mucous membranes, and can precipitate inflammatory bowel disease and allergies.*

Too much toxic waste, if eliminated via the wrong channels, devitalises the tissues in that area which then become a breeding ground for bacteria. A healthy skin has its own balanced eco-system where pathogenic micro-organisms, like the staphylococcus aureus, are contained by non-pathogenic species (non-disease causing micro-organisms). It is the balance between the different species that prevents disease. This balance is upset when tissue becomes toxic allowing pathogenic bacteria to thrive. Antibiotics, so often prescribed for skin conditions, aggravate the overall picture. A skin infection may seem to clear with antibiotics as they kill off all bacteria, good and bad. However, fungi and yeasts will continue to thrive uninhibited (usually kept in check by the good bacteria) and the more pathogenic strains of bacteria will be the first to re-colonise.

*A high toxic load in the colon recycles to the liver. Toxic colon = toxic liver.*

These effects also occur in the colon which can support, in total, around 1½ kg of bacteria. A balanced ecology is critical to colonic health and the integrity of the mucous membranes. Persistent antibiotic abuse leads to a toxic colon, which in turn leads to a toxic liver, toxic lymph and toxic skin. This is why antibiotic treatment never provides long-term results. Although you may look better on the outside, conditions worsen on the inside, and new, more chronic forms of illness may start to occur in the colon, digestive system, lymphatic system, lungs and kidneys.

The link between the external skin and internal membranes is clearly seen with the eczema/asthma picture. Suppression of eczema invariably leads to asthma and during the healing process the asthma will resolve only to apparently revive the eczema, much to the horror of many parents. However, if healing is allowed to continue then this condition will also resolve itself. On the other hand, if the asthma is also suppressed, congestion and toxicity rises and symptoms may appear in the mental area resulting in ADHD or hyperactivity. This progression can be seen thus:

irritation of skin ⟶ irritation of lungs ⟶ irritation of brain

These three conditions share the same deep major mineral imbalance where an inherited acidic constitution inhibits the correct utilisation of calcium. The high sodium, high calcium dietary trends exacerbate this picture eroding the magnesium status further. It is important to incorporate magnesium-rich foods and limit the amount of dairy under such conditions.

## The internal skin (mucous membrane) lines the internal passageways from the nose through the sinuses to the lungs; from the mouth to the stomach and out through the colon; from the fallopian tubes to the uterus and vagina and from the kidney tubules to the bladder and urethra. These linings secrete mucus which keeps them lubricated and traps bacteria and other substances, preventing them from entering the body. Mucus is also a medium for the disposal of toxic waste carrying toxins from the body to the outside, much like the skin eliminates body waste. For example, carcinogens from smoking may be detected in malignant cervical cells.

Mucus is also produced during an immune response to allergy or infection where it carries dead cells, bacteria and other pathogens to the surface. Prolonged irritation from repeated exposure to allergens or infection will result in an overproduction of mucus which can stagnate and become a breeding ground for infection itself. This may lead to inflammation of the delicate mucous membranes which may ulcerate and bleed. These conditions arise in the respiratory tract as chronic sinusitis, bronchitis and laryngitis; in the digestive tract as ulcers, ulcerative colitis, and diverticulitis; in the kidneys as cystitis and nephritis; and in the reproductive tract as pelvic inflammatory disease, vaginitis and chronic candida. (The chronic discharge seen in candida is usually due to immune reactions to undigested sugars which leak from the digestive tract into the systemic circulation where they initiate an immune response.)

Chronic inflammation may lead to excessive scar tissue formation causing fibrosis, the blocking of tubes and airways (chronic obstructive airways disease) or increased permeability of the mucous membranes which allows pathogens and allergens to readily breach these defences. At the gut, some forms of enteritis, such as that caused by campylobacter, can lead to damage of the mucosal lining of the gut, and the toxins move inwards to not only affect the joints (enteropathic arthritis) but also the skin (arthritic psoriasis). You can begin to appreciate the role of mucosal integrity as a main barrier to the outside world and the guarding of inner health.

*Inflammation in the colon moves "downstream" giving rise to chronic inflammatory diseases of the joints and skin.*

It is worth mentioning that toxins are passed from mother to baby during pregnancy. The foetus becomes a receptacle sharing the toxic burden if the mother cannot eliminate toxins efficiently. The foetal liver is immature and unable to deal with toxins. In addition, it has the role of making foetal blood cells until the bone marrow matures and takes over this function in the last trimester. The onset of childhood leukaemia may be related to toxic conditions in the foetal liver during pregnancy. Toxins are also passed from mother to baby in the breast-milk. Milk is a ten-fold concentration of the blood plasma - so circulating toxins will also concentrate ten-fold. I do not advocate detoxification plans during pregnancy or breast-feeding as this increases the circulating toxic load which would be passed to the baby. It is better to embark upon a detoxification program six months (minimal) prior to conception.

*The kidneys carry the acidic burden of the body; a prolonged acidic burden is a key factor in the erosion of kidney vitality.*

*The health of the kidneys underpins our cellular vitality; they control the pH and sodium/potassium balance, both of which are fundamental to cellular health.*

**The kidneys** eliminate water-soluble compounds, such urea and uric acid (both end-products of protein metabolism) urobilin (bile pigment), creatinine (end-product of tissue breakdown), phosphates, sulphates and oxalates. They are also the principle organs controlling our acid/alkaline (pH) and sodium/potassium balance and, as we know, both the pH and the sodium/potassium balance are the most important determinants of cellular health. In fact they are inseparable; the higher the levels of sodium within the cells, the greater the acidity, and by reducing the sodium levels you also reduce acidity (and vice-versa!). We could say that the pH of the body is the bottom line. If the pH shifts just 0.3 points either side of pH 7.4 (slightly alkaline), then death would ensue as the body's enzyme systems cannot operate outside this narrow range. The enzymes straighten out, and once they've lost their shape they cannot function. Being that we produce a colossal equivalent of 1.5 litres of strong acid daily as a waste product of our metabolism, the body must have efficient methods of disposal.

In TCM (Traditional Chinese Medicine), the Kidney element (which refers to both the adrenal glands and the kidneys) "house" the constitution and is the source of our Yin and Yang. In other words the integrity and functional capacity of our kidneys reflects the stamina and strength of the body as a whole. Once the kidneys weaken, our physical substance (Yin) becomes deficient and its function (Yang) fails. So from this perspective, any acceleration of the ageing process, where our biological age outstrips our chronological age (we get sicker earlier than we should) is measured in terms of Kidney integrity. As we know, increased acidity coupled with hardening and inflammation underpins most of our chronic degenerative diseases.

*Stress has a deeply erosive effect on the adrenal glands and kidneys. Prolonged stress can diminish the adrenal output of corticosteroid hormones which may exacerbate chronic inflammatory disease.*

When we translate this into modern terms, we can see a strong correlation between Eastern and Western perspectives. It is the kidneys that maintain the optimum environment of the whole body through their control of pH and the sodium/potassium status; they regulate calcium and vitamin D metabolism, and hence the health of the bones; they detoxify water soluble toxins and the end-products of metabolism; they regulate blood volume and blood pressure, promoting a diuretic effect in high blood pressure and stimulating constriction of the arteries and an increase in blood volume in low blood pressure; and they regulate oxygenation by stimulating the bone marrow to increase their production of red blood cells and hence the uptake of oxygen in low oxygen-states. The adrenal glands work in concert with the kidneys where they communicate closely with regard to blood pressure and the sodium/potassium balance, but additionally, they have a major responsibility in directing the nervous system in "fight and flight" reactions (adrenaline), conversing with the liver in the regulation of energy and blood sugar levels (glucocorticosteroids), modifying the inflammatory response (cortisone) and supplementing our sex hormones (DHEA, androgens), which becomes important for women during and after the menopause.

You will begin to appreciate how the Western diet, high in protein, salt and stimulants (tea, coffee and alcohol), will have an erosive effect on the kidneys over a prolonged period of time. Prolonged stress will also have a negative impact on our kidneys and adrenal glands. The effects of an ageing kidney will specifically manifest as general hardening arising from acidity in the body (arthritis, inflammatory disease), high blood pressure, hardening of the arteries and heart disease, cardiac asthma and fluid retention. The kidneys also affect bone integrity (osteoporosis) and specific types of bone disease and anaemia can arise from chronic kidney conditions.

**The liver** is the principal organ of elimination and I often refer to it as the main drain as it is here that toxins are prepared for elimination. The liver converts fat-soluble substances to water-soluble substances for excretion either by the kidneys or by the liver via the bile. Bile is the main secretory product of the liver and is the medium for the disposal of its toxic waste. Many compounds are detoxified by the liver and passed to the bile.

Bile contains water, bilirubin (bile pigments), bile acids, lecithin and cholesterol. Bile acids and lecithin are both strong emulsifiers, which not only keep cholesterol in solution inhibiting the formation of gall stones, but also assist in the digestion of fats. Bile acids are themselves synthesised from cholesterol by the liver, so an increased rate of synthesis results in a reduction of cholesterol levels. Hence the liver is the main organ for controlling cholesterol. Steroid hormones, alcohol, drugs and bilirubin (from dead red blood cells) are some of the products degraded by the liver and secreted into the bile for elimination via the colon.

Hepatic production of bile is critical to the detoxification process; when this becomes compromised, symptoms of liver congestion will arise and generalised congestion may occur in the other eliminative channels. This is why we always look to determine how well the liver can cope on any detoxification plan. If it is congested then it won't cope at all; but if there are relatively few indicators of congestion then strong detoxification should pose no problem. It is possible to tell from the case history the level of liver congestion by the various symptoms that appear throughout the medical history.

*Toxin removal is secured by a healthy bile production.*

**Jaundice** in the new-born is a typical manifestation of an immature liver which cannot cope with the breakdown products of red blood cells that naturally occurs after birth. The yellow pigment, bilirubin, should be cleared by the liver. If not, it will cause jaundice, or a yellowing of the skin, which can be very serious if left untreated. Not much thought is given to infant jaundice as treatment is simple and effective; the baby receives photo-therapy until the jaundice resolves. However, a healthy baby with a more efficient liver can cope with the breakdown of red blood cells and the elimination of bilirubin.

*Jaundice is due to the inefficient clearing of bilirubin (a breakdown product of red blood cells) by the liver via the bile.*

**Cradle cap** may also be a sign of liver congestion. The head is the only place of elimination via the skin in a small baby and it will carry the load if there is liver congestion. Many children of school age still exhibit these symptoms of elimination.

**Recurrent tonsillitis** occurs when the glands become involved resulting in infection. You may remember that toxic lymph enters the liver via the subclavian vein, so the final detoxification of the lymph is dependent on liver function. Recurrent symptoms in the glands usually indicates a toxic liver and toxic lymph.

*Lymph is ultimately cleansed by the liver. Recurrent infection in the lymph nodes may indicate liver congestion.*

**Fat intolerance** occurs with inadequate bile production. Bile emulsifies dietary fats, breaking them down into smaller globules so that the digestive enzymes can work on a greater surface area. Undigested fat leads to loose, foamy stools, and losses of the fat-soluble vitamins (A, D, and E) and calcium.

*A deficiency of digestive enzymes may be a fundamental cause of both food intolerance and allergy.*

**Food intolerances** may cause local symptoms in the gut, such as indigestion, bloating, cramping, spasms, diarrhoea and irritable bowel. These may be caused by a deficiency of digestive enzymes. Lactose intolerance, for example, is due to a deficiency of the enzyme lactase which digests milk sugar which causes chronic diarrhoea, whereas bloating and flatulence is more likely caused by undigested sugars (due to a deficiency of the disaccharidases – or sugar-splitting enzymes). These sugars then pass to the colon and undergo fermentation. Yeasts, such as candida, will aggravate this situation. If the bowel becomes toxic then pathogenic bacteria may also proliferate into the small intestine which is sterile under normal conditions. The by-products of pathogens and incompletely digested foods circulate to the liver and compound its congestion.

*An allergic reaction involves immune cells. Commonly, there is an elevation of the antibody, Immunoglobin E, which stimulates the release of histamine from mast cells.*

**Food allergies** usually arise from incomplete digestion of proteins in the gut, although a range of chemicals present in food and food additives can also be a major trigger. The two main culprits are dairy and wheat, and again we are looking at a deficiency of digestive enzymes, namely the dipeptidases (enzymes that split small protein chains). These partially digested chains and/or chemicals then pass into the circulation. Under normal circumstances these products should be taken up by the liver and degraded before they reach the systemic circulation. However, with liver congestion, these particles escape and cause allergic reactions at the skin (**eczema, hives**) and mucous membranes (**asthma, rhinitis**).

In both instances - food allergy and intolerance - the cells lining the gut supply the enzymes responsible for the end-stage digestion of foods and the deactivation of certain food chemicals. Digestive deficiency simply means that the gut has lost this integrity and you can appreciate how the removal of offending foods without repairing gut integrity through better nutrition and detoxification will only give short-term relief. Digestive deficiency can both cause and compound liver congestion, as the liver is a "first pass" for these by-products, which increase its toxic load.

**Constipation** may also be a consequence of inadequate bile production as bile is our natural laxative.

**Toxic bowel** may arise as a consequence of liver congestion. There is a two-way relationship between the liver and colon. If the liver fails to support the digestion this will lead to stagnation in the gastrointestinal tract. Toxins are then reabsorbed from the colon and circulated back to the liver. It is interesting that abnormal liver function tests are almost always detected in diseases of the gastrointestinal tract. Eventually, as congestion deepens, constipation may give way to diarrhoea. Bowel function becomes altered and organic change occurs leading to the alternating **diarrhoea/constipation** cycle of **irritable bowel syndrome**. Impacted stools, which have a slow transit time, may cause infection and inflammation of the bowel wall as seen in **colitis** and **diverticulitis**.

**Skin conditions**, such as **eczema, psoriasis** and **dermatitis** are also directly linked to liver congestion. These conditions may be caused by food allergies but additionally, the liver is responsible for the manufacture and packaging of fatty acids that are circulated to the tissues. Some of these fatty acids are used in the synthesis of cell membranes conferring strength and integrity to the cell wall. Of particular interest is the essential fatty acid, linoleic acid, which is converted to its active form, gamma-linolenic acid (GLA), by the liver. Deficiency in this essential nutrient leads to cell permeability and eczematous lesions. Evening primrose oil is a natural source of GLA and is often prescribed for skin conditions.

*When treating skin conditions factor in food allergy and essential fatty acid deficiency.*

However, provided that there are adequate nutrient supplies (C, B3, Mg, Zn) and not too many saturated fats in the diet the liver should be able to convert linoleic acid to GLA. Rather than treating on a purely symptomatic basis, it is more advantageous to improve the nutritional status of the liver and reduce its burden in order to correct the cause. By adopting this approach you will also restore health on all levels.

**Low blood sugar** is also associated with liver congestion. Stable energy levels are dependent upon the blood glucose concentration. When this dips we feel hungry and usually grab for a snack that will raise the blood sugar levels quickly (see chapter 6 *Regeneration & blood sugar control*). However, we should be able to last between meals without suffering cravings and low energy. The liver is under hormonal regulation which monitors fluctuations in blood sugar levels. When the blood sugar concentration falls, the liver is mobilised into converting its glycogen (stored glucose) to glucose and releasing this into the circulation. If the liver is functioning well then we should not even notice the energy curve as the release of stored glucose compensates before signals hit the brain. However, many people have inadequate blood sugar control due to liver congestion.

**Hormonal imbalances** also indicate liver congestion. In Chinese medicine the liver is regarded as the planner of cycles. As far as the sex hormones are concerned **menstrual irregularities, short gestation cycles (premature birth, miscarriage)**, symptoms caused by hormonal imbalances **(infertility, cancers, pre-menstrual syndrome), early menopause** - all indicate liver congestion. Although the liver does not produce the sex hormones, it does control their activity. A healthy liver manufactures proteins (sex hormone binding globulins [SHBG]) that bind the sex hormones inactivating them. Only the 2-3% that remain free are biologically active. In addition, the liver degrades and clears all hormones. Both these activities regulate the quantities of active circulating sex hormones which controls hormonal activity, regulates menstrual cycles, improves fertility and diminishes the side effects of hormonal imbalance. Hence detoxification programs that relieve the toxic load of the liver have an enormous impact on hormonal regulation.

*The liver also controls thyroid hormone activity, inactivating it through binding and degradation, and activating it through conversion to its active form, T3*

**Heart disease** and the accumulation of fatty deposits in the arteries are not commonly associated with liver congestion. It is assumed that eating less fat and refined carbohydrate is the sum total of preventative measures we can take. But the imbalance in fat handling starts long before fatty deposits accumulate; it begins when the liver becomes compromised in its capacity to convert cholesterol to bile acids for excretion. This is how the body eliminates cholesterol. It is true that high fat/high sugar diets promote the synthesis of cholesterol but, as always, it is a two-fold equation:

*Bile acids are a degradation product of cholesterol. By stimulating bile acid production, you also lower your cholesterol.*

$\uparrow$ cholesterol (high fat/sugar diet) + $\downarrow$ conversion to bile acids $\rightarrow$ cholesterol deposits in arteries

So liver congestion contributes to atheroma in the arteries which results in **heart disease, kidney disease** and **strokes**.

**Gall stones** are another indication of faulty cholesterol metabolism. Some cholesterol is secreted into the bile unchanged but the greater proportion is converted to bile acids. Bile acids act like detergent keeping the cholesterol emulsified. If the ratio between cholesterol and bile salts in solution is disturbed (i.e. too much cholesterol, too little bile acids) then cholesterol clumps to form stones.

**Glandular fever and hepatitis** are common illnesses that specifically involve the liver. Any incidence of these diseases in the case history (particularly in the absence of therapeutic treatment to revitalise the liver) will indicate compromised liver function.

I have given a brief overview covering a large number of indicators of liver congestion. For some, this may suffice, but I suspect that many readers would like to gain greater insight into these conditions, how they arise and how they can be best addressed by following the principles of detoxification and dietary healing. Hopefully, in the remaining sections of this chapter you will gain sufficient understanding of your condition so that you may help yourself.

## REVERSING LIVER CONGESTION

The detoxification diet will start the process of cleansing and regeneration. But this, in itself, may be inadequate to create an impact particularly at the beginning of treatment if the liver is very congested. This is when specific work may be needed to prepare the liver for a strong elimination.

*Quite simply, three avenues need to be addressed:*
- removal of the accumulated liver fat;
- stimulation of the production of bile; and
- revitalisation of the liver detoxification pathways.

*Make sure you understand your condition, your level of toxicity and your liver capacity before you start on your program.*

Before toxins can be secreted into the bile they are made water-soluble via the liver detoxification pathways and then eliminated in the bile. If the production of bile is sluggish extreme toxicity will arise within the body causing chronic disease. Under these circumstances, the liver will be unable to handle the volume of toxins that may be released on a deep cleanse and toxic coma can ensue from the influx of toxins into the circulation. It is very important to understand this sequence of events and the need to spend some time in advance preparing the liver before embarking on a deep cleanse if you have a chronic illness. It is possible, and even advisable under some circumstances when time is of the essence, to immediately start on a very deep cleanse (stronger than the one advocated in this book). However, it should not be undertaken lightly or without professional guidance as aggravations can be severe and may require appropriate management.

The following three major sections will provide you with sufficient information to understand the mechanics of liver detoxification and help you make discriminative choices in treatment. I have found that when my patients understand their starting point (what is my current state of health

# Common factors that burden the liver

In order that we don't continue to undermine our liver function it's wise to be aware of some of the common factors that burden the liver. Below is a list outlining the major influences on liver congestion.

- Dietary imbalance of the four major minerals (sodium and calcium excess, potassium and magnesium deficiency) and diets that promote losses of the cell minerals (stimulants, refined foods, fats etc.) lead to liver congestion. As with all the body cells, the liver cells are also vulnerable to these disturbed ratios;

- Specific nutrient deficiencies - selenium, magnesium, vitamin E, B12, B6, folic acid, linoleic acid and choline. Magnesium is important in the conversion of cholesterol to bile acids and the secretion of bile into the liver ducts;

- High fat and highly refined carbohydrate foods promote the synthesis of cholesterol and lead to the accumulation of liver fat causing congestion;

- Protein deficiency from prolonged fasting, starvation, anorexia or diets lacking quality protein results in the deposition of fats in the liver. The liver normally exports fats using protein as a packaging material. Protein is also important for the manufacture of conjugating elements required in detoxification pathways;

- Alcohol abuse leads to fatty liver and cirrhosis;

- All medical drugs, but of the most common:
  - Paracetamol destroys liver tissue
  - Oral contraceptives and hormone replacement therapy (HRT) interfere with bile salt secretion and excretion
  - Tetracycline antibiotics inhibit the export of fats from the liver
  - All antibiotics cultivate a toxic environment in the bowel which will lead to a toxic liver

- Chemicals – these include agricultural and industrial chemicals, and food additives.

and how did I get here?), they can start to appreciate what is required of them and how long their journey may take. It is much easier to swap elements of your life-style to support your healing journey, and to stay with it for the required length of time, when you understand the route you are taking, how you're going to get there and how long it's going to take. Monitoring outcome is also helpful, so if you wish to follow your progress with blood tests or scans, make sure you have these done before you start your program and continue to monitor at intervals.

*Detoxification programs are long-term for chronic conditions. Progress needs to be monitored regularly to make sure you are reaching your desired goals.*

# Removal of liver fat

*If you consume more fat and carbohydrate than you need, they are stored as fat both in the fat tissues and the organs - including the liver.*

**By reducing the amount of dietary fat** and refined carbohydrates (which are converted to fat by the liver and fat cells if taken in excess), we can ensure that the burden on the liver is reduced. The liver assumes a major role in fat management. Although it receives a relatively small proportion of dietary fat (this goes straight to the tissues for energy and storage) it is still busy making fats and packaging them ready for shipment out to the tissues. Diets high in fat and refined carbohydrates increase this fat handling burden and also stimulate the synthesis of cholesterol by the liver. Any excess dietary fat that is not cleared by the circulation is returned to the liver, and similarly excess carbohydrates are also converted to fats (triglycerides) by the tissues and the liver – which is why you get fat if you eat too much sugar. In addition, stress, stimulants and low blood sugar levels cause the release of fatty acids (as an energy supply) into the circulation from the body's own reserves, which increase the liver's metabolic burden.

*If you are deficient in nutrients the liver may be unable to export fats and they will remain in the liver increasing congestion.*

Fat handling creates one of the biggest metabolic burdens for the liver, and the nutrient requirements for the handling of fats are high. In short, fats are expensive. When we consume fats and oils as naturally found in foods, they come with their full complement of nutrients required for their metabolism. Once they are extracted from their food-state, they are stripped of these nutrients and will pull on the body's existing nutrient resources. So high fat diets can induce nutrient deficiencies. Magnesium is particularly vulnerable, as it is required for the metabolism and removal of fats and cholesterol from the liver. Although high fat and high carbohydrate diets are two of the biggest culprits in liver congestion and heart disease, it is a two-edged sword as the nutrient deficiencies they induce also exacerbate the symptoms of disease.

*A lipoprotein is the vehicle for the transport of fats from the liver.*

## The Packaging of Fats by the Liver

Before fats can be shipped out of the liver they need to be packaged into a water-soluble form for transport. You can imagine that unless they are processed in this way they would clump together and clog the arteries before reaching their destination. The liver packages the triglycerides and cholesterol as the fatty core, and builds a coat of lecithin (phospholipids) and small proteins (apoproteins) to surround it. The outer covering is hydrophilic (water-loving) and therefore enables these small fat globules to move easily in the blood. These fat packages are known as lipoproteins.

*Lecithin synthesis*

**Figure 5.4**  A lipoprotein molecule

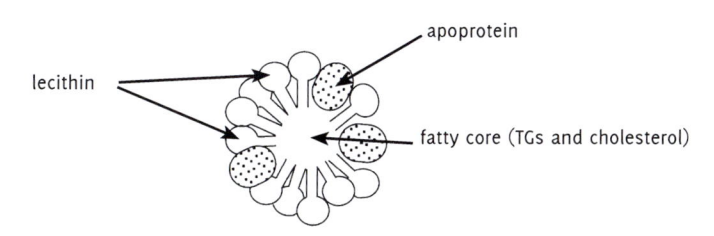

A lipoprotein has a fatty core of cholesterol and triglycerides surrounded by a hydrophilic layer (water-loving) of lecithin molecules and apoproteins. Apoproteins are responsible for activating the enzymes involved in the breakdown of lipoproteins for the transfer of cholesterol and triglycerides into the cells.

Lecithin is unique in that one end of its molecule mixes with water and the other, with fat. It is similar to a triglyceride in that it has fatty acids attached to a glycerol nucleus. The triglyceride has three fatty acids attached to the glycerol nucleus while the lecithin molecule has only two. One of these fatty acids is linoleic acid.

*Lecithin is a good emulsifier as it is both hydrophilic and hydrophobic.*

**Figure 5.5**  Comparison between a triglyceride and phospatidyl choline

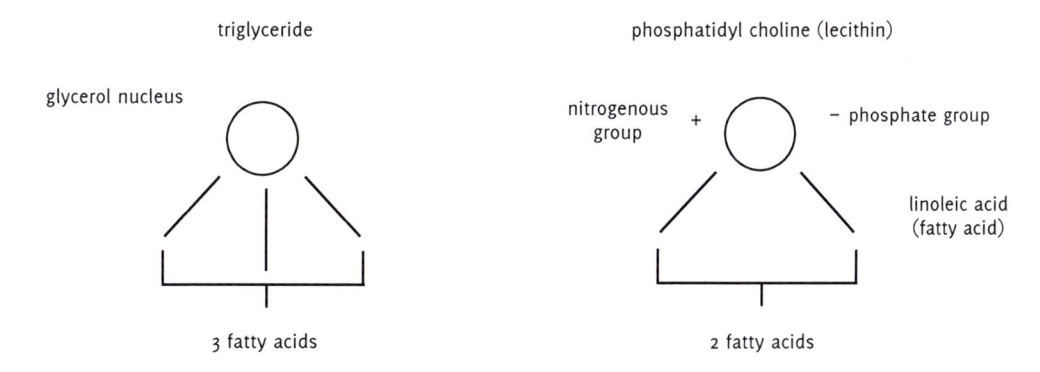

A triglyceride is composed of three fatty acids attached to a glycerol nucleus. Lecithin has two fatty acids attached to the glycerol nucleus, the third position taken by a positively charged nitrogenous group and a negatively charged phosphate group. One of the fatty acids is the essential fatty acid, linoleic acid. Lecithin is hydrophilic at the charged pole and hydrophobic at the opposite pole.

The other position is taken by two charged molecules, a negatively charged phosphate group and a positively charged nitrogenous group, usually choline and sometimes inositol - hence the chemical name for lecithin is phosphatidyl choline. It is the charged head that mixes with water while the fat-soluble tails are repelled toward the fatty core. The apoproteins are also hydrophilic. The finished product is called a lipoprotein and is shipped out of the liver as a VLDL (very low density lipoprotein).

*Hydrophilic: water-loving*

*Hydrophobic: water-hating*

## Nutrients which reduce liver fat – the lipotrophics

Here we are concerned with the nutrients required by the liver for the manufacture of the apoproteins and lecithin. These nutrients are known as lipotrophic factors, or simply reducers of liver fat.

*VLDLs export fats from the liver. They have a very high fat content.*

**Magnesium and vitamin B6** plus good quality protein are required for the manufacture of the apoproteins by the liver. Protein and nutrient deficiencies, as in starvation and poor diet, will lead to fatty infiltration of liver tissue and congestion. However, if the diet provides sufficient nutrients fats will not only be transported into the circulation but they will also be metabolised by the tissues once they reach their destination. The apoproteins act as cofactors and activators of enzyme systems involved in the breakdown of lipoproteins before they transfer their triglycerides and cholesterol to the cells. They become smaller as they offload their cargo: VLDLs become IDLs (intermediate density lipoproteins) and finally LDLs (low density lipoproteins). LDLs carry a high cholesterol load and when levels are elevated are known as "bad cholesterol". Any deficiency or abnormality of the apoproteins leads to abnormal blood fat ratios and their accumulation in the circulation, which is a risk factor for heart disease. You can appreciate the importance of the liver's role in the correct packaging of fats to the overall management of fats by the rest of the body.

*The apoproteins ensure the metabolism of the lipoproteins, the off-loading of their cargo and their removal from the circulation.*

It is worth mentioning here that the tetracycline antibiotics exert negative effects as they inhibit the manufacture of the apoproteins by the liver. Consequently fats cannot be exported and fatty infiltration of the liver occurs. Tetracyclines are often prescribed over long periods for skin conditions and have an extremely adverse effect on liver function. General toxicity will increase in the body as a consequence of this medication.

**Lecithin** is the other essential lipotrophic nutrient and is widely found in foods. The raw ingredients for making lecithin are choline, inositol and linoleic acid. The co-factors required are vitamin B12, B6 and folic acid. Linoleic acid is the fatty acid that takes up one of the positions on the glycerol nucleus. If the diet is rich in these nutrients then the liver can package and mobilise fats to the tissues.

*Linoleic acid is an essential fatty acid (w6 series). Deficiencies compromise lecithin synthesis.*

If you look at table 5.1 *Distribution of cholesterol and lipotrophic factors in foods* you can see the distribution of the lipotrophic factors, choline, inositol and lecithin, while table 5.2 *Saturated and unsaturated fatty acid levels in foods* shows the distribution of linoleic acid. Rich sources of linoleic acid are found in the unrefined cold-pressed oils such as sunflower oil and safflower oil. If taken in this raw state, the high levels of linoleic acid will favour lecithin production. However, most commercial polyunsaturated oils are subjected to high temperature extraction which alters the molecular structure of the oil so that it mimics and behaves as a saturated fat. Olive oil is not a rich source of linoleic acid, and once heated loses its biological properties and behaves as a saturated fat.

*Diets high in saturated fats, while low in the unsaturated essential fatty acids, promote fat deposition in the liver.*

Consequently diets high in saturated fats, damaged polyunsaturated fats (PUFAs) and refined carbohydrates promote the formation of triglycerides by the liver, while diets high in lipotrophic factors promote the formation of lecithin. Problems occur when this balance is upset and the ratio of saturated fats is much greater that the phospholipid (lecithin) component (remember that refined carbohydrates promote saturated fat synthesis and damaged PUFAs behave as saturated fats). It is then that fats start accumulating in the liver which not only cause congestion due to fatty infiltration but also promote oxidative and free radical damage to liver cells.

**Figure 5.6** Precursors to triglyceride, cholesterol and lecithin synthesis

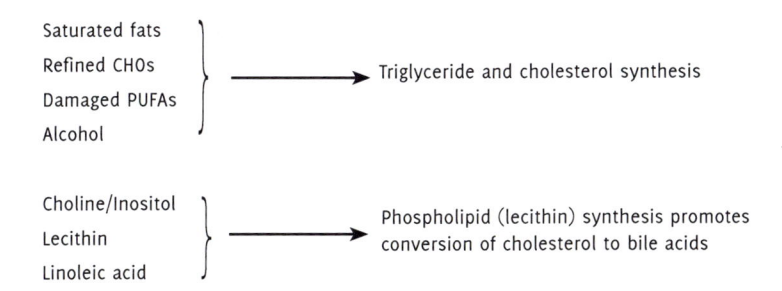

Saturated fats, Refined CHOs, Damaged PUFAs, Alcohol → Triglyceride and cholesterol synthesis

Choline/Inositol, Lecithin, Linoleic acid → Phospholipid (lecithin) synthesis promotes conversion of cholesterol to bile acids

By ensuring that your diet favours the production of lecithin over triglyceride and cholesterol, you will support the transport of fats and inhibit the build-up of fats both in the liver and in the circulation.

Free radicals are highly unstable compounds which attack polyunsaturated fats. The higher your PUFA intake, the greater the risk of damage. They act like sparks which come out of a fire burning holes in the carpet. Free radicals attack cell membranes setting up a chain reaction where one spark initiates a whole sequence of attack along the cell membrane and within the cell itself. The cell eventually loses its integrity and dies. The most important nutrients required by the liver for the deactivation of free radicals are vitamin E, selenium and glutathione. They are known as anti-oxidants and act like a fireguard protecting tissues from oxidation and rancidity.

# Cholesterol handling

Elevated cholesterol occurs when cholesterol production is greater than its elimination. This can arise as a consequence of a diet high in saturated fat and refined carbohydrates (which promotes cholesterol synthesis) or a failure by the liver to convert cholesterol to bile acids for excretion (see fig. 5.7 *The recyclable pool of bile acids*). It is usually a combination of both factors. Conversion of cholesterol to bile acids is dependent upon certain nutritional factors: lecithin (or its precursors - choline, linoleic acid), magnesium, vitamin C, B12, and B6. In addition to nutritional deficiencies, impairment in this conversion is caused by oral contraceptives and hormone replacement therapy (male and female sex hormones).

*High fat/high CHO diets induce nutrient deficiencies; both compromise the capacity for the conversion of cholesterol to bile acids.*

You will notice from table 5.2 *Saturated and unsaturated fatty acid levels in foods* that shellfish and cheese are high in cholesterol while low in lipotrophic factors. This is one of the reasons why shellfish is omitted from the diet. Most other natural foods, like eggs and liver, while high in cholesterol, also provide substantial amounts of choline and/or lecithin which offset any imbalance that may otherwise occur.

## 5 Liver cleansing

**Case history 5.2**

# Stephen was 46 years old and worried about his high cholesterol levels. Many of his relatives had died from heart attacks and so naturally he was concerned about his own health. Six months prior to our appointment he had attended a lecture on nutrition and decided to remove all animal protein and take plenty of fruit, salad and whole grains. However, he was disappointed to find that although his cholesterol level had fallen it was still in the upper level of normal.

I asked Stephen about his diet. He told me that would eat nothing but fruit until lunchtime when he would have a wholemeal salad sandwich. In the afternoon the sweet cravings began and he would eat a Danish pastry followed by several fruesli bars. He frequently suffered chocolate cravings and while he tried to keep his coffee consumption to a minimum he would still consume at least two cups daily. His main meal was around 9 pm when he returned home from work, which consisted of soup or rice and vegetables.

Stephen's past history revealed that he had had a tonsillectomy at 12 years and suffered with acne during his teens. He still suffers with skin irritations and athlete's foot which have been medically treated but continue to flare. Over the past few years Stephen had begun to experience breathing difficulties.

It was obvious from dietary factors alone that Stephen had a deep magnesium deficiency and that his current dietary changes had done nothing to redress this imbalance. In addition, Stephen's blood sugar levels were very unstable resulting in cravings during the afternoon. The body's response to stress and low blood sugar levels is to mobilise fats for energy which, over a period of time, leads to raised blood fats and liver congestion. The consumption of fruit in the morning aggravates this picture further as fruit does nothing to raise or stabilise blood sugar levels and in addition, fruit sugar (fructose) is preferentially metabolised toward triglyceride synthesis. Blood sugar levels are naturally low in the morning, and if liver stores of glucose are not replenished, the body will break itself down for energy and regeneration will not take place.

We introduced magnesium-rich foods (whole grains, nuts and legumes) into the diet. These foods not only provide a valuable source of protein (lacking in Stephen's present diet) but are also rich in fibre which is essential for liver cleansing and stimulating the conversion of cholesterol to bile acids for its elimination (see fig. 5.7 *The recyclable pool of bile acids*). Stephen started to eat three meals a day, never skipping breakfast, omitted dairy from the diet and incorporated two fish meals a week, preferably of the more oily fish like salmon or tuna. I recommended magnesium, vitamin C and the EPA marine lipids (omega 3 series) at that initial treatment.

Over the next five months Stephen adopted most of the dietary principles and gradually the liver began to detoxify. Liver congestion had been apparent since childhood and following the tonsillectomy his skin had taken the burden. Recurrent fungal infections indicate a highly acidic picture which favours the growth of pathogens, including fungus which may manifest on the skin and internal membranes. Stephen's skin irritations were associated with stress and took the form of an itchy, dry rash which was suppressed with various medical creams. However, Stephen's case had taken a new path, and more recently he was experiencing breathing difficulties. As the disease-state deepens, the link between liver congestion, the skin and lungs becomes increasingly apparent.

Cholesterol values in foods

After five months Stephen's cholesterol levels had fallen to 4.6 [reference range <5.5mmol/L], his rash and fungal infection had resolved and he had no breathing difficulties. During treatment I introduced selenium, vitamin E and phosphatidyl choline to stimulate liver cleansing and much later I recommended zinc to aid skin integrity. As an ongoing plan I suggested that Stephen should continue to take the EPA fish oils, maintain a high fibre diet, paying special attention to the magnesium-rich foods.

Table 5.1 Distribution of cholesterol and lipotrophic factors in foods   mg/100g

|  | Choline | Inositol | Lecithin | Cholesterol |
| --- | --- | --- | --- | --- |
| **Animal Sources** |  |  |  |  |
| Beef heart | 1,720 | 1,600 |  |  |
| Beef | 600 | 260 | 650 | 70 |
| Liver | 650 | 340 | 850 | 300 |
| Egg yolk | 1,700 |  |  | 1,500 |
| Whole egg |  |  | 350 | 550 |
| Fish |  |  | 580 | 70 |
| Oysters |  |  |  | 200 |
| Shrimp |  |  |  | 125 |
| Crab |  |  |  | 125 |
| Lobster |  |  |  | 200 |
| Milk | 30 |  |  |  |
| Cheese |  |  |  | 100 |
| Butter |  |  | 150 | 250 |
| **Vegetable sources** |  |  |  |  |
| Lecithin oil | 800 | 360 |  |  |
| Brewers yeast | 300 |  |  |  |
| Cereals | 240 | 320 | 750 |  |
| Wheat | 80 | 100 | 2,800 |  |
| Wheat germ | 505 | 690 |  |  |
| Nuts | 220 | 180 | 1,000 |  |
| Legumes | 120 | 160 | 1,200 |  |
| Green vegetables | 80 | 100 |  |  |
| Root vegetables | 40 |  |  |  |
| Fruits | 44 | 210 |  |  |
| Citrus fruits | 85 | 200 |  |  |
| Molasses |  | 180 |  |  |

**Table 5.2** Saturated and unsaturated fatty acid levels in foods - g/100g

| | Linoleic Acid | Saturated Fat |
|---|---|---|
| **Dairy/eggs** | | |
| Cheese | 0.7 | 18.9 |
| Milk | 0.08 | 2.04 |
| Yoghurt | 0.04 | 0.8 |
| Eggs | 1.2 | 3.4 |
| **Fats/Oils** | | |
| Butter | 1.8 | 50.4 |
| Lard | 10.0 | 39.3 |
| Coconut oil | 2.0 | 91.0 |
| Corn oil | 57.5 | 12.7 |
| Olive oil | 8.1 | 14.1 |
| Peanut oil | 30.8 | 17.2 |
| Safflower oil | 73.5 | 9.4 |
| Soybean oil | 34.7 | 14.6 |
| Sunflower oil | 71.0 | 12.0 |
| **Meat** | | |
| Beef | 0.9 | 16.4 |
| Lamb | 1.3 | 16.6 |
| Liver | 0.7 | 8.5 |
| Chicken | 1.4 | 1.7 |
| **Grains** | | |
| Barley | 0.4 | 0.1 |
| Buckwheat | 0.4 | 0.2 |
| Wheat | 0.4 | 0.2 |
| **Nuts/seeds** | | |
| Almonds | 9.7 | 4.2 |
| Brazils | 25.3 | 17.1 |
| Cashews | 7.2 | 9.1 |
| Coconut | 0.6 | 31.1 |
| Hazelnuts | 3.3 | 2.3 |
| Peanuts | 14.7 | 9.7 |
| Pecans | 17.6 | 6.3 |
| Pumpkin seeds | 19.5 | 8.4 |
| Sunflower seeds | 30.7 | 6.0 |
| Walnuts | 38.2 | 5.0 |

# Stimulating bile production

**The more toxins you release** from your cells the more critical the capacity by the liver to produce bile becomes. The production of bile is essential for the elimination of toxins. As we have discovered, bile is synthesised from cholesterol so a supply of nutrients to facilitate this process is required. Magnesium remains a key mineral in both the production and secretion of bile. Secretion is an active process where bile is pumped across the hepatic cell membrane into the bile ducts and, as with so many of our energy-dependent processes, magnesium is required for this energy transfer. Elevated levels of the natural sex hormones and also synthetic sex hormones, such as oestrogen, progesterone and testosterone, are known to affect bile salt metabolism adversely either by inhibiting the secretion of bile into the bile ducts or inhibiting its propulsion along the ducts and out of the liver.

Nutrient deficiencies, diets that promote triglyceride synthesis over phospholipid (lecithin) synthesis, abuse of alcohol and stimulants, the contraceptive pill, HRT and specific antibiotics all lead to liver congestion and a compromised bile production. Under these circumstances the elimination of toxins will be compromised.

Making good nutrient deficiencies and altering the diet by dramatically decreasing the fat content will start the process rolling. Liver fat will gradually be reduced, and liver cells and enzymes will regenerate returning full functionality to the liver. The liver is the only organ in the body that has such an immense regenerative capacity. It is possible, even after partial excision, for the liver to regenerate to its original size in a very short time, although you may not see a total restoration of function. Alcohol, for example, destroys the liver in such a way that regeneration is accompanied by scarring. It is the scar tissue that "hardens" the liver (cirrhosis) which then becomes a cause of disease itself.

## The role of fibre

In addition to these obvious dietary changes there is another fundamental way to increase bile production - by increasing the soluble fibre content of the diet. Soluble fibre is found in fruits as pectin, and as the viscous gums and mucilage found in cereal grains, nuts, seeds and legumes which is released on cooking. The gum in oats accounts for its mucilaginous texture when cooked, and the starchy thick water produced after cooking brown rice or barley is rich in soluble fibre. In addition, psyllium, linseeds and guar gum are all sources of soluble fibre.

*Sex hormone therapy, as in the contraceptive pill or HRT, may compromise bile salt metabolism and the secretion of bile.*

*Synthetic sex hormone therapy can exacerbate gall stone formation in a person who is predisposed.*

*Insoluble fibre promotes regular bowel movements but binds and depletes iron, calcium and zinc. It does not bind bile salts.*

Soluble fibre is not the same as the insoluble fibre found in wheat bran. Insoluble fibre is used to promote bowel regularity for lower intestinal health, whereas soluble fibre performs an entirely different role; it binds and carries bile salts and toxins via the colon to the outside. Under normal conditions, 95% of the bile salts (along with the toxins) are reabsorbed from the digestive tract and recycled by the liver, so hepatic synthesis contributes only 5% daily to the total bile acid pool. If you can reduce the recyclable pool by promoting its excretion, you will encourage an increased production of bile acids by the liver.

**Figure 5.7** The recyclable pool of bile acids

*Soluble fibre performs the role of binding bile salts in the gut, preventing their reabsorption.*

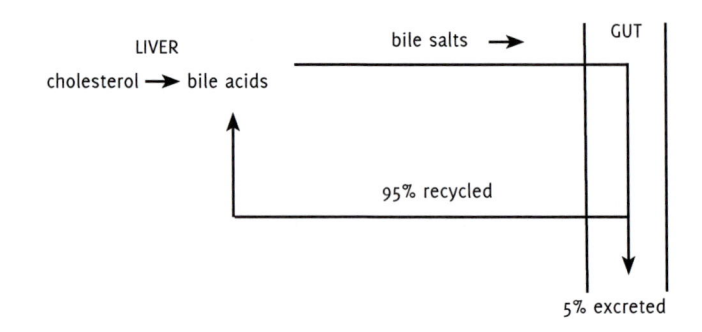

```
                                    bile salts →        GUT
      LIVER
  cholesterol → bile acids
                 ↑
                 |
                 |_____ 95% recycled _____
                                                    ↓
                                               5% excreted
```

Bile acids are produced from cholesterol and eliminated in the bile as bile salts. They participate in the digestion and absorption of fats and are reabsorbed in the small intestine. The body is economical in its recycling of bile acids, thus preserving the bile acid pool.

*If you wish to reduce your cholesterol and improve your detoxification, then ensure your diet is high in soluble fibre.*

The inclusion of significant quantities of soluble fibre (such as brown rice cooked by absorption method so that none of the cooking water is discarded) in the diet will reduce the recyclable pool of bile salts through its bile salt binding capacity. This has a two-fold effect: toxins, which tend to be re-absorbed along with the bile salts, are removed from the body more effectively, and the liver is stimulated to take up more cholesterol from the circulation for conversion to bile salts, thereby reducing cholesterol levels. Insoluble fibre does not have these protective effects and additionally can cause nutrient deficiencies of iron, calcium and zinc. Wheat bran should not be a dietary recommendation of choice because its negative effects can outweigh any positive ones. Other grains are more balanced in their ratio of soluble to non-soluble fibre. Oat bran, for example, can reduce cholesterol levels dramatically while increasing faecal bulk and accelerating transit time through the colon.

LDLs, or low density lipoproteins, are the specific blood fats which contain cholesterol. High levels of LDLs indicate high cholesterol and increased risk of heart disease. Bacterial action on soluble fibre in the colon releases inositol, which is absorbed and inhibits cholesterol synthesis in the liver and, by default, lowers total cholesterol levels.

**Figure 5.8** Effect of soluble fibre in the reduction of cholesterol

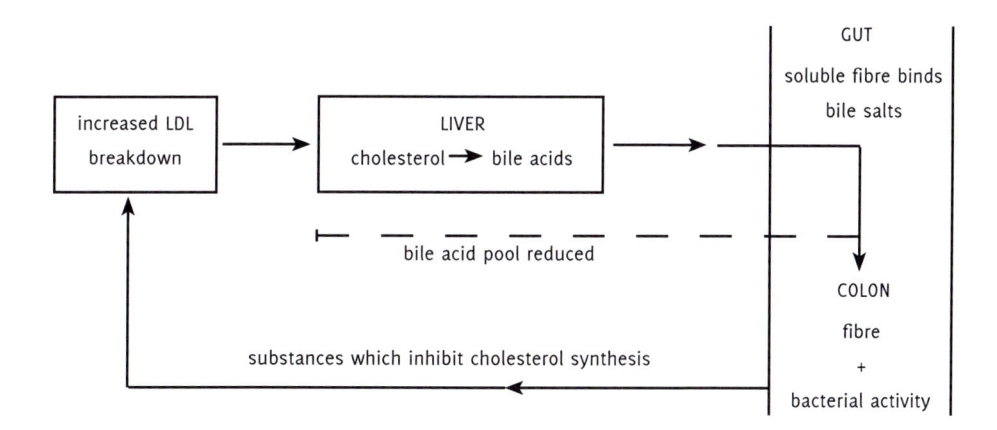

```
                                                            GUT
                                                      soluble fibre binds
                                                          bile salts
  ┌─────────────┐       ┌──────────────────┐
  │ increased LDL│──────▶│     LIVER        │─────────────┐
  │  breakdown   │       │cholesterol→bile acids│          │
  └─────────────┘       └──────────────────┘              │
         ▲                                                 │
         │  ─ ─ ─ ─ ─ ─ ─ ─ ─ ─ ─ ─ ─ ─ ─ ─ ─ ─ ─ ─ ─ ─ ─│
         │           bile acid pool reduced               │
         │                                                 ▼
         │                                               COLON
         │                                               fibre
         │                                                 +
         └───── substances which inhibit cholesterol synthesis ◀── bacterial activity
```

Soluble fibre has a dual action on lowering cholesterol. It binds bile salts, reducing the recyclable bile acid pool and therefore stimulates the liver to convert more cholesterol to bile acids. In addition, bacterial activity on fibre in the bowel releases inositol, which is absorbed and inhibits new cholesterol synthesis in the liver. As the liver is one of the main organs where cholesterol is produced, this will have an overall cholesterol-lowering effect.

The inclusion of foods high in soluble fibre is critical to the detoxification process, hence the use of brown rice as the staple carbohydrate. Potatoes do not perform the same function, nor are they as rich in minerals as cereal grains and true vegetables. They are a storage organ and predominantly provide starch, not fibre. You may eat them on the diet but they should not replace the brown rice. Choosing a carbohydrate that is rich in soluble fibre ensures the removal of a greater percentage of bile acids along with their toxins.

The traditional drink of lemon barley water (not the commercial brands) is an excellent remedy for the removal of toxins and for balancing the pH in the tissues to aid the healing process. The soluble fibre from cooking the barley is present in the liquid and the lemon juice has a strong alkalinising effect on tissue fluids. A patient of mine supplied this recipe for lemon barley.

### Recipe for lemon barley

½ cup of barley
1 litre of purified or distilled water
Juice of 6 lemons (or more to taste)
Honey to sweeten

Cover and simmer the barley in the water for around one hour. Strain and discard the grains. Add the lemon juice and honey.

**Case history 5.3**

# Jenny was 44 years old and came to see me with menstrual difficulties. She suffered from heavy bleeding and eighteen months ago had haemorrhaged so badly that she was hospitalised and given progesterone treatment to control the bleeding. Heavy menstrual bleeding is associated with oestrogen dominance which occurs with anovulatory cycles (failure of ovulation). Progesterone is normally produced by the ovarian follicle after ovulation. After her condition stabilised she came off the treatment but 6 months later the symptoms recurred. She went back on the hormone therapy but felt unwell. Jenny decided to try a naturopathic approach.

When I took her case history, Jenny told me that she had never suffered menstrual difficulties up until two years ago. At eighteen she had her first child and then took the contraceptive pill for fifteen years. After her second pregnancy at 34 years she became extremely ill suffering with gall stones and had her gall bladder removed. Jenny told me that although her second child was full-term she had felt unwell during the pregnancy and was hospitalised at the end of the pregnancy with vomiting. Her baby was physically under-developed at birth and now suffers asthma. Jenny went on to have a third baby with no complications but he later developed eczema.

I then asked Jenny about her past medical history. She told me that she had recurrent tonsillitis (treated with antibiotics) up until the age of 20 years when they were removed. She had also had her appendix removed. Jenny had no other medical problems other than extreme pre-menstrual tension with irritability, fatigue, fluid retention and chocolate cravings. Her family history revealed that her grandmother had suffered gall stones and later died of heart failure. There was also a history of eczema in the family.

This was such a clear case of liver congestion starting with the repeated tonsillitis, antibiotic abuse, culminating in gall bladder disease. For someone like Jenny, who has an inherited predisposition to gall stone formation, the contraceptive pill would not only exacerbate this condition but increase congestion in the liver and subsequently lead to lowered tissue vitality eventually affecting the heart. (Oestrogen and progesterone affect bile salt secretion by the liver cells and invariably cause centrilobular liver cell damage with the retention of bile in those who are genetically predisposed). If Jenny had continued to take the progesterone treatment offered then the liver would have been compromised further leading to the possible formation of stones in the bile ducts.

We started on the detoxification plan immediately and reduced fats to a minimum supplementing with the lipotrophic factors, choline and inositol, along with vitamin C. Within two months the premenstrual tension had disappeared and as the liver continued to reduce its toxic load her blood sugar levels stabilised and the menstrual cycle became regular. However, during the seventh month the heavy bleeding returned. At this stage I supplemented with manganese which has proved successful in addressing progesterone/oestrogen imbalance. By the following month Jenny's period was normal and we continued on manganese supplementation for the next four months. There was no recurrence of heavy bleeding and Jenny remains in good health.

# Additional help in releasing liver congestion

**The coffee enema** is a well-known practice in detoxification. There is no better stimulant for flushing bile than the coffee enema. This is due to a number of pharmacologically acting substances in the coffee. The combination of theobromine, theophylline and caffeine stimulates the relaxation of smooth muscles causing dilatation of blood vessels and bile ducts. Hence bile flow is increased. The volume of toxins conjugated in the bile is also increased. This is due to the activity of other substances in the coffee, the palmitates, which activate the enzyme system glutathione-S-transferase, seven-fold. This selenium-dependent enzyme system is responsible for neutralising free-radicals and grabbing toxins for conjugation as they are delivered to the bile for elimination. The mopping up of free-radicals effectively inhibits the formation of carcinogens, and therefore by stimulating this enzyme system, the coffee enema performs a liver-protective role.

*The coffee enema is liver-protective. It not only stimulates the neutralisation of free radicals, but also increases the speed of elimination of toxins from the liver.*

The coffee enema is unsurpassed in its capacity to stimulate the conjugation of toxins and the flushing of toxic bile and it has literally been a life saver to many hundreds of people undergoing extreme detoxification. For example, on the Gerson cancer therapy the specific prescription of diet, juicing and supplementation causes enormous releases of sodium, water and toxins from the cells, which would result in toxic poisoning of the system if not eliminated via the bile. Dr. Gerson recommended that these enemas be taken at four hourly intervals, and up to five daily, to relieve the toxic burden.

*Judicious use of the coffee enema may enable you to progress at a faster pace on your detoxification program.*

Cancer is a very deeply congested picture and thankfully we do not all have to adopt such extreme measures to maintain our health. However, I have found that the use of enemas in certain cases proves very beneficial in the detoxification process and has enabled some patients to progress at a faster rate than they would normally have been able to do so by alleviating their extreme symptoms of toxicity experienced even on a comparatively mild cleanse.

The effects of taking a coffee enema are not the same as drinking coffee. Rectal administration allows the coffee to be absorbed by the mesenteric vein and be taken directly to the liver via the portal vein. The enema is retained for 15 minutes during which time it stimulates the liver cells to cleanse the blood, removing toxins. The entire blood circulation will be recycled through the liver about five times during this period enabling a thorough cleanse. The dilatation of the bile ducts encourages a flushing of the toxic bile which enters the gastro-intestinal tract. The volume of fluid retained in the lower colon stimulates peristaltic activity which accelerates the propulsion of bile down the length of the intestine to the outside. It is important to remember that the enema is given for the stimulation of the liver and not for the function of the intestines. I would also add that the administration of enemas is not dangerous and has been practised safely for hundreds of years both in the home and in hospitals. Enemas do not stop normal bowel function, nor do they make the bowel lazy. The bowels will continue to operate independently even when taking the enemas and start functioning on their own after they are discontinued.

*The coffee enema is specifically used for liver cleansing - not bowel cleansing. It is both safe and non-habit forming. The bowel will function independently of the enema.*

## 5  Liver cleansing

*Rule of thumb: 750ml vegetable juice per coffee enema.*

### Method and preparation of the coffee enema

Coffee enemas are very easy to do yourself. I would recommend that if you are considering using them that you seek some advice from a professional. You must also ensure that the diet includes vegetable juices if you are using coffee enemas on a regular basis, as they will deplete minerals (caffeine is a diuretic) much like drinking coffee. As a rule of thumb I would recommend taking 3 vegetable juices (total volume, 750ml) per enema. You will need to purchase an enema kit (douche can kit) available at most pharmacies that stock surgical supplies. You will need a hook on the bathroom door so that you can hang the kit up and the coffee can then drain down through the tube and into the rectum.

#### Recipe:

¼ cup organic fine-ground medium roast coffee
1 litre distilled water
Boil for 3 mins, uncovered
Simmer for 15 mins, covered
Strain through fine mesh and make up to 1 litre
Serve luke-warm!

The coffee enema is prepared by putting 3 rounded tablespoons (1/4 cup) of medium roast, fine ground organic coffee into one litre of purified or distilled water. Bring to the boil for 3 minutes, uncovered. Then simmer, covered, on very low heat for 15-20 minutes. Cool and strain through a fine mesh and make up the quantity to 1 litre with purified/distilled water. Pour the filtered enema, lukewarm or body temperature, into the bucket/bag and hang on the door (make sure the nozzle end is closed). Lie on your right side and place the nozzle into the rectum releasing the flow. Inject and retain for 15 minutes (while remaining on your right side) before emptying the bowel as normal. You may make a concentrate for four enemas by taking 1 cup of coffee to 1 litre of water and preparing as above. For each enema, take 250ml of the concentrate and dilute with 750ml of water. You may store this in the refrigerator for up to 4 days.

## Herbal enemas

may be effective for those who are sensitive to caffeine. A tea may be made from the infusion of an equal mixture of Burdock Root, Clover Blossoms, Raspberry leaves, Yellow Dock Root and Chamomile flowers. Take two tablespoons of the mixture and pour 1 litre of boiling purified water over the herbs. Leave to infuse for 15 minutes before straining. Again, administer at body temperature.

### Method and preparation of the chamomile tea enema

The chamomile tea enema may be taken when the bowel is irritated, or if the coffee enema is stimulating too great a release of toxic bile from the liver resulting in vomiting or diarrhoea. The instructions are similar to the preparation of the coffee enema, but instead you take one cup of organic chamomile flowers and simmer, covered, in 1 litre of water for 15 minutes. Strain, and make the solution up to 1 litre. This will give you a concentrate for four enemas.

**The castor oil enema** is a strong purgative and liver stimulant. Dr. Gerson made use of the castor oil treatment (castor oil by mouth followed 4 hours later by the castor oil enema where castor oil is added to the normal coffee enema) for a stronger elimination. However, it is not normally necessary to go to such lengths (unless you have cancer) as the coffee enema will more than adequately fulfil the role for liver detoxification.

However, castor oil packs can be used as a gentle stimulant both for the liver and colon. They are particularly useful in conditions of colon toxicity, such as constipation, diverticulitis, colitis, irritable bowel syndrome and cancer. A toxic colon pollutes the rest of the body, especially the blood circulation, the lymph and the liver.

*The castor oil pack softens and disperses congestion and eases muscle tension, spasms, griping and colic.*

They assist the enemas as the absorption of castor oil through the skin into the lymph system softens and disperses congestion and tension and slowly helps release blockages in bowel pockets. If placed over the liver area (found on the right side of the body directly over and just under the lower rib cage) it will stimulate liver function and ease pain and spasms associated with gall stones.

The instructions for preparing the castor oil pack can be found on p85, chapter 4 *Vitality & healing*.

# Optimising liver detoxification pathways

*Toxins that are not removed from the system cause inflammation. Inflammation is the natural response by the body to toxins.*

**Finally, we come to the last aspect** of guaranteeing adequate liver detoxification. Under normal circumstances, if you ensure a diet rich in fruit and vegetables, high in fibre and low in saturated fat, while ensuring that you have plenty of the lipotrophic factors (including the co-factors B12, folic acid and B6) then your liver should function optimally both in the secretion of bile and the elimination of toxins via the bile.

However, with the rise in pollution we are finding that the liver often becomes overloaded with toxins which may saturate individual liver detoxification pathways and, as a consequence, may lead to a range of health problems. Quite simply, if the liver cannot detoxify and eliminate poisons they will create havoc both in the liver and throughout the body. Toxins are irritants, and irritants cause reactions; some toxins initiate immediate effects as experienced by those who are chemically sensitive, whilst others induce inflammatory reactions. Some inflammation is self-evident, such as immune reactions which occur in eczema, asthma, arthritis and autoimmune disease, whilst other inflammatory processes remain silent. The silent inflammation is the most insidious as it involves a self-perpetuating cycle whereby the immune cells unsuccessfully try to remove the irritant and in the process generate an uncontrolled production of free radicals which destroy the surrounding tissue. In an effort to patch up the damage healthy cells secrete growth factors that stimulate the formation of scar tissue.

*Scar tissue is just a symptom of the body healing itself.*

And it is here that the problem begins. The greater the oxidative damage (or the longer the self-perpetuating inflammatory cycle), the greater the replacement of healthy tissue by scar tissue - much like the darning of a sock where the darn has no function other than to fill the hole. This relentless oxidative toll "plasticises" the body: in the brain, amyloid plaque is formed (Alzheimer's Disease), in the arteries, atheromatous plaque; in the joints, an overgrowth of cartilage; and in insulin-resistance or diabetes (high glucose in the circulation) the superfluous glucose cross links with proteins along the blood vessel walls forming advanced glycosylation end products (AGEs). Eventually the small capillaries fur up inhibiting circulation causing capillary and nerve damage along with necrosis.

In health the liver should remove anything surplus to requirements or toxic to the body; this includes endogenous substances (made by the body itself, such as cholesterol, hormones, chemicals and the end products of digestion) and exogenous substances (environmental toxins such as heavy metals, agricultural and industrial chemicals, preservatives, dyes, colourings and medical drugs). If toxins remain in the body, then the immune system will attempt to remove

# The liver and chemical pollution

the toxins from wherever they are lodged, and if unsuccessful will eventually lead to a "named disease" or may act as a carcinogen causing cancer. So the implications of inadequate liver detoxification on our health are enormous.

## How much pollution am I subjected to on a daily basis?
Environmental toxins are ubiquitous, so no matter where you live you are going to have a degree of exposure from the air you breathe, the water you drink and the food you eat. In some areas we may have little control, but in others we can self-determine our degree of exposure through healthy choices and environmentally friendly practices. Let's identify some of the major culprits.

*Heavy metals exacerbate inflammation and oxidative damage.*

### Heavy metals
Did you know that in excess of 1,500 tonnes of mercury is belched into the atmosphere on an annual basis and that mercury is liberally applied as an anti-fungal agent on crops that are prone to mould such as strawberries, tomatoes and red capsicums? Heavy metals have an affinity for fatty tissue, such as the brain, nervous system and bone marrow. Here they block enzyme receptor sites, paralyse enzymes, switch on inflammation while simultaneously switching off the antioxidant enzymes responsible for mopping up free radicals, and putting out the fire of inflammation. You can appreciate how these heavy metals lead to widespread oxidative tissue destruction leaving in their wake uncontrolled scar tissue formation.

### Xeno-oestrogens
(environmental oestrogens) stem from a variety of sources both agricultural and industrial, including herbicides and pesticides. Our bodies accumulate these oestrogen mimics, which not only have a negative impact on the fertility of both sexes, but may also lead to abnormalities in foetal sexual development and programming. This may be a strong factor influencing fertility (or lack of) in both sexes, the feminisation of males, and may account for the surge in reproductive disorders in females (endometriosis and polycystic ovarian syndrome to name but two) along with the rise in the hormone-sensitive cancers such as breast, uterine, cervical, ovarian and prostate cancers.

Oestrogen mimics are not only derived from agricultural chemicals but also leach from plastics and polystyrene and are by-products from the bacterial activity on detergents and personal care products in water treatment plants. In addition, we have to contend with other endocrine-disrupting chemicals such as the family of phthalates, used to increase plastic flexibility and found in children's toys, vinyl, nail polish and used as a fixative for perfume, deodorants and hair sprays. These chemicals inhibit testosterone production affecting the sexual development of male children. Some pesticides and fungicides contain anti-androgenic compounds which also inhibit or block testosterone activity, whilst others alter the body's clearance of naturally produced hormones. One example is the pesticide Atrazine which converts testosterone to oestrogen and is responsible for the feminisation of frogs in the USA.

*There is no such thing as a "bad" gene. Genes are selected for their survival value. To focus exclusively on a gene as a major risk factor for breast cancer ignores other and more pressing causes.*

### PCBs and dioxins
are among the list of millions of chemicals in different combinations being added to the environment each year. Many of these chemicals are persistent (meaning that they are not biologically degradable) such as:

*Liver cleansing*

- the PCBs, which cause neurological impairment in children, thyroid problems, immune deficiency, infertility and cancer; and
- the dioxins, a by-product from the burning of fossil fuels and the herbicides 2,4-D and 2,4,5-T, which cause infertility, feminisation of males, immune deficiency and the lymphomas.

Food additives, such as preservatives and colourings, increase the daily toll on the liver. Any food that has a shelf life (will not go "off" for a prolonged period of time) will be packed full of chemical preservatives. When processed food is eaten at every meal (this includes bakery products, processed meats and fish, canned and frozen foods) this is akin to chronic exposure where the relentless toll on the liver will slowly undermine its functional and detoxification capacity over a prolonged period of time.

## How can I restore my detoxification capacity?

In restoring the capacity to detoxify there are three main considerations:

- Are we meeting our **nutrient requirements** for the liver to power its detoxification pathways?
- Are we placing an undue **toxic burden** on the liver that is greater than its capacity to detoxify and eliminate?
- Do we have **enzyme deficiencies** in our detoxification pathways due to genetic variance?

Making good nutritional deficiencies and reducing the toxic burden is the simplest approach and for many, this may be enough. But with the rise in toxic pollution, we are finding that those who are poor detoxifiers (due to genetic variance) are more at risk not only from chronic inflammatory disease including autoimmune disorders such as Alzheimer's, Parkinson's, motor neurone disease, arthritis, allergy and fibromylagia, but also mental disorders such as ADHD, autism, psychosis, depression and seizures. Fortunately, deficiencies in these pathways can be determined and alternative steps may be taken to support the pathways and reduce the toxic load.

In order to gain greater insight into the mechanism of toxicity and its impact on the whole body, I am going to take you through the steps of liver detoxification and help you understand the link between the various health conditions and specific deficiencies in the detoxification pathways.

# Traditional Chinese Medicine: a bird's eye view

## Liver Yin deficiency and the Hyperactive Yang

Traditional Chinese Medicine (TCM) has the best bird's eye view on this scenario. In TCM a liver disharmony invariably lies at the root of many chronic diseases including mental disease. When the liver is deficient (Liver Yin deficiency) and unable to fulfil its tasks, the burden is passed to the rest of the body leading to over-activity (predominance of Yang) in other organs and tissues as they try to deal with the excess load. Yin represents the integrity of the organ, and Yang, its function. When the Yin becomes deficient in one area, the Yang may become in excess in another area trying to compensate for this under-activity. On a simpler level, Yin represents Water, and Yang represents Fire. Yin keeps Yang in check, as Water keeps Fire in check. Therefore inflammation, allergy and hyperactive states may be viewed as a predominance of Yang due to deficient Yin. This situation of excess Fire usually has its origins in Liver Yin deficiency. The liver should protect other tissues and organs from toxin accumulation and disease. Eventually, the Yang may consume itself, commonly referred to as "burn-out", or the last flicker of flame (Yang) before the wood (Yin) is completely burned.

## Liver Yin deficiency and the mental state

In TCM, a Liver Yin deficiency affects the Heart. The Heart is said to "house the Mind". The Mind refers to the overall state and capacity of the brain, our memory, our ability to process thoughts, to concentrate, to relax or switch off and get a good night's sleep, and our mood. In Western terms, if the liver does not detoxify poisons they can accumulate in the brain exerting extremely toxic effects that negatively affect our mood and concentration. The effects of certain foods and food additives on the sensitive individual are well documented. Of interest are the **phenolic compounds** derived from specific foods and additives (colourings, preservatives) and produced as a by-product from bacterial and fungal overgrowth in the bowel, and the **opioids** from incompletely digested fragments of milk and wheat proteins. These toxins may directly interfere with the production and transmission of our brain chemicals (serotonin, dopamine and noradrenaline) leading to depression, insomnia, attention deficit disorder (ADHD), behavioural problems and in severe cases, autism. The brain has its own inbuilt detoxification mechanisms to neutralise these compounds (similar to some of the liver detoxification pathways) but problems arise when the toxic burden exceeds the detoxification capacity. Again, this may simply be due to nutritional deficiencies or toxin overload, which are relatively easy to address, but if due to genetic variance (involving deficiencies in the enzyme pathways) then the situation becomes more difficult to resolve and may require life long compliance to dietary programs and nutritional supplement regimes.

## 5  Liver cleansing

*Liver detoxification is a two-phase process. It is only when these two phases are out of step that problems may occur.*

### How does my liver detoxify?
The liver filters your entire blood volume every three minutes. Its job is to neutralise and eliminate all chemicals, both endogenous and exogenous. These toxins will either be eliminated via the kidneys or the bile. You can appreciate how a healthy bile flow is integral to the elimination of toxins.

When toxins enter the liver most will undergo a two-phase process. Phase 1 takes up the toxin and will either directly neutralise it (such as caffeine), make it water soluble for excretion by the kidneys, or modify it preparing it for entry into the Phase 2 pathways. Phase 1 activity generates free radicals and modified toxins (intermediate metabolites), both of which are highly reactive. In other words, Phase 1 metabolites can create much damage through oxidative stress in the liver unless they are inactivated or "mopped up". Having a plentiful supply of the antioxidant vitamins and minerals (A, C, E, the bioflavonoids, selenium and zinc) will neutralise the free radicals, while the speedy transfer of reactive metabolites to the Phase 2 enzyme pathways will ensure that any potentially damaging activity will be short-lived. Problems occur when Phase 1 produces more reactive metabolites than Phase 2 can detoxify. This may be due to an overactive Phase 1, an underactive Phase 2 or a combination of both.

**Figure 5.9**   The two phases of liver detoxification

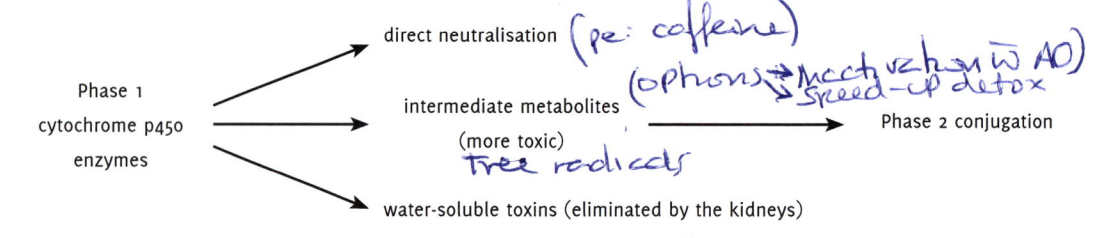

```
                              → direct neutralisation (re: caffeine)
Phase 1                                                (options → inactivation w AO)
cytochrome p450               → intermediate metabolites ─────────→ Phase 2 conjugation
enzymes                         (more toxic)            speed-up detox
                                 free radicals
                              → water-soluble toxins (eliminated by the kidneys)
```

It is important that Phase 2 keeps abreast of Phase 1. A slow Phase 2 may lead to the build-up of reactive metabolites which will cause liver damage.

# Phase 1 liver detoxification

## How can I tell if my Phase 1 is working adequately?

### The underactive Phase 1

**Caffeine, alcohol and nicotine** sensitivities are real giveaways that indicate deficiencies in this phase. Generally, it is easier to tell if your Phase 1 is under-active rather than over-active. So if you are sensitive to caffeine and not able to get to sleep for hours after the last cup of coffee, feeling the stimulating effects long after the event, or if the adrenal rush leaves you jittery and nervy for longer than you would expect – then you can safely assume deficiencies in the Phase 1 enzyme pathways that detoxify caffeine, adrenaline, alcohol and nicotine. You may have overworked these enzyme systems for a prolonged period of time leading to "burn-out" or exhaustion of these pathways.

*Increased sensitivity to caffeine, alcohol and nicotine can indicate a slow Phase 1 pathway.*

**Food sensitivities** to certain foods such as **cheese, nuts, chocolate, red wine** and **oranges** may also indicate deficiencies in the Phase 1 pathways. These foods contain "amines" which are derived from proteins and have strong pharmacological effects on the vascular system and brain, leading to symptoms such as high blood pressure, palpitations, headache and hyperactivity. Under normal circumstances these "amines" are oxidised and inactivated by the Phase 1 cytochromes, the mono-amine oxidase enzymes (MAOs) and diamine oxidases (DAOs). These enzymes are found at the gut wall, in the liver and brain. But with a deficiency of these enzymes or their suppression (due to medications such as the MAOIs - a group of drugs used in depression known as mono-amine oxidase inhibitors) these amines may not be deactivated and their influence will be felt in the nervous system and in the brain. See table 5.3 *Amines: Food sensitivities and symptoms*.

**Chemical sensitivities** to environmental toxins, such as **exhaust fumes, paints, strong odours** and **perfumes** may also be indicated in Phase 1 deficiencies although this is harder to deduce from symptoms alone. These toxins induce Phase 1 enzymes but if this pathway is unable to accommodate the onslaught they may pass unchanged back into the tissues to be detoxified by the p450 cytochromes found in other organs such as the brain, kidneys, adrenal glands, digestive tract, lungs and skin, and even the ovaries and testes. A new set of problems then arises. In tissues other than the liver, the p450 enzymes may convert toxins to their more reactive intermediate forms, but without mechanisms within the cell to complete the detoxification (no Phase 2), as would occur in the liver, we see a widespread rise in free radical activity which may lead to chronic inflammatory tissue changes.

*MCS: multiple chemical sensitivity occurs when the liver can no longer detoxify chemicals and they pass straight back into the circulation.*

*Liver cleansing*

### Table 5.3 Amines: Food sensitivities and symptoms

Foods high in the amino acids **phenylalanine, tyrosine** and **tryptophan** will give rise to the main amine culprits – **phenylethylamine, tyramine** and **tryptamine**. All these amines can cause vasoconstriction leading to **high blood pressure, migraine** and **asthma**; and may increase the synthesis of the excitory brain chemicals – noradrenaline, adrenaline and serotonin which can lead to **hyperactivity, mental disturbances** and **psychosis**. High levels of histamine are found in a wide variety of fermented and processed foods which can mimic allergic-type reactions.

| Food Culprits | Symptoms |
|---|---|
| **Tyramine** and **phenylethylamine** (derived from tyrosine and phenylalanine, respectively) are probably the greatest culprits.<br>Foods high in tyramine include: *cheese, red wine, sherry, beer, yeast, game, liver, salted fish, sour cream, cream, yoghurt, soy sauce, vanilla, chocolate* and *broad beans*. | The tyramine syndrome includes: **headache, pallor, nausea, restlessness, apprehension, sweating, palpitations, high blood pressure, fever, chest pains, hyperactivity** and **psychosis**. |
| **Tryptamine** and **serotonin** (derived from tryptophan). Foods high in tryptophan include: *bananas, kiwi fruit, pineapple* and *nuts*. | These amines may cause breathing difficulties/ **asthma**. They can also aggravate mental states **hyperactivity** and **psychoses** – hence the common sayings "going bananas" or "nutty" relating to the known aggravating effects of these foods. |
| **Histadine.** Foods high in histadine include: fermented foods and drinks, such as *alcohol, ripened mature cheese, processed meats, ferments, pickles, vinegar,* fish, particularly *mackerel, herring, tuna and shell fish,* and various fruits and vegetables such as *tomatoes, spinach, eggplant, avocado, strawberries, oranges, pineapple* and *kiwi fruit*. | Allergic type reactions may be caused by foods high in histadine which includes a range of symptoms: local and/or systemic **swelling, rashes, itching** and **mucus secretion** which can result in **hives, eczema, asthma** and, if severe, **anaphylactic shock**. |

*Extra-hepatic: tissues outside the liver*

Of particular interest are the aldehydes, a group of intermediate metabolites produced by Phase 1 reactions in the liver and in extra-hepatic tissues. Aldehydes on the loose make you feel drowsy and fatigued. So the greater the induction of Phase 1 enzymes by environmental fumes and toxins (including alcohol), the more aldehydes you will produce. In addition, environmental exposure to **formaldehyde gas** (given off by new soft furnishings and carpets) or increased endogenous production from an intestinal overgrowth of **Candida Albicans** in a compromised individual will increase the toxic toll and cause many of the symptoms of Multiple Chemical Sensitivity (MCS) and chronic fatigue syndrome (CFS). Eventually we may see depletion of the Phase 1 enzymes. Under these circumstances we need to reduce the toxic exposure on the whole body, not just the liver, and to seek ways to support the Phase 1 enzymes. (Table 5.4 *Supporting Phase 1 liver detoxification*.)

**Figure 5.10** Consequences of the under-active Phase 1

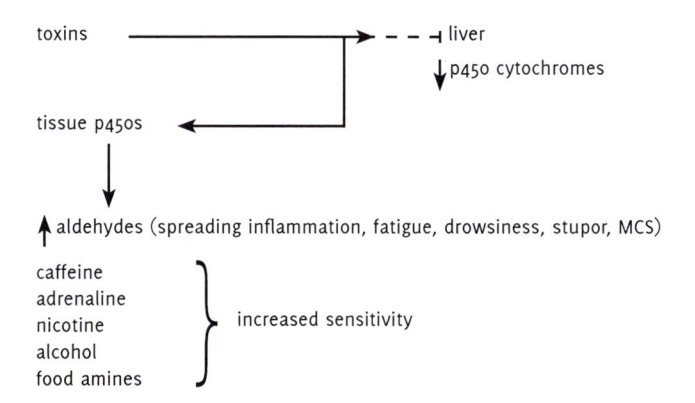

```
toxins ─────────────────► ─ ─ ┤ liver
                   │          ↓ p450 cytochromes
                   │
tissue p450s ◄─────┘
    │
    ▼
↑ aldehydes (spreading inflammation, fatigue, drowsiness, stupor, MCS)
  caffeine    ⎫
  adrenaline  ⎪
  nicotine    ⎬ increased sensitivity
  alcohol     ⎪
  food amines ⎭
```

Toxins that are not detoxified by the hepatic p450 cytochromes will pass back into the circulation to be detoxified by tissue p450 cytochromes. This leads to a range of symptoms due to the rise in intermediate metabolites, specifically the alcohols and aldehydes, and an increased sensitivity to stimulants, alcohol and food "amines".

## The overactive Phase 1

It may be difficult to determine Phase 1 overactivity from symptoms alone. An overactive Phase 1 is determined when the production of intermediate metabolites exceeds their rate of clearance by the Phase 2 pathways. People with this imbalance are known as pathological detoxifiers. Under these circumstances, the intermediate toxins are only slowly taken up and conjugated by the Phase 2 pathways. This means that the liver cells are exposed to a prolonged toxic onslaught of reactive chemicals and free radicals which poison the liver, cause inflammatory changes, scarring (cirrhosis), liver disease, and increase the susceptibility to liver cancer. If the toxins spill into the systemic circulation they may give rise to widespread inflammatory disease and chemical sensitivities.

*Pathological detoxifier: Phase 1 activity is increased relative to Phase 2 activity.*

**Figure 5.11** Consequences of the over-active Phase 1

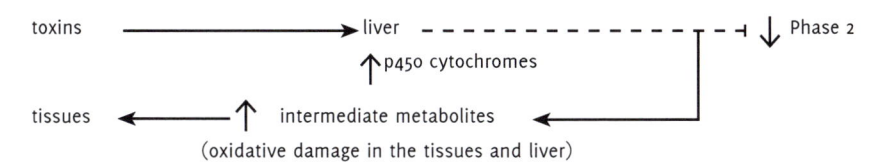

```
toxins ─────────────► liver ─ ─ ─ ─ ─ ─ ─ ─ ─ ─ ┬ ─ ┤ ↓ Phase 2
                     ↑ p450 cytochromes         │
                                                │
tissues ◄─── ↑ intermediate metabolites ◄───────┘
      (oxidative damage in the tissues and liver)
```

An overactive Phase 1 is relative to Phase 2 activity. If Phase 2 pathways are slow, then intermediate toxic metabolites will accumulate causing inflammatory damage in the liver. They may escape into the circulation giving rise to inflammatory disease and chemical sensitivities.

Obviously, under these circumstances our first priority is to reduce toxic exposure and ensure maximum supply of antioxidants to the liver in order to protect it from free radical damage. In addition to nutritional antioxidants, some herbs not only have very strong antioxidant properties, such as **St. Mary's thistle**, **green tea**, **turmeric** and **schizandra**, which protect the liver, but St. Mary's thistle and **globe artichoke** also stimulate the regeneration of liver cells.

Figure 5.12    Protecting the liver from an overactive Phase 1

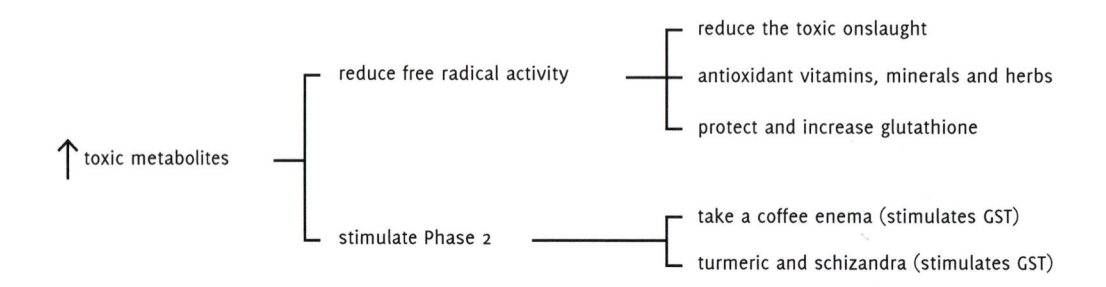

```
                                              ┌─ reduce the toxic onslaught
                     ┌─ reduce free radical ──┼─ antioxidant vitamins, minerals and herbs
                     │  activity              └─ protect and increase glutathione
↑ toxic metabolites ─┤
                     │                        ┌─ take a coffee enema (stimulates GST)
                     └─ stimulate Phase 2 ────┤
                                              └─ turmeric and schizandra (stimulates GST)
```

By ensuring the neutralisation and speedy passage of toxins via the Phase 2 pathways, the liver and extra-hepatic tissues are protected from oxidative stress. The Phase 2 glutathione pathway can be stimulated by the activation of the glutathione-S-transferase enzyme system (GST) which transfers toxins down this pathway.

Of additional concern with an over-active Phase 1 is the potential depletion of glutathione, a powerful antioxidant. Glutathione is known as a "suicide substrate" as it conjugates directly with some p450 reactive metabolites and may therefore be used up. As one of the main Phase 2 pathways is dependent on glutathione, it is imperative that these stores are maintained or this pathway will become slow. Glutathione can be protected by a plentiful supply of antioxidants, such as vitamin C, alpha lipoic acid and N-acetylcysteine, and the use of herbs, such as St. Mary's thistle and schizandra, all of which help to regenerate glutathione.

It is also possible to stimulate Phase 2 pathways. Of particular interest is the enzyme, glutathione-S-transferase (GST), which transfers the Phase 1 intermediate metabolites to the Phase 2 glutathione pathway. As we know, the coffee enema can stimulate this enzyme system sevenfold, and I know of no more effective method to reduce a toxic load than via this method. But it's important to remember that this mechanism is still dependent upon adequate supplies of glutathione; the coffee enema will not replenish these stores, but only facilitate the removal of toxins using this pathway. Restoration of the liver and its nutritional supplies remain of prime importance.

Two herbs worth mentioning in this context are turmeric and schizandra. Both stimulate GST activity, but will not work as quickly or effectively as the coffee enema. Interestingly, turmeric has the capacity to regulate Phase 1 and Phase 2 activity. It reduces Phase 1, while stimulating Phase 2 and therefore is a useful herb for pathological detoxifiers.

Finally, if you suspect that you may be a pathological detoxifier then it may be worthwhile investigating which of your Phase 2 pathways may be slow. In the next section, we shall discover some clues that may be indicators of deficient Phase 2 liver detoxification.

Table 5.4  Supporting Phase 1 liver detoxification

| Underactive | Overactive |
|---|---|
| *Symptoms:*<br>Environmental chemical sensitivities<br>Alcohol, caffeine and nicotine sensitivity<br>Increased sensitivity or toxic reactions to drugs<br>Food sensitivities and allergies<br>Poor stress tolerance<br>Drowsiness and fatigue after eating | *Symptoms:*<br>Environmental chemical sensitivities<br>Abnormal liver function tests<br>Liver damage; cirrhosis<br>Increased susceptibility to toxin-induced diseases such as cancer<br>Rapid clearance of caffeine, alcohol, nicotine |
| *To Do:*<br>**Reduce toxic exposure** to chemicals and foods that are known to aggravate your condition<br><br>**Ensure quality protein:** protein deficiency decreases Phase 1 activity, but equally, high protein may exhaust this pathway<br><br>Ensure nutrient co-factors for the Phase 1 enzymes: **B vitamins** (B3 [niacin] also accelerates clearance of aldehydes), **vitamin C and the bioflavonoids; Co-enzyme Q 10, magnesium, iron**<br><br>Increase your intake of the **cruciferous vegetables** (broccoli, cauliflower, sprouts, cabbage, bok choy); they supply indoles which enhance Phase 1 activity<br><br>The herbs **caraway, dill** and **citrus peel** are high in limonene which supports Phase 1 activity<br><br>The liver regenerating herbs may prove useful: **St. Mary's thistle, licorice, schizandra** and **globe artichoke**. Licorice and schizandra increase p450 activity.<br><br>Take plenty of **fresh organic vegetables and fruits** for their antioxidant value. Additional antioxidant minerals and vitamins may help quell inflammation in the rest of the body.<br><br>If you have a **toxic colon** or an overgrowth of **Candida** then take appropriate steps with prebiotic and probiotic formulae. Toxins from the bowel recirculate to the liver and increase its burden, and both aldehydes and phenolic compounds (by-products of fungal metabolism) will aggravate CFS, MCS and mental disorders.<br><br>Be aware that certain **drugs** such as the benzodiazepines, antihistamines and stomach-acid secretion blocking drugs will inhibit Phase 1 activity. **St. John's wort** will induce Phase 1 enzymes and therefore should not be taken in conjunction with medical drugs as it may accelerate the drug's clearance and thus reduce its effectiveness. | *To Do:*<br>**Reduce toxic exposure** to chemicals and foods<br><br>Protein intake: don't **exceed protein** requirements, ensuring quality rather than quantity. High protein increases Phase 1 activity and may eventually exhaust this pathway.<br><br>Replenish with **antioxidant nutrients** to curb free radical damage to liver cells: **selenium, magnesium, zinc, vitamins A, C** and **E, bioflavonoids** and **alpha lipoic acid**<br><br>Protect your **glutathione** levels (a major player as an antioxidant and in Phase 2 conjugation reactions): **St. Mary's thistle, schizandra** and **alpha lipoic acid** regenerate glutathione. N-acetylcysteine (NAC) renews the glutathione pool. The **cruciferous vegetables** are a good source of glutathione.<br><br>Regenerate and protect your liver: the herbs **green tea, schizandra, turmeric** and **St. Mary's thistle** protect against oxidation and free radical damage; St. Mary's Thistle and **globe artichoke** regenerate liver cells; and the catechins in green tea protect against carcinogens and liver cancer<br><br>**Grapefruit juice, turmeric, clove oil, quercetin, chilli peppers** and **calendula** suppress Phase 1 activity<br><br>Stimulate the Phase 2 uptake of toxins: **coffee enemas, schizandra** and **turmeric**, plus the **cruciferous vegetables** stimulate the enzyme, glutathione S transferase (GST), which transfers toxins for conjugation in the Phase 2 glutathionation pathway.<br><br>If in doubt about your liver clearance capacity then check your **Phase 2 pathways** with a FLDP – if clearance is defective, then intermediate metabolites will build up. |

# Phase 2 liver detoxification

*FDLP: functional liver detoxification profile; a laboratory test which measures the capacity of Phase 1 and Phase 2 pathways.*

**How can I tell if my Phase 2 is working adequately?** This is not so easy. If you are in doubt about your liver's capacity then I would recommend a functional liver detoxification profile (FLDP) to assess the capacity of these pathways. These tests are available through your health practitioner. It may be worth having this profile done as it can make a difference in understanding the cause of any problem and will facilitate the choice of appropriate treatments – as we shall see.

Liver detoxification works like a bus terminal. Between 50 and 100 buses (p450 cytochrome oxidase enzymes) are involved in taking toxins (passengers) via the Phase 1 route to a central terminal where they disembark and are transferred to one of the six major bus routes. During the transfer time, if the passengers have too long to wait they become unruly (reactive or intermediate metabolites). As they queue the toxins create havoc and oxidative damage. Unruly free radical damage can be controlled by the antioxidants, but it is essential that the toxins are quickly transferred onto the next waiting bus where they are bound (conjugated). If some of the bus services are slow or too full (saturated) then other buses will take these passengers which means that their regular passengers may have to wait. Once the toxins are on the bus they are inactivated, made water soluble and eliminated via the bile. The Phase 2 pathways are known as conjugating pathways where the toxin is bound to a specific neutralising compound.

*Saturation of a pathway will occur if the pathway is too slow or if overloaded with toxins.*

There are six main conjugation pathways, and as we have seen, some pathways (bus routes) can act as supplementary pathways for saturated or "slow" pathways. For example, the *glucuronidation* pathway can pick up the excess for the *sulphation* or *glycination* pathways when they are overtaxed.

**Figure 5.13** The six main conjugating pathways in Phase 2 liver detoxification

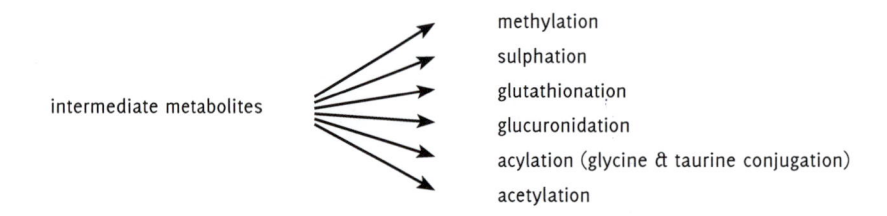

intermediate metabolites →
- methylation
- sulphation
- glutathionation
- glucuronidation
- acylation (glycine & taurine conjugation)
- acetylation

Intermediate metabolites from Phase 1 detoxification will be transferred via enzyme systems for conjugation by the Phase 2 pathways.

Problems may arise when there is either a shortage of conjugating substances, such as glutathione or sulphur, or deficiencies in the enzyme systems that transfer the reactive metabolites to their conjugating partners. There should be no shortage of the actual conjugating compounds used in each pathway as they are supplied by dietary protein and glucose. Methionine, an essential amino acid (found in cereal grains, animal protein and nuts), supplies methyl groups for *methylation*, sulphur for *sulphation* and cysteine as a building block for glutathione (*glutathionation*). The amino acids glutamic acid, glycine, taurine and cysteine, supply the *acylation* pathways (these are amino acid conjugation pathways which include glycine and taurine conjugation), while glucose supplies the *glucuronidation* pathway and acetic acid supplies the *acetylation* pathway. Provided that there are enough enzyme co-factors (all the B vitamins, but most importantly B5, B6, B12, folic acid and choline, plus the minerals magnesium, selenium and zinc) and that enzyme activity is not defective, then these pathways should run smoothly. Problems arise when the toxic load is greater than can be accommodated by Phase 2 pathways which leads to a depletion of the conjugating substances and a "bottleneck" of specific pathways.

*There is no shortage of nutrients required for liver detoxification on a balanced diet. Quality carbohydrate and protein will supply all the conjugating elements and required co-factors (minerals and vitamins).*

**Figure 5.14** Methionine and its related pathways

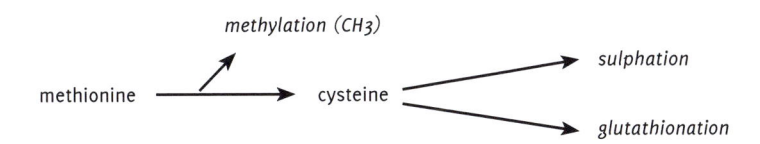

methionine → cysteine → *methylation (CH3)*, *sulphation*, *glutathionation*

Methionine is the parent compound for methylation, sulphation and glutathionation. Provided that there are sufficient vitamin and mineral co-factors present, by taking a diet that not only delivers adequate quality protein but also carries no toxic burden, then these liver detoxification pathways should suffer no deficit.

*Rich sources of methionine include most grains, animal protein and eggs.*

In a non-toxic world there would be little problem, but with increasing toxicity the first casualties are those who are genetically "slow" detoxifiers. These people are more likely to accumulate heavy metals, toxic metabolites (endogenous and exogenous) and xeno-oestrogens, and go on to experience a whole raft of symptoms from hormonal imbalance to neurological and inflammatory disease. For example, a high percentage of individuals suffering from motor neurone disease, Alzheimer's, Parkinson's, autism and ADHD are poor sulphators. This means that their sulphation pathway is slow which will increase their vulnerability to these specific diseases should they encounter increased toxin exposure, particularly from chemicals and heavy metals.

The following section covers the main indicators that may alert you to deficiencies in your Phase 2 pathways.

# Main indicators of Phase 2 deficiencies

## Fat intolerance and/or gall stones

*Bile acids emulsify dietary fat to aid its absorption, and emulsify cholesterol to prevent the formation of gall stones.*

If you have difficulty digesting fats then you may not be producing enough bile acids or your glycination or taurine conjugation pathways may be slow. Bile acids (formed from cholesterol) are conjugated with either glycine or taurine which makes them water soluble. They then enter the bile and act like detergent, emulsifying any cholesterol which prevents the formation of gall stones. The bile is stored in the gall bladder and is squirted into the small intestine in response to food leaving the stomach and entering the duodenum. In the small intestine the bile salts emulsify dietary fat which promotes its digestion and absorption.

**Fig 5.15** Conjugation of bile acids

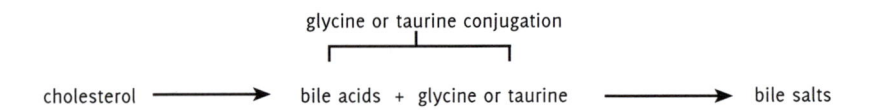

cholesterol ⟶ bile acids + glycine or taurine ⟶ bile salts

(glycine or taurine conjugation)

*Cholestasis: inhibition of bile flow often leading to jaundice*

Bile acids are conjugated with either glycine or taurine to form bile salts which have an important role in the emulsification of cholesterol and dietary fats. Any deficiencies in either the conversion of cholesterol to bile acids, or in their subsequent conjugation may result in gall stone formation and intolerance to dietary fats.

*Elevated oestrogen inhibits bile salt metabolism leading to cholestasis.*

A small percentage of women may experience problems in bile salt metabolism related to their oestrogen levels. Normally the liver clears oestrogen, but for some women this pathway is sluggish. The subsequent elevation of oestrogen, particularly during pregnancy and with endometriosis, places a stress on the liver and interferes with bile salt metabolism. This leads to cholestasis (inhibition of bile flow) and for some, the formation of gall stones and jaundice. The best way to alleviate this problem is to support your *methylation* pathway (S-adenosyl methionine [SAMe] is the supplement of choice here) which converts oestrogen to a safe form, and your *sulphation* pathway. Both the sulphation and *glucuronidation* pathways clear oestrogen.

## Figure 5.16  Elevated oestrogen and its effect on bile salt metabolism

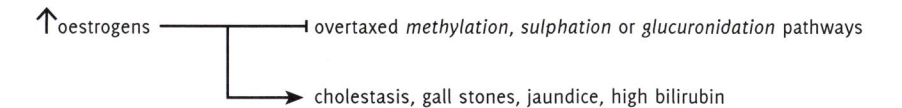

↑oestrogens ⟶ overtaxed *methylation*, *sulphation* or *glucuronidation* pathways

⟶ cholestasis, gall stones, jaundice, high bilirubin

Oestrogens are chemically altered via the methylation pathway and cleared by the sulphation and glucuronidation pathways. When these pathways are overtaxed, elevated oestrogens will inhibit bile salt metabolism leading to cholestasis, gall stone formation and jaundice.

## High homocysteine

If you have high cholesterol and high blood pressure, your GP may wish to assess your homocysteine levels. Homocysteine is an intermediate by-product of methionine metabolism, and elevated levels are a risk factor for heart disease. It contributes to inflammatory change in the arteries and is associated with vascular disease, stroke, heart attack and dementia. High homocysteine indicates deficiencies in either the *methylation* pathway or the *glutathionation* and *sulphation* pathways, all of which are relatively easy to correct. If you look at figure 5.17 The *methionine-homocysteine-cysteine pathway*, you will see that once methionine has donated its methyl group ($CH_3$) it becomes homocysteine.

*Elevated homocysteine contributes to inflammatory changes in the circulatory system.*

Homocysteine can be regenerated to methionine by the addition of a methyl group. This requires an adequate B12 and folic acid status. Other methyl donors include trimethlyglycine (TMG), dimethylglycine (DMG) and choline.

*Methylation: the addition of a methyl group ($CH_3$) to a compound.*

### Figure 5.17  The methionine-homocysteine-cysteine pathway

methionine —(Mg + ATP)→ SAMe —→ [$CH_3$ (methylation)] —→ homocysteine —(B6 (P5P), Mg)→ cysteine NAC

{ sulphate *Mo*, glutathione *Se*, metallothionein *Zn*, alpha lipoic acid, taurine }

homocysteine —(+$CH_3$)→ methionine

B12 (methylcobalamin), folate (5-MTHF)
choline, betaine (TMG), DMG

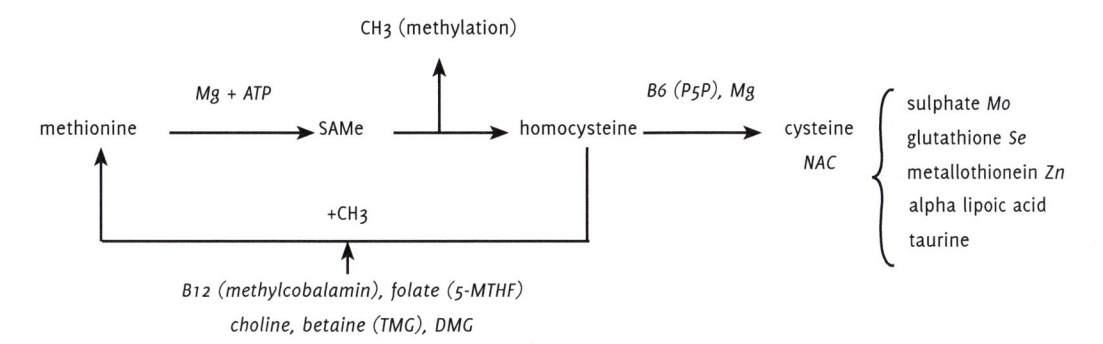

Methionine is converted to its active form, SAMe (S-adenosylmethionine), and once it has donated its methyl group to supply methylation pathways it becomes homocysteine. Homocysteine may either be regenerated to methionine (in the presence of adequate B12 and folate) or is channelled via the cysteine pathway to donate its thiol group for sulphation or for the synthesis of glutathione, taurine, alpha lipoic acid and metallothionein. The nutritional co-factors required are indicated in italics: P5P, pyridoxal-5-phosphate [activated B6]; TMG, trimethylglycine [betaine]; DMG, dimethylglycine; NAC, N-acetylcysteine; 5-MTHF, 5-methyltetrahydrofolate; Mo, molybdenum; Zn, zinc.

## 5 Liver cleansing

*Thiol: a compound containing a functional group composed of a sulphur and a hydrogen atom (-SH). It is an antioxidant and a chelator of heavy metals.*

Alternatively, homocysteine can continue its journey and be channelled through the sulphation and glutathionation pathways where it donates thiols (sulphur-containing groups), the active conjugating group. Other detoxification and free radical scavenging enzyme systems in the body, such as metallothionein and alpha lipoic acid, also require thiols. Thiol groups are important for the conjugation and detoxification of heavy metals and many harmful chemicals both in the liver and the tissues. These pathways require B6.

Making good vitamin B12, folate and B6 deficiencies will protect against elevated homocysteine levels. Folate in its active form is found in green leafy vegetables and legumes; B12 is found in animal foods (vegetarians and the elderly need to guard against B12 deficiency) and B6 is found in all whole foods, except dairy.

## High bilirubin

*Bilirubin is cleared by the glucuronidation pathway. Oestrogen also uses the glucuronication pathway.*

A chronically elevated unconjugated bilirubin may indicate that you have either Gilbert's syndrome, a common genetic condition where the enzyme responsible for conjugating bilirubin (a breakdown product of haemoglobin in red blood cells) via the *glucuronidation* pathway has a slow reaction rate, or that the glucuronidation pathway is being used as a supplementary pathway for the removal of toxins that would ordinarily be conjugated by the sulphation, methylation or glycination pathways. If the glucuronidation pathway becomes over-taxed, it may be unable to meet the conjugation demands for bilirubin and levels will rise. The simplest way of alleviating this problem is to support your sulphation, methylation and glycination pathways. High levels of circulating oestrogens can also throw a spanner in the works, as the glucuronidation pathway is an important pathway for the removal of oestrogens.

**Figure 5.18** Defects in bilirubin clearance via the glucuronidation pathway

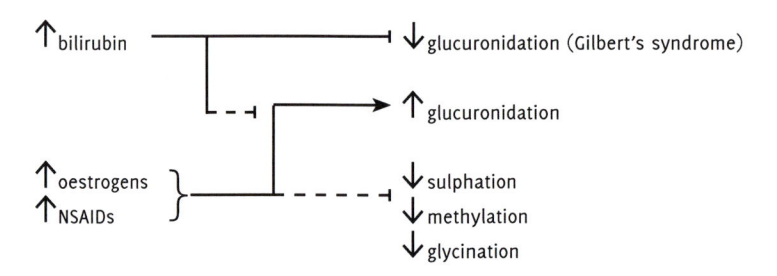

↑bilirubin ──────────── ↓glucuronidation (Gilbert's syndrome)
                        ↑glucuronidation
↑oestrogens }           ↓sulphation
↑NSAIDs     }           ↓methylation
                        ↓glycination

Elevated bilirubin occurs in both down-regulation of the pathway as seen in Gilbert's syndrome, and up-regulation of the pathway due to over compensation for slow or depleted sulphation, methylation or glycination pathways. Under these circumstances, elevated oestrogens or chronic use of NSAIDs (non-steroidal anti-inflammatory drugs) may saturate the glucuronidation pathway leading to elevated unconjugated bilirubin levels.

## Oestrogen dominance

Oestrogen dominance is associated with **endometriosis, fibroids, fibrocystic breasts, heavy or painful periods, erratic menstrual cycles, infertility, menstrual migraine/headaches** and **cancer**

*Oestrogen metabolism*

**of the reproductive organs.** Although the liver does not produce sex hormones, it controls their activity and their elimination. In Chinese medicine the liver is referred to as the "planner of cycles". The female cycle depends upon the rise and fall of oestrogen. It is the communication between the pituitary gland (located in the brain) and the ovaries, which governs the cycle. At the beginning of the cycle oestrogen levels are low; this signals the pituitary to release FSH (follicle stimulating hormone), which targets the ovaries and stimulates their production of oestrogen which, in turn, matures the ovum or egg. Oestrogen levels peak, and this signals a LH (luteinizing hormone) surge from the pituitary; the follicle releases the matured egg and starts to produce progesterone. From here on, oestrogen levels fall while progesterone rises. The cycle repeats itself when oestrogen levels fall sufficiently to stimulate the release of FSH by the pituitary gland.

*The liver detoxifies oestrogen. Inadequate clearance results in oestrogen dominance, a self-perpetuating cycle.*

**Figure 5.19** Oestrogen and its role in regulation of the female cycle

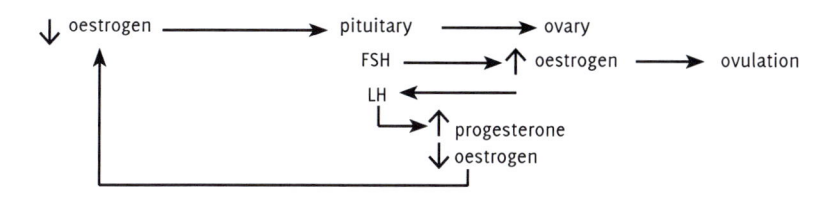

```
↓ oestrogen ──────→ pituitary ──────→ ovary
                      FSH ────────→ ↑ oestrogen ──────→ ovulation
                      LH  ←────────┐
                       └─→ ↑ progesterone
                           ↓ oestrogen
```

Low oestrogen at the beginning of the cycle exerts "positive feedback" at the pituitary which then releases FSH. FSH stimulates the ovarian follicle to produce oestrogen that matures the egg, which is subsequently released. When oestrogen levels peak, LH (luteinizing hormone) is released from the pituitary which stimulates the follicle to produce progesterone. Oestrogen levels continue to fall until positive feedback once again stimulates the pituitary to initiate the next cycle.

You can imagine that if oestrogen levels remain slightly elevated (through non-clearance) then the pituitary effectively becomes "switched off". It is the rise and fall of oestrogen that stimulates the release of the pituitary hormones, FSH and LH, and it is these hormones that control ovulation and hence fertility. Additionally, if ovulation fails to occur, progesterone is not produced and we see a self-perpetuating state of oestrogen dominance. The contraceptive pill works by maintaining a steady hormone state which inhibits the natural rise and fall of oestrogen and hence ovulation.

*The pill interferes with the rise and fall of oestrogen and thus inhibits ovulation.*

Oestrogen dominance essentially describes a state where oestrogen is dominant to progesterone, or unopposed by progesterone, and unfortunately this invariably becomes a self-perpetuating cycle. It occurs in the following conditions:

- Over-production of oestrogen by the body, as in endometriosis and polycystic ovarian syndrome;
- Exposure to xeno-oestrogens (environmental oestrogen-mimics in our food and water);
- During peri-menopause (the pre-menopausal stage) marked by increasing anovulatory cycles;
- Infertility due to anovulatory cycles; or
- Inadequate oestrogen clearance by the liver.

*Oestrogen dominance merely implies an excess of oestrogen relative to progesterone.*

## 5  Liver cleansing

*Iodine decreases oestrogen receptor sensitivity and therefore protects against breast cancer, fibrocystic breast disease and may improve ovulation rates in polycystic ovarian syndrome (PCOS).*

As a consequence of oestrogen dominance, hormone-sensitive tissues may become over-exposed to oestrogen. Not only is the fertility cycle upset leading to infertility, but excessive stimulation of oestrogen responsive tissues (cervix, uterus, ovaries, breasts and in men, the prostate gland) may lead to the overgrowth of tissue (**fibrocystic breast disease, fibroids, endometrial hyperplasia, genital warts, prostatic hypertrophy**) and **cancer.** It is worth mentioning that many of the xeno-oestrogens cause a rise in "bad" oestrogens that are strongly proliferative or carcinogenic.

Under these circumstances oestrogen metabolism and clearance via the liver and colon becomes the main consideration in treatment and we can now begin to understand why, in TCM, the liver is the planner of cycles. Application of progesterone merely further taxes the liver and will not rectify the problem.

In hepatic clearance of oestrogen there are two aspects to consider:
- liver conversion of "strong" oestrogens, which have proliferative activity and are implicated in cancer, to their weaker and more protective forms; and
- successful elimination via the liver and colon.

### Oestrogen metabolism via the liver

*Cruciferous vegetables (Brassica family) include arugula, broccoli, cauliflower, brussels sprouts, cabbage, watercress, bok choy, radish, turnip, kohlrabi and kale. They contain sulphur groups and indoles – both are anti-cancer nutrients.*

Phase 1 pathways convert oestrogens to either a *weakly* oestrogenic (good form) or strongly oestrogenic form (bad form). High protein diets tend to promote the metabolism of oestrogens to their strongly active form (16-OH oestrogens), while diets high in cruciferous vegetables (indoles) support conversion to the weaker form (2-OH oestrogens) which is more protective against cancer. Nutritional supplements containing indole 3 carbinole (I3C) or diindolylmethane (DIM), a bioavailable form of the indole phytonutrient, will not only promote the 2-OH pathway but also reduce activity at oestrogenic receptor sites. The *methylation* pathway will further convert oestrogens to either 2-methoxy-oestrone (anti-carcinogenic) or 4-methoxy-oestrone. (See figure 5.20 *Oestrogen metabolism and clearance.*)

In order to protect against the formation of the more dangerous 4-OH and 16-OH oestrogen metabolites you need to ensure that you support the Phase 1, 2-OH pathway and the Phase 2 methylation pathway for conversion to the anti-cancer oestrogen metabolites. Oestrogens are ultimately detoxified and eliminated via the *glucuronidation* and *sulphation* pathways. The glucuronidation pathway is the most important liver detoxification pathway for oestrogen where oestrogen conjugates with glucuronic acid, and clearance via this pathway will significantly reduce serum oestradiol levels. You may recall that this pathway is also used for the clearance of bilirubin, and therefore high bilirubin levels can indicate defects in oestrogen clearance, particularly when there are symptoms of oestrogen dominance.

### Oestrogen elimination via the colon

*Constipation is a risk factor in oestrogen dominance.*

However, liver detoxification is only half the story; oestrogen may be reabsorbed from the colon back into the systemic circulation. Successful elimination is dependent upon a short transit time through the colon. Constipation and/or diets high in animal protein and fat that lack fibre may predispose or exacerbate oestrogen dominance because the longer the food hangs around in the colon, the greater the activity of intestinal bacteria that produce the enzyme beta-glucuronidase.

This enzyme cleaves the oestrogen-glucuronide bond and liberates free oestrogen back into the body! Vegetarian diets that are high in fibre are generally considered protective against oestrogen dominance as they accelerate the transit time and therefore tend to support effective elimination of the glucuronide-oestrogen conjugates. Calcium D Glucarate, found in oranges, grapefruit and broccoli, is a potent inhibitor of beta-glucuronidase and helps to ensure oestrogen elimination. It can be taken as a supplement, and studies using this product indicate a 70% reduction in oestrogen-mediated abnormal cell proliferation.

*Nutrients which assist oestrogen metabolism and elimination include Ca D Glucarate, I3C and folinic acid.*

**Figure 5.20** Oestrogen metabolism and clearance

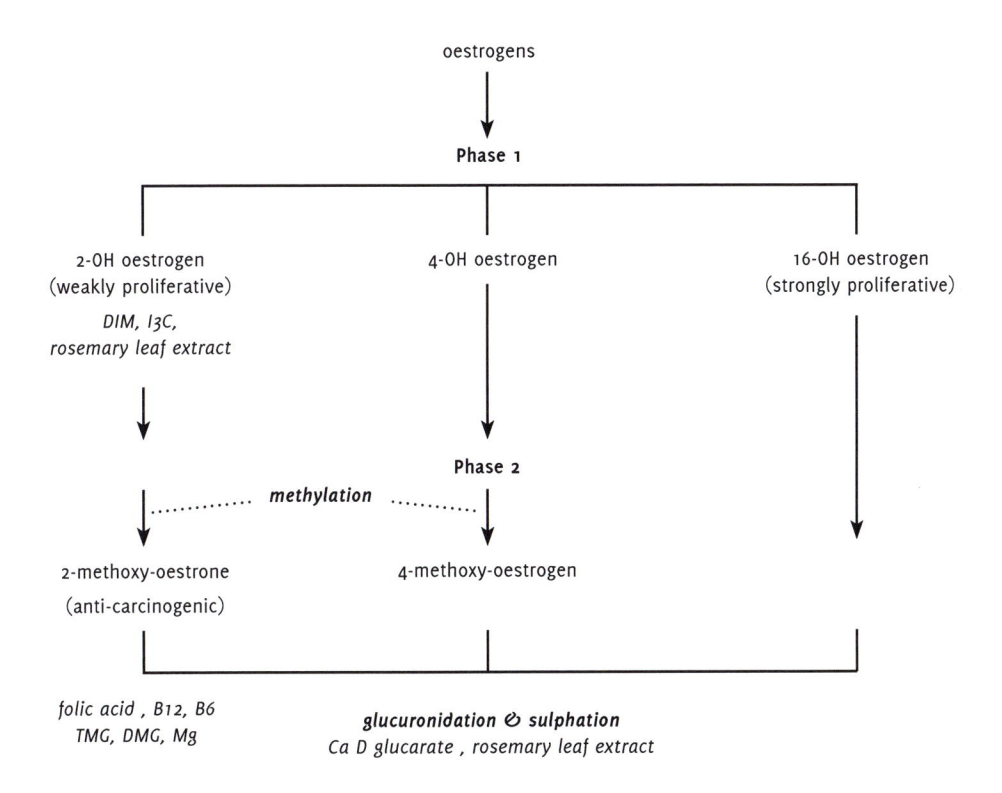

```
                    oestrogens
                        │
                        ▼
                     Phase 1
    ┌───────────────────┼───────────────────┐
    │                   │                   │
2-OH oestrogen      4-OH oestrogen      16-OH oestrogen
(weakly proliferative)                  (strongly proliferative)

DIM, I3C,
rosemary leaf extract
    │                   │                   │
    │                   ▼                   │
    │                Phase 2                │
    │....methylation....│                   │
    ▼                   ▼                   │
2-methoxy-oestrone   4-methoxy-oestrogen    │
(anti-carcinogenic)                         │
    └───────────────────┴───────────────────┘

folic acid, B12, B6        glucuronidation & sulphation
TMG, DMG, Mg               Ca D glucarate, rosemary leaf extract
```

Strongly proliferative forms of oestrogen are promoted by high protein diets, while weakly proliferative forms are promoted by diets high in vegetables, particularly the cruciferous group. Methylation further converts these oestrogen metabolites to an anti-carcinogenic form (2-methoxy-oestrone). Oestrogens are finally eliminated via the glucuronidation and sulphation pathways. A short transit time via the colon supports effective elimination.

# Food sensitivities and allergies

A person can develop sensitivities to many naturally occurring compounds found in foods. We have seen how the enzymes in the gut and the liver (the MAOs) quickly detoxify the "amines" during Phase 1 detoxification, but most of our food sensitivities and allergies implicate deficiencies in the Phase 2 pathways, specifically the *methylation* and *sulphation* pathways.

## Food allergies

*Mast cells may become sensitised to a range of substances including chemicals and bacterial toxins, and also extremes of temperature.*

Technically speaking, an allergic response involves an immune reaction where specific antibodies (immunoglobulins [Ig]) are activated in response to the allergen. The two main classes of immunoglobulins associated with food intolerance are IgG and IgE. If IgE is triggered by contact, ingestion or inhalation of the allergen, we see a release of endogenous histamine from mast cells leading to hypersensitive reactions such as increased secretion from the mucous membranes (**conjunctivitis, rhinitis, sinusitis** and **asthma**) and a range of itchy skin conditions, such as **hives** and **eczema**. Many foods are capable of triggering an IgE response but the food groups to watch for are dairy, wheat, nuts, soy and eggs. To complicate things, in an allergic individual these mast cells are capable of spontaneously releasing histamine to other triggers such as heat (as in exercise), sudden cold, alcohol, paints, fumes, colourings, additives, salicylate and phenol-rich foods, and bacterial and plant toxins.

*Immune tolerance (negative immune response) to ingested foods is programmed at the gut. It is believed that altered conditions in the gut (infection, inflammation or a state of dysbiosis) excite positive immune responses which lead to a state of allergy.*

Histamine is detoxified by *methylation* so it is important to support this pathway by ensuring adequate dietary B12 and folate and by reducing your exposure to known triggers. Although you may not be able to alter your genetic predisposition for hypersensitivity, if you have developed allergies to specific substances after childhood, it may be possible to redress the situation. By supporting your general immunity, improving your digestive capacity and ensuring that your liver detoxification pathways remain unburdened, then the hypersensitive branch of the immune system may become less active and less irritated. It is not uncommon for allergic reactions to surface following periods of general stress, gastro-intestinal infection, antibiotic medication or exposure to infectious illness, all of which weaken the digestion and stress the immune system. In fact, you may find that these types of events precede general food sensitivity states where it can be almost impossible to determine which food or substance is doing what and why.

## Food sensitivities

Substances that act as irritants can be divided into three groups:

*Consider three factors in food sensitivity: integrity of the gut/digestion, integrity of the liver and the degree of immune sensitivity.*

- Synthetic chemical additives including colourings (tartrazine), preservatives (benzoates, sulphites and sorbates), nitrates and glutamates;
- Naturally-occurring food chemicals such as the phenols and the chemically-related salicylates; and
- Partially digested proteins and sugars which escape into the system from the digestive tract.

In an allergic individual any of these substances can also trigger allergic reactions. Sensitivity to a food or additive depends on how well you digest your food and how competently your liver can detoxify the by-products. If you develop any sensitivity then you need to address the possible causes in order to reverse the problem.

- **Synthetic chemicals**

    Most common colourings and preservatives are detoxified via the *sulphation* (tartrazine) and the *glycination* (benzoates) pathways. So, quite simply, if these pathways are slow or saturated, then these toxins will create havoc in the system. Symptoms may mimic allergic reactions or give rise to gut-related problems such as **cramping** and **irritable bowel**, and cause **headaches, mental** and **behavioural disturbances** (ADHD), **dizziness**, or act as a nervous system stimulant leading to **anxiety, sweating** and **palpitations**.

- *Naturally-occurring chemicals in foods: the phenols and salicylates*
Phenolic and the chemically-related salicylate compounds usually occur together in fruits, vegetables, nuts, flavourings and spices. They are strongly anti-oxidant, protecting the plant from injury, and include the bioflavonoids found in the brightly coloured orange, yellow, red and purple fruits, vegetables and spices. However, if you can tolerate aspirin, which is a salicylate, then you are not likely to be intolerant to salicylates in foods unless, as I mentioned earlier, your system is already over-irritated by hypersensitive IgE reactions - then salicylates could compound this further.

Both phenols and salicylates can have a negative effect on brain function. They are structurally similar to our brain chemicals, dopamine and noradrenaline, and can act as false neurotransmitters. By occupying receptor sites on nerve terminals in the brain they can prevent our normal signals from getting through. In short, they neutralise the signal. This is why foods that contain these compounds can lead to a range of **behavioural disorders** including **ADHD, poor concentration, autism, psychosis** and **depression**.

*Hyperactive children often react badly to salicylate and phenolic compounds in foods as they may disrupt brain signalling.*

Both phenols and salicylates should be digested in the gut. Under normal conditions, enzymes break down the plant wall and start the digestion of the phenols and salicylates. If the digestion is inefficient, these compounds enter the system, but provided they can be detoxified through the *sulphation* or the supplementary *glucuronidation* pathways, then no problems will arise. (These fruits and vegetables may not prove so problematic when cooked as the cell wall is broken down during cooking.) But when more phenols are absorbed than these pathways can cope with, we start to see reactions. If you are a genetically "slow" sulphator or if this pathway is saturated, then phenols will enter the systemic circulation and affect the brain. The brain has its own sulphation detoxification system for phenols (PST: phenol sulphotransferase pathway) but if these pathways are also diminished or saturated, then these compounds will accumulate and inhibit the normal transmission of signals.

*Digestive enzymes that contain cellulase or xylanase may help in the digestion and inactivation of phenols and salicylates.*

*Check for dysbiosis as this can be a significant source of phenols.*

Fungal and bacterial overgrowth in the intestine (dysbiosis) can compound this problem. Yeasts and bacteria, such as candida and clostridia, produce phenolic metabolites that increase the phenolic load. Invariably, children with salicylate or phenol sensitivity may fail to respond to dietary manipulation until any fungal or bacterial overgrowth is resolved.

*Inorganic iodine is a powerful anti-microbial agent. Iodine deficiency may exacerbate dysbiosis.*

- *Products of partial digestion: exorphins from milk and wheat proteins*
Casomorphin and gliadorphin are peptides derived from milk and wheat protein respectively. They are alike in structure, each containing a similar sequence of seven amino acids which may resist digestion in certain individuals. If they are absorbed they may attach to opiate receptors in the brain and affect speech and auditory integration

which affects responsiveness and communication skills. If you suspect an intolerance to these exorphins, it can be confirmed by detection of these peptides in the urine, while a blood test can reveal the presence of anti-gliadin and anti-casein antibodies.

## Other sensitivities

*The cells of the gut wall complete the digestion of foods. A damaged mucosa leads to digestive impairment.*

Nowadays, we have the capacity for testing an extensive range of food sensitivities. By the time one experiences a wide variety of food intolerances it is safe to say that the digestion is usually very impaired and that we may have a "leaky gut". Although the digestive juices from the stomach, liver and pancreas play a fundamental role in the enzymatic splitting of food into smaller components, it is the enzymes that are tethered to the cells lining the small intestine which complete digestion. This is where the disaccharidase enzymes, maltase, sucrase and lactase, split the disaccharides (two sugar units), maltose, sucrose and lactose respectively, into single sugars, and the dipeptidases split dipeptides (two amino acid units) into single amino acids.

*A "leaky gut" arises as a consequence of local inflammation which may be triggered by infection, food allergies or dysbiosis.*

When sugars and proteins are not fully digested they may trigger a local allergic reaction and a release of histamine which makes the small intestine permeable (leaky) to these partially digested foods. Once entering the systemic circulation they may evoke allergic or immune reactions in the allergic individual. Alternatively, these undigested foods may pass to the large intestine and undergo either fermentation or putrefaction by the bowel flora. Putrefaction of proteins produces indoles as a by-product, while sugars ferment producing strong acids. The fermentation process gives rise to **bloating** and **gas**, while the acids can be extremely irritating to the wall of the colon and lead to **inflammation**, **mucus colitis**, **irritable bowel syndrome**, **diarrhoea**, **constipation** and **griping spasms**. Unlike the fermentation of sugars, the fermentation of dietary fibre by bacterial cellulase produces the by-products glutamine and short chain fatty acids (SCFAs), both of which fuel the growth of colonocytes (cells lining the colonic wall) which promote a healthy bowel wall that ensures no end products of digestion can leak back into the system, and also protect the bowel against cancerous change.

In a state of **dysbiosis,** pathogenic organisms feed off undigested matter and produce a variety of metabolites, including phenolic compounds, aldehydes, alcohols and acids. They do not provide fuel for the colonocytes, and the colonic wall loses its integrity and may become leaky.

*In Traditional Chinese Medicine, fibromyalgia is a condition of "damp-heat" – toxins settling in the muscles causing inflammation and pain.*

Yeasts produce tartaric acid, a muscle toxin which may be implicated in **fibromyalgia**. Arabitol is another metabolic by-product of yeast which is converted to arabinose (a pentose sugar) by the liver before undergoing further metabolism. However, if this pathway is defective then arabinose enters the system and may cause widespread inflammation through its capacity to bind and cross link proteins, significantly altering the shape and function of both structural proteins and enzymes. Any subsequent effort by the immune system to remove the offending sugars may lead to a chronic state of inflammation. Additionally, there is the risk of triggering **autoimmune reactions** to the modified cross-linked cellular proteins.

In protein maldigestion, partially digested proteins that enter the system may elicit an immune response directly where antibody-antigen complexes are formed which lodge in the tissues and become a foci for chronic inflammation.

**Figure 5.21** The implications of gut dysbiosis

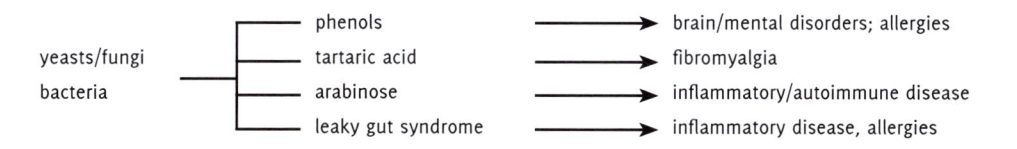

```
                      ┌── phenols            ──→  brain/mental disorders; allergies
yeasts/fungi          ├── tartaric acid      ──→  fibromyalgia
bacteria     ─────────┤── arabinose          ──→  inflammatory/autoimmune disease
                      └── leaky gut syndrome ──→  inflammatory disease, allergies
```

Dysbiosis leads to poor integrity of the bowel wall and a leaky gut. Undigested proteins and sugars may escape into the system causing a variety of inflammatory conditions. Additionally, yeast and fungal metabolites may enter the systemic circulation and exacerbate mental conditions, allergies and inflammation.

Both immune complexes and pentose sugars (specifically fructose and arabinose) are invariably implicated in inflammatory disease such as **eczema, psoriasis, arthritis, Alzheimer's, autoimmune disease (rheumatoid arthritis, systemic lupus erythematosus [SLE], thyroiditis, insulin-dependent diabetes mellitus [IDDM])**. We often see remission of symptoms when the offending foods are eliminated from the diet.

*Diabetics should steer clear of sweeteners that contain fructose, such as modified corn starch, as these sugars are notorious for embedding in the capillary walls. The nutritional supplement lipoic acid will block the embedding of these sugars and is a supplement of choice in diabetes.*

Gluten intolerance is also becoming more commonplace. Gluten is found in wheat, oats, rye and barley and sensitivity occurs when IgA activity (the major immunoglobulin of the gut) is impaired. The gliadin fraction of the gluten molecule is toxic for all of us and unless bound and destroyed by IgA will lead to inflammatory changes and destruction of the lining of the small intestine thereby reducing its digestive and absorptive capacity. This will give rise to **coeliac disease, diarrhoea, weight loss** and **nutritional deficiencies**.

## Tips for addressing food sensitivities

- Remove the known offending foods;
- Support your digestion using digestive enzymes that break down proteins (dipeptidases), sugars (disaccharidases) and the plant cell wall (cellulase, xylanase), and fats (lipases);
- Treat pathogenic bacterial and fungal overgrowth (ensure iodine sufficiency);
- Restore the beneficial bacteria with probiotics (the lactobacillus and bifidobacterium species) as these colonies not only keep pathogenic strains in check but also support the maintenance of a healthy bowel lining, protecting against leaky gut syndrome;
- Take prebiotics (glutamine, arabinogalactans, fructo-oligosaccharides [FOS], galacto-oligosaccharides [GOS]) which not only encourage repopulation of healthy bowel flora, but provide fuel to support the maintenance of a healthy bowel lining; and
- Support your sulphation and glucuronidation pathways by reducing their burden and making good any suspected nutritional deficiencies required for this pathway. (See figure 5.22 *Supporting your sulphation pathways*.)

**Figure 5.22** Supporting your sulphation pathways

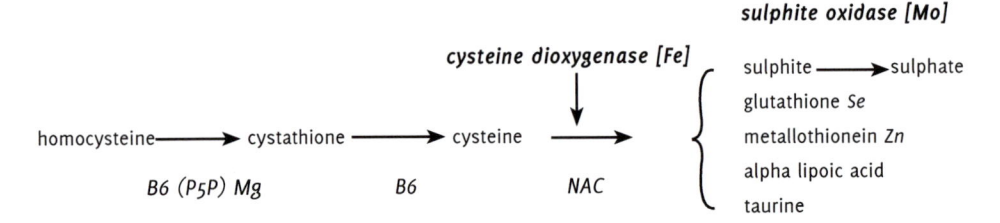

```
                                                              sulphite oxidase [Mo]
                                    cysteine dioxygenase [Fe]    ⎧ sulphite ⟶ sulphate
                                              ↓                  ⎪ glutathione Se
homocysteine ⟶ cystathione ⟶ cysteine ⟶                          ⎨ metallothionein Zn
                                                                 ⎪ alpha lipoic acid
         B6 (P5P) Mg         B6            NAC                   ⎩ taurine
```

A deficiency of nutrients or a deficiency in enzyme capacity or saturation of the sulphation pathways will lead to inadequate clearance of both toxins and heavy metals. In enzyme deficiency (slow sulphation) a "bottle neck" effect may occur when it may be advisable to supplement with an activated product such as N-acetylcysteine (NAC) or sulphate to facilitate the pathway. Those with intolerance to sulphur dioxide or with chemical sensitivities often have slow sulphation capacity and are more likely to accumulate heavy metals. Mo, molybdenum; Fe, iron; P5P, pyridoxal 5 phosphate (activated B6); Mg, magnesium; Se, selenium; Zn, zinc.

## Heavy metal toxicity

*Heavy metals have an affinity for fatty tissue, therefore the brain, nervous system and the bone marrow are the most vulnerable organs*

Heavy metals, such as mercury, lead, cadmium, copper and aluminium, have an affinity for tissues that are high in fat: the brain, the bone marrow (where we make our blood and immune cells) and the nerves (the myelin sheath is 70% fat). It is these organs that bear the greatest burden. So in any condition that involves the brain or mental illness (**Alzheimer's disease, ASD** [autistic spectrum disorders: Asperger's, Rett's, autism], **ADHD Parkinson's, depression, psychosis and seizures**), nerve degeneration (**multiple sclerosis, motor neurone disease**) or **bone marrow disorders** and **immune suppression**, one should look for heavy metal involvement. Heavy metal toxicity may also exacerbate existing inflammatory conditions such as **arthritis** and **autoimmune disease.**

*Sulphur is the best chelating agent for heavy metals.*

Heavy metals enter the cells and attach to sulphur groups on proteins and enzymes, disrupt their function, paralyse the antioxidant systems and initiate a self-perpetuating cycle of free radical damage and inflammation. Once pro-inflammatory genes get switched on, they stimulate cell division, inhibit cell death and may initiate **cancer**. So heavy metals can act as co-factors in the development of cancer.

*Inorganic iodine promotes excretion of heavy metals such as lead, mercury, cadmium and aluminium.*

Heavy metal detoxification normally occurs through the *sulphation* and *glutathione* pathways - iron and aluminium being two exceptions to this rule. Mercury, lead, copper and cadmium have a high affinity for sulphur and are oxidised with the sulfhydryl (thiol) groups found in the sulphur-containing amino acids, methionine and cysteine, and their metabolites, N-acetylcysteine (NAC), taurine, glutathione, alpha lipoic acid and metallothionein, all of which contribute to the detoxification and elimination of heavy metals. (See figure 5.22 *Supporting your sulphation pathways*.) The rate-limiting step for sulphation is cysteine availability, and unless there are inherent enzyme deficiencies in these pathways, by taking quality protein and ensuring adequate vitamin B status, all should proceed well. Chemical agents, such as DMSA (dimercaptosuccinic acid) may also be used for the chelation and excretion of heavy metals via the urine.

Selenium is a key trace mineral protecting against mercury toxicity through its capacity to regenerate glutathione. Additionally, it can directly bind mercury forming an inactive complex, which prevents the movement of mercury into the tissues. The insoluble complex is then stored in the liver and spleen. The other essential trace mineral is molybdenum, a co-factor for the enzyme sulphite oxidase, required in sulphation-conjugation reactions of toxins including heavy metals.

*Heavy metal toxicity induces selenium deficiencies: selenium binds with heavy metals and consequently becomes depleted.*

Unfortunately, heavy metals can tie up the sulphation pathways and exacerbate any existing health problems linked to poor sulphation, such as food and chemical intolerance, inflammatory disease and behavioural disorders. Patients often need to work on reducing their heavy metal load before they see any improvement. For this reason, oral chelating agents, such as DMSA, are often used over a prolonged period of time. However, these products do not fix inadequate or poor sulphation rates, they merely chelate mercury as it is released from tissue proteins where it is bound. So it is advisable to simultaneously support these pathways using products such as NAC and ensure dietary inclusion of garlic, cilantro (coriander leaf) and chlorella. NAC is readily absorbed and will chelate heavy metals when released from the tissues. This spares dietary cysteine for other sulphation activities, such as liver detoxification. Patients also need to be mindful of their copper load, as copper is not only antagonistic to molybdenum but also zinc. Zinc stimulates the synthesis of metallothionein, a circulating protein that not only prevents the uptake of heavy metals from the gut, but also detoxifies heavy metals within the body.

So a word of caution: when embarking on any treatment that draws heavy metals out of the tissues, make sure that there is enough available chelating agent or cysteine (as NAC) to bind the metals. If not, you will not only increase the load on the sulphation pathways, which may exacerbate any other current symptoms, but you also run the risk of redistributing the heavy metals into the central nervous system if they cannot be eliminated. I would recommend supplementation of NAC and lipoic acid for the duration of your heavy metal detoxification therapy along with sulphur-rich foods. You also need to protect against the re-absorption of heavy metals via the nerve endings in the gut. Chlorella, an intestinal toxin-absorbing agent, is renowned for its ability to bind every existing toxic metal within the gut and hence ensure its successful elimination. (See pp 149-150 *Tips on mercury removal*.)

*It is difficult to measure mercury toxicity as the bulk is "locked" in the tissues; only "free" mercury can be measured.*

# Depression

In Traditional Chinese Medicine a poorly functioning liver is often related to depression. From a Western perspective it is easy to see the connection. As we know, circulating toxins such as food by-products, if not detoxified by the liver can enter the brain and create havoc. The brain has both *methylation* and *sulphation* pathways so there is a backup mechanism for the detoxification of these toxins, but in the genetically predisposed, where these pathways may be down-regulated (or if these pathways are saturated) then we may see depression.

Depression is related to either an underproduction of the "feel good" brain chemicals, serotonin, dopamine and noradrenaline, or poor transmission capacity. Anti-depressant medications will boost levels of these chemicals by either increasing their output, or reducing their rate of breakdown. This means that higher levels of chemicals remain in the brain for a longer period of time.

## 5 Liver cleansing

*Nutritional deficiencies of B12, B6, folic acid, zinc, iodine and magnesium may contribute to depression.*

From a nutritional perspective, the parent molecules for neurotransmitter synthesis are the amino acids **tryptophan** and **tyrosine**. Both pathways require **vitamin B6** and **magnesium**. Tryptophan is the direct precursor for serotonin synthesis, and tyrosine the direct precursor for dopamine, noradrenaline and adrenaline synthesis. So B6 and magnesium deficiencies can directly lead to depression. Oestrogen dominance can suppress dopamine production which also leads to depression.

**Figure 5.23** Neurotransmitter synthesis from parent molecules and the co-factors involved

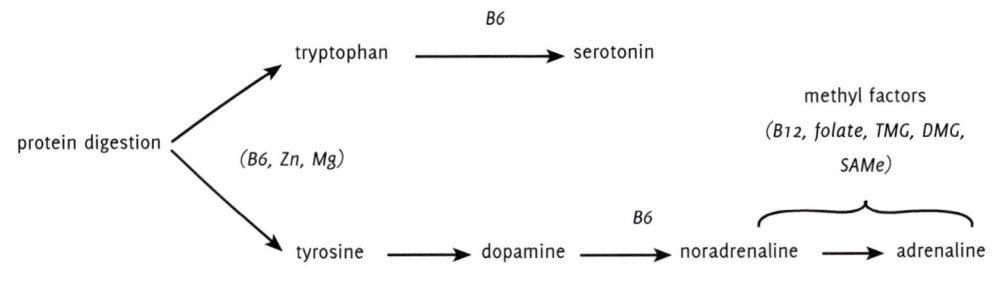

*Iodine deficiency is linked to insulin resistance and depression. Iodine increases insulin sensitivity and by default increases the uptake of tryptophan and its subsequent conversion to serotonin.*

```
                            B6
              tryptophan ────────→ serotonin
             ↗
                                        methyl factors
                                        (B12, folate, TMG, DMG,
protein digestion                              SAMe)
             ↘   (B6, Zn, Mg)
                                    B6
              tyrosine ──→ dopamine ──→ noradrenaline ──→ adrenaline
```

Good quality dietary protein will deliver ample amounts of the protein precursors, tryptophan and tyrosine, for neurotransmitter synthesis. Making good Mg, Zn, B6, B12 and folate deficiencies will ensure adequate neurotransmitter production.

*Long-term stress may lead to depression as stress hormones oppose the action of insulin in the brain. Insulin enables the uptake of tryptophan by the brain cells prior to its conversion to serotonin.*

The activation of neurons and production of neurotransmitters require methylation. If you support methylation by ensuring adequate magnesium, B12 (as methylcobalamin) and folic acid, or by supplementing DMG or TMG (which are B12/folic acid independent methylation pathways), then concentration and mood can improve if the depression is due to these specific nutrient deficiencies. SAMe (activated methionine) is the nutritionist's anti-depressant of choice. It not only directly donates methyl groups (without any requirement for B12, folic acid or magnesium), but can also support sulphation by donating its sulphur group. (See figure 5.17 *The methionine-homocysteine-cysteine pathway*.) If your poor concentration and brain fog is related to phenolic compounds and aldehydes which interfere with brain signal transmission, then supporting sulphation will go a long way to assist in their detoxification.

## ASD (Autistic Spectrum Disorders)

This is an umbrella group of disorders covering a wide spectrum - autism, Asperger's syndrome, Rett's Disorder, Pervasive Developmental Disorder [PDD] and Child Disintegrative Disorder [CDD] - that share common characteristics: impairment in social functioning and cognitive development, loss of reciprocal social interaction and communications skills, and repetitive patterns of behaviour. The degree of impairment and the specific manifestation of symptoms determine the position of the disorder on the spectrum.

In addition, there are some shared biochemical characteristics, confirmed by metabolic tests and subsequent response to treatment which indicate abnormalities in both the *methylation* and *sulphation* pathways of the liver and the brain, with the greatest response to any single treatment being the chelation of mercury.

Working backwards, we know that mercury ties up sulphation pathways and is neurotoxic to the brain, so our concern tends to focus on prenatal and neo-natal exposure when the brain is rapidly developing, tripling in size during the first year. As many vaccinations contain thimerosal, a mercury-containing preservative, it becomes increasingly difficult to ignore the correlation between the increasing vaccination schedule for the young infant and the rise in incidence in ASD. The danger time for an infant is immediately following vaccination, particularly with the significant mercury overload of multiple vaccinations at 2-3 months of age, which create a spike in exposure that exceeds the recommended upper limit of safety 138-fold. Between 1990 and 1994 the cumulative mercury exposure from vaccination during a child's first year climbed from 100mcg to 190mcg. During that same period we witnessed a dramatic rise in incidence in ASD in the USA from 12 per 10,000 to 20 per 10,000. A decade later, by 2004, this figure had risen to 60 per 10,000; a five-fold increase in 14 years. It is interesting that the majority of these children develop normally through their first year. The first signs of regression in autism usually appear between 12 to 24 months, and in CDD, between 36 to 48 months, although regression may occur anywhere up to 10 years of age. For children with genetically impaired pathways, even minute amounts of mercury can be toxic, while for others, the cumulative effects of poisoning may take months or years to manifest.

*It appears that "spikes" in exposure to mercury are more damaging than incremental exposure to the developing brain of the baby. The effects of poisoning are not immediate but may take months or years to manifest.*

Hair analysis as an indicator for mercury toxicity in these children may be of little value as levels may not represent the chronic load but only the capacity to excrete it. For example, hair mercury levels in a group of autistic children were 0.47 parts per million (ppm) versus 3.63 ppm in controls, a significant difference, and yet these children were found to carry far greater loads which they were unable to excrete. A study that measured the mercury excretion rates of children with ASD undergoing chelation therapy showed a six-fold increase over controls. Additionally, it has been found that the majority of these children have abnormal amounts of metabolites in their blood and urine which indicate slow reaction rates of enzymes involved in the methionine-sulphation pathway. By supplementing with high doses of the active vitamin co-factors required (folinic acid, TMG), some of these reaction rates were significantly enhanced with a corresponding improvement in symptoms.

*It is difficult to measure mercury toxicity from hair analysis. A reliable indicator is urinary excretion following chelation therapy.*

Other common problems include:
- multiple food sensitivities to salicylates, phenols, dairy, wheat and food additives;
- fungal or bacterial overgrowth in the bowel;
- mineral deficiencies (specifically zinc and iodine); and
- dysregulation of the immune system leading to increased immune reactivity.

You will by now be familiar with the vicious cycle of inadequate digestion leading to the absorption of partially digested foods and their effects on the tissues and brain, and how these substances can elicit allergic reactions, antibody formation and even act as "white noise" in the brain inhibiting brain signal transmission. Not only do many of these children have decreased methylation reactions in the brain, and consequently decreased neurotransmitter output, but also reduced activity of the enzyme phenol sulfotransferase (PST) which detoxifies phenolic compounds. This means that we have a combined low neurotransmitter output with poor signal reception.

*A low neurotransmitter output combined with poor signal reception compounds the situation.*

In ASD we are seeing a complex metabolic disorder, where genetic factors play a major role. However, it seems that chronic exposure to toxic metals (including mercury) and environmental pollutants may tip the balance in very early childhood, which is then compounded by negative reactions to foods, gut dysbiosis and a skewing of the immune system.

If you follow figure 5.24 *Consequences of impaired methylation and sulphation pathways in ASD*, you can see at a glance the relationship between impairments in these enzyme pathways, heavy metal exposure, food and chemical intolerance and the impact on the brain.

**Figure 5.24** Consequences of impaired methylation and sulphation pathways in ASD

*folinic acid*
*methylcobalamin*
*SAMe, TMG, DMG, P5P*

↓ NTs    ←    brain
                ↓ methylation
                ↓ sulphation         neurotoxic

*inhibition of signal transmission*

reactions to:
- phenols/salicylates
- colourings/preservatives
- exorphins (dairy/wheat)
- multiple chemicals
- bowel flora by-products (phenols)

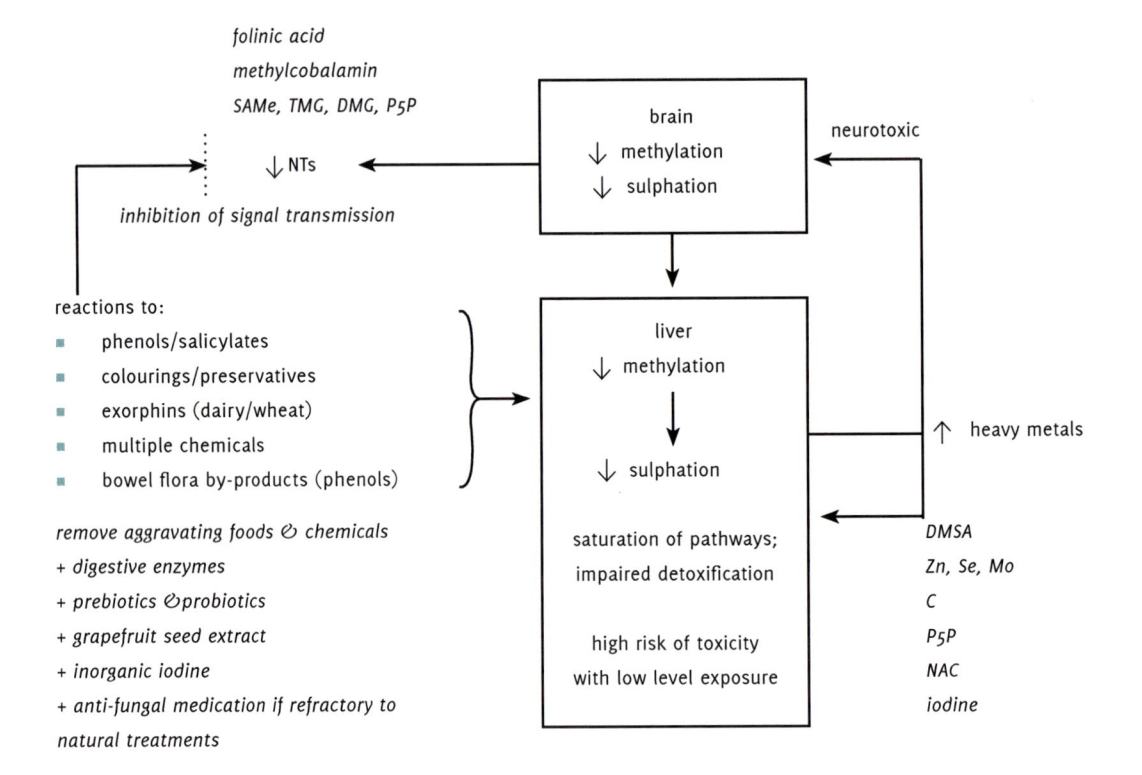

liver
↓ methylation
↓ sulphation                          ↑ heavy metals

saturation of pathways;              DMSA
impaired detoxification              Zn, Se, Mo
                                     C
high risk of toxicity                P5P
with low level exposure              NAC
                                     iodine

*remove aggravating foods & chemicals*
*+ digestive enzymes*
*+ prebiotics & probiotics*
*+ grapefruit seed extract*
*+ inorganic iodine*
*+ anti-fungal medication if refractory to natural treatments*

Phenolic compounds and other toxic metabolites, when not detoxified by the liver or brain can inhibit neurotransmission in the brain. This, coupled with poor rates of neurotransmitter production, leads to learning difficulties, behavioural disorders and poor communication skills. Accumulation of heavy metals (which share the same detoxification pathways as many food chemicals) exacerbate any degenerative changes in the brain. Supporting the methylation pathway (B12 as methylcobalamin, folate as folinic acid, B6 as pyridoxal-5-phosphate [P5P], s-adenosylmethionine [SAMe]) not only assists in the production of neurotransmitters, but also facilitates the channelling of methionine down the cysteine pathway for the synthesis of sulphate, gluthathione and metallothionein. This pathway is important in the detoxification of heavy metals and phenolic compounds. Additionally, prolonged treatment with other chelating agents, such as DMSA, may be required to remove the excess mercury.

# Tips on mercury removal

Mercury has an extended biological half-life of 70 days in the circulation and 20 years in the brain and nervous system. It is easier to remove mercury immediately following acute exposure when it is still in the circulation – say, after dental amalgam removal – rather than from long-term chronic exposure. If you suspect that heavy metals may be a cause of your problems and a challenge test supports this (urinary mercury is measured before and after a high dose of chelating agent), then chelation therapy would be the best answer – but this needs to be managed by a professional.

- **Chelation** is the use of a chemical substance to bind molecules, such as metals or minerals, and hold them tightly so they can be removed from the body. The two products which may be selected are DMSA (dimercaptosuccinic acid) or DMPS (dimercaptopropanesulphonate); both bind free mercury tightly in the tissue fluids and excrete it via the kidneys. These agents do not draw mercury from their bound state in the tissues, but only bind what is free; therefore, treatment may be long term and expensive.

- **Dental amalgam removal** may be more advantageous when undertaken incrementally – as low-dose is preferable to high-dose mercury exposure. If your sulphation pathway is slow, then you may need to think twice about removal and opt only to do this when the filling needs to be replaced. Your dentist will give you a detoxification protocol which will need to be continued for six to eight months. It is inadvisable to remove amalgams during pregnancy, as exposure in utero carries the highest risk for the unborn child.

## General Tips

- **n-acetylcysteine (NAC)** will support your glutathione and sulphation pathways, both of which are important for heavy metal detoxification. It can chelate mercury directly, but binding is loose and uncommitted – so if another metal comes along, mercury may be dumped.

- **alpha lipoic acid** tightly binds and detoxifies mercury, and is an excellent antioxidant supplement that has many actions. It is fat soluble, crosses the blood-brain barrier and chelates mercury in the central nervous system.

- **zinc** is important for the production of metallothionein, another heavy metal binder. Metallothionein also inhibits heavy metal absorption from the gut.

- **iodine,** in the form of inorganic iodine (Lugol's solution), promotes the excretion of all heavy metals, including aluminium and the halides, bromide and flouride. One drop of Lugol's solution delivers 6.25mg elemental iodine. Therapeutic dosages lie between 12.5mg – 50mg per day. It is recommended that you seek professional advice before embarking on iodine supplementation. Avoid ingestion of fluoride and chlorine as these elements oppose and deplete iodine.

- **selenium** chelates mercury but will not detoxify it. Instead, it forms insoluble complexes which are stored in the liver. Consequently mercury depletes selenium, which in turn has a negative impact on the selenium-dependent glutathione system. So make sure your selenium intake is adequate. Garlic is the best source of bio-active selenium – and it is high in sulphur as well.

- **cilantro**, or coriander leaf, mobilises cadmium, lead, aluminium and mercury from the tissues. However, it may loosen more than can be removed, resulting in redistribution to the nervous system. It's better to go slowly and surely than attempt major removal. The dose is 2–10 drops of the tincture, 2–3 times daily. It is best not to use this for the first month after amalgam removal as you wouldn't wish to increase the mercury load.

- **chlorella** is the best intestinal chelator of all toxins and heavy metals, in its unprocessed and non-absorbable form. The biggest problem with heavy metal detoxification via the liver (bile) is its reabsorption by the nerves in the gut. The maintenance dose is 1g, three times daily, 30 minutes before meals, increasing to 3g, three times daily during heavy metal detoxification programs as in dental amalgam removal. The release of bile is stimulated by food intake; therefore by taking chlorella 30 minutes prior to eating it will be in the right place to receive the heavy metals from the bile. Do not take with vitamin C. Other natural intestinal binding agents include apple pectin and chitosan.

- **reduce the burden on your liver** and free up your sulphation pathway by reducing environmental exposure to all heavy metals.

- **thimerosal-free vaccines** - if you wish to vaccinate, ask your GP for thimerosal-free vaccines. These have been available in the USA since 2001, although the DPT (diphtheria, pertussis, tetanus) vaccine may not be mercury free.

# Nutritional deficiencies in the detoxification pathways

**To recap**, the problems we face with detoxification stem from a fundamental imbalance in the amount of toxins produced and the liver's capacity to eliminate. Reduction of toxin load along with supplementation of nutrients required for detoxification may be all that is required to facilitate the process; but if pathways are down-regulated due to genetic variance, then the situation may need professional guidance.

You'll appreciate by now that there is a great deal that you can do armed with the right knowledge. If you look back at figure 5.17 *The methionine-homocysteine-cysteine pathway* you will see at a glance all the vitamin and mineral co-factors required by the enzymes to support the Phase 2 pathways. As methionine is the parent compound for several pathways, including sulphation and glutathionation, then providing you have adequate protein intake and the co-factors magnesium, B12, folic acid and B6, then you are half way there. Remember, by supporting glutathionation and sulphation pathways, you will automatically support glucuronidation, a pathway that is often exploited by deficiencies in other pathways. By reducing your toxic exposure (both exogenous and endogenous) and by taking additional supportive measures appropriate to your specific condition, you can fine-tune and be more discriminative about your choice of treatment.

*Intermediate, or active nutrients include: folinic acid (folic acid), methylcobalamin ($B_{12}$), pyridoxyl-5-phosphate ($B_6$) and N-acetylcysteine (cysteine).*

If you suspect that the problem may lie in genetic variance and down-regulation of enzyme pathways (often indicated by Functional Liver Detoxification Profile), then you may need to consider supplementation with an intermediate nutrient that allows you to bypass the impaired step. Here are a few examples:

- It is estimated that around 35% of the population may have impaired folate metabolism. For these people the activated form of folic acid, **5-methyltetrahydrofolate** (5-MTHF) or folinic acid, is more easily assimilated into the folate metabolism than its synthetic form, folic acid, and would therefore be a supplement of choice.
- Similarly, cyanocobalamin, or vitamin B12, is metabolised to its active form, **methylcobalamin**, by the liver. This is the only form that can be utilized by the brain and nervous system. Therefore individuals that suffer from depression, ADHD or ASD, may benefit more from this form of B12 than cyanocobalamin.
- Poor glutathionation and sulphation capacity can also prove a stumbling block. Supplementing with **N-acetylcysteine** (NAC), an activated form of cysteine, may bypass the impaired step to stimulate glutathionation production and support sulphation.

If you refer to table 5.5 *Supporting Phase 2 detoxification pathways* you can see at a glance the types of disorders that may indicate deficiencies in the specific pathways concerned and the various nutritional remedies suggested.

## 5 Liver cleansing

**Table 5.5** Supporting Phase 2 detoxification pathways

### Methylation

| Symptoms | Nutrients | Foods/herbs |
|---|---|---|
| • Allergy (high histamine)<br>• Oestrogen dominance<br>• Homocysteine, heart disease<br>• Depression<br>• Anxiety (high adrenaline)<br>• ADHD, ASD<br>• Fatty liver<br>• Alcoholism<br>• Multiple Chemical Sensitivity | Methionine<br>Mg<br>B12, folate,<br>Choline, carnitine<br>TMG, DMG<br>SAMe | Sulphur containing foods: broccoli, brussels sprouts, cauliflower, red/green cabbage, watercress, onions, garlic, leeks, radish, quality protein<br>*Licorice* |

### Sulphation

| Symptoms | Nutrients | Foods/herbs |
|---|---|---|
| • Allergies<br>(food additives: benzoates, sulphur dioxide, tartrazine; foods: salicylates, phenols, amines)<br>• Drugs: paracetamol /aspirin/NSAIDs<br>• Oestrogen dominance<br>• Thyroid hormone imbalance<br>• Inflammatory disease<br>• Anxiety/high adrenaline<br>• Heavy metal accumulation<br>• Candida, clostridia<br>• ADHD, ASD<br>• Gall stones (taurine conjugation) | Methionine, cysteine, taurine<br>B12, folate, B6<br>Mg, Mo, Zn, Fe<br>NAC, lipoic acid, taurine<br>MSM<br>Glucosamine sulphate and chondroitin sulphate for joint disease and arthritis; these supplements will spare the sulphate pool.<br>NSAIDs deplete the sulphate pool and may therefore exacerbate the cause of the arthritis. | Sulphur containing foods: broccoli, brussels sprouts, cauliflower, red/green cabbage, watercress, onions, garlic, leeks, radish, quality protein<br><br>Fresh *coriander leaf* and chlorella will assist in heavy metal detoxification. |

### Glutathionation

| Symptoms | Nutrients | Foods/herbs |
|---|---|---|
| As for sulphation pathway including:<br>• High Phase 1 activity<br>• Liver toxicity, cirrhosis, hepatitis, cancer, abnormal iver function tests<br>• Chemical and solvents, petrol<br>• Drug sensitivity: penicillin, tetracycline, paracetamol | As for sulphation including:<br>Se, glutathione, glycine, glutamine<br>B2, B3, B6<br>Lipoic acid<br>NAC | Foods as for sulphation<br>*Turmeric, schizandra, milk thistle* |

### Glucuronidation

| Symptoms | Nutrients | Foods/herbs |
|---|---|---|
| • Elevated bilirubin<br>• Gilbert's syndrome<br>• Jaundice<br>• Oestrogen dominance<br>• Under-active/saturation of glycination and sulphation pathways<br>• Anxiety – high adrenaline<br>• Drugs: a wide range of drugs including aspirin, paracetamol, diazepams, steroids | Calcium D glucarate<br>SAMe | Grapefruit, broccoli, oranges, Brussels sprouts<br><br>*Licorice, kombucha tea, green tea, rosemary leaf extract* |

### Glycination

| Symptoms | Nutrients | Foods/herbs |
|---|---|---|
| Allergy to benzoates, salicylates/ aspirin<br>Gall stones, jaundice | Mg, Zn B3, B6<br>Glycine | Glycine is widely available in foods |

# Tips on supporting liver detoxification

- Make sure your diet is low in saturated fats and refined carbohydrates while high in lecithin and the lipotrophic factors (choline, inositol and linoleic acid).

- Do not cook with poly-unsaturated oils as heating renders these oils toxic to the system. It is better to use a virgin olive oil (which is mono-unsaturated) or small amounts of unsalted butter or ghee. Of course it is best to reduce oils to a minimum on a deep cleanse.

- Absolutely no alcohol. Both high fat diets and alcohol promote the formation of "bad" oestrogens.

- Lecithin as a nutritional supplement may be used. Commercial lecithin is high in neutral lipids and low in phosphadidyl choline. Purified lecithin in the form of phosphatidyl choline is more effective and will pass to the liver without being broken down. Choline supplements are also available but choline is degraded in the gut by bacterial activity often giving rise to a fishy odour.

- Flaxseed oil is a rich source of linolenic acid, although only 5%-10% may be converted to the beneficial DHA (docosahexanoic acid) and EPA (eicosapentanoic acid) fatty acids that are found in fish oils. This series of fatty acids (omega 3 series) are beneficial against inflammatory conditions (including allergy), and support brain signalling transmission and eyesight. Like all polyunsaturated fatty acids they are destroyed upon heating. If you suffer any inflammatory condition or loss of brain power/eyesight it may be wise to supplement with these oils. Flaxseed oil has beneficial cholesterol-lowering effects and small amounts speed up the reduction and absorption of tumours in cancer patients.

- Ensure that your diet is rich in linoleic acid (omega 6 series). The body requires a balance between the omega 6 and omega 3 series in a ratio of 4:1. Linoleic acid promotes the production of lecithin which assists in the removal of fats from the liver and the reduction of cholesterol both in the liver (via its conversion to bile acids) and in the circulation. Evening Primrose Oil contains active linoleic acid (GLA – gamma-linolenic acid). This is an expensive preparation and needs to be taken over many months. For long-term improvement in health it may be wiser to make good deficiencies of magnesium, zinc, B6, B3 and vitamin C to enable the conversion of linoleic acid to active GLA and to take unrefined safflower or sunflower oil as a salad dressing in the diet – both of which are rich in linoleic acid.

- Nutritional supplements such as selenium and vitamin E will guard against oxidative damage particularly in liver cells. This damage may be widespread when the diet has been rich in polyunsaturated oils. Supplementation with these nutrients actively removes brown deposits of rancid fat in the liver.

- Ensure adequate B12, folic acid and B6 status. These vitamins ensure smooth functioning of the liver detoxification pathways.

- Increase your intake of specific phytonutrients – the indoles and the D-glucarates – found in cruciferous vegetables (e.g., cabbage, cauliflower, brussels sprouts, kale and turnips). These nutrients not only assist in carcinogen and oestrogen elimination but may slow down or arrest tumour growth.

- Increase the amount of sulphur in your diet from foods such as broccoli, cabbage, brussels sprouts, watercress, onions, garlic, leeks and radish.

- Make sure your diet is high in soluble fibre as this increases bile turnover and aids in the elimination of toxins.

- Stimulants must be avoided as these add to liver congestion by increasing the metabolic burden of the liver.

- Stabilise the blood sugar levels by eating regularly. The body cannot regenerate when blood sugar levels falls. Low blood sugar increases fatty congestion of the liver and stimulates the release of hormones which break down body tissue, increasing the metabolic burden on the system.

- Watch your protein intake. Quality vegetable protein is preferred (combining legumes with grain, or legumes with nuts/seeds), but amounts should be kept to minimum i.e. 1g protein/kg body weight. (See chapter 3, table 3.1 *Percentage of carbohydrates, fats and proteins in foods*.)

- Buy organic produce whenever you can and check the country of origin. Although the use of DDT was banned in the USA in 1972, it continues to be produced and exported to Third World countries.

- Avoid all foods with additives. This includes preservatives, colourings and enhancers.

- Choose 'safe' personal care products. Most creams, cosmetics, perfumes, deodorants and shampoos contain hormone-disrupting chemicals which are absorbed directly through the skin.

- Avoid using chemicals in the home, garden or workplace.

- Avoid plastics and vinyls (including plastic toys for children).

- Follow the basic rules for detoxification programs: remove all added salt, increase the potassium content of the diet (fruits and vegetables), reduce the acid-forming foods and ensure protein quality rather than quantity.

Relieving the burden on the liver is the most beneficial step you can take towards health.

I can assure you that strain on the liver can largely be alleviated by diet – by what you leave out more than what you put in.

Nutritional products and herbs may facilitate the liver's processes, but the ultimate burden lies with diet, stress and chemicals.

You cannot detoxify or heal when your blood sugar levels are low.

Low blood sugar leads to the release of hormones that actively break down the body's tissue for energy supply.

# 6

# Regeneration & blood sugar control

# 6 Regeneration & blood sugar control

**Most people admit** that dieting would be easy if it wasn't for those insatiable cravings that hit mid-afternoon when all your will power turns into "want" power. Even people with the strongest intentions can succumb to the coffee and biscuit temptation while resolving that tomorrow they will do better. But by the next day the cravings return creating guaranteed despondency, and you manage to convince yourself that the diet wasn't really worth the effort allowing you to promptly return to old eating habits.

In order to succeed on any diet we have to manage our cravings, and diets that do not address the root cause of these will ultimately fail. This becomes a high priority for two reasons: firstly, strict adherence to the detoxification plan over a sustained period of time is critical in order to initiate the momentum required for detoxification, and secondly, regeneration of healthy new tissues is dependent upon efficient blood sugar control. Fluctuating blood sugar levels, or more precisely, low blood sugar, not only cause cravings but also lead to the release of hormones that actively break down body tissue for energy supply. In other words, instead of regenerating new tissue your body begins to "eat itself" just to fulfil its basic energy requirements.

Under these circumstances dieting becomes destructive. Most people start a diet to look and feel better and yet there is a large percentage that, in the long-term, actually feels worse after dieting. Not only may they look ill but they also feel devitalised and, more disappointingly, see no change in their overall health picture. Invariably they return to the same old eating patterns. I have also seen this situation in people who are keen detoxifiers drinking volumes of vegetable juices while sustaining themselves on a raw food diet.

Perhaps the fault lies in the assumption that if you go on a diet, a detoxification plan or otherwise, that the body automatically regenerates leading to an improvement in health. However, unless your diet includes foods that stabilise blood sugar levels and is rich in nutrients essential for tissue repair and maintenance, then it will be impossible to diet or even detoxify without incurring debts at the expense of the body's integrity. The simple fact is that there can be no regeneration when blood sugar levels are low, but if you stabilise your blood sugar you will not only be able to keep to the diet but improve your health dramatically.

## How can I tell if my blood sugar levels are low?

In order to answer this you will need to answer the following questions:

- Do you suffer from cravings for tea, coffee, coca cola, alcohol, cigarettes, sugar, sweets, cakes, biscuits or chocolate?
- Are the cravings worse around 4pm in the afternoon?
- Do you suffer from food cravings, particularly prior to menstruation?
- Do you skip breakfast and/or lunch and rely on quick pick-me-ups, such as coffee or tea, to get you through the day?
- Do you become moody, irritable or suffer headaches if you get hungry?
- Do you suffer from palpitations, hot or cold sweats, shaking or panic attacks?
- Do you suffer from fatigue or sudden loss of energy?

If you have answered yes to any of these questions then it is likely that your blood sugar levels are poorly controlled.

## Why does my blood sugar become unstable?

Symptoms of low blood sugar occur after long periods of dietary abuse brought on by excessive intake of refined carbohydrates (sugar, sweets/chocolate, refined bakery products), stimulants (tea, coffee, cola) and poor dietary habits, such as severe dieting and the skipping of meals.

In health the body is able to regulate the amount of sugar (or glucose) in the blood within a very narrow range independent of the type of diet you eat. It is only when the blood sugar falls below a certain level that the hunger centre in the brain tells you that you need to eat. Usually this occurs some four to five hours after your last meal.

However, if the blood sugar levels fail to stabilise between meals then you suffer constant cravings that are difficult to ignore. The urge to eat is so strong because the detection of a low blood sugar concentration signals a critical situation for the brain and nervous system. Glucose is the main source of energy for these tissues and consequently any deficiency in the energy supply induces a major shift in liver metabolism to produce ketones, an alternative energy supply from keto-acids (a breakdown product of fats and proteins) as seen in diabetes and fasting. Our cravings, when seen in this light, aren't merely an inconvenience but a very effective mechanism ensuring that we eat.

*Glucose is the preferred source of fuel for the brain and nerves. Hunger is the alarm signal when supplies become low.*

# Regulation of blood sugar

**The liver** has a central role to play in the regulation of blood sugar. One of the functions of the liver is to store glucose derived from dietary carbohydrate immediately following a meal, which can then be released between meals into the circulation as readily available energy for the brain and nervous system.

*Insulin is a storage hormone; it enables the cells to take up glucose and store it as an energy substrate.*

Upon digestion of our food, the glucose from carbohydrate passes into the circulation and is taken to the liver. A proportion is taken up by the liver and converted to stored glucose, or glycogen, and the rest is taken to the cells. The initial rise in blood sugar experienced after a meal stimulates the pancreas to release insulin. This is the hormone which enables the body tissues to take up glucose for energy or storage. The muscles store glucose as glycogen while the fat cells convert it to fat.

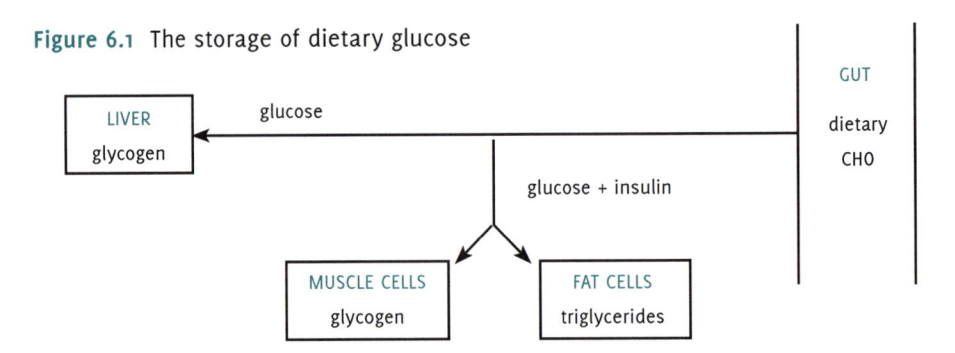

**Figure 6.1** The storage of dietary glucose

```
                                                            | GUT
    ┌──────────┐   glucose                                  |
    │  LIVER   │◄────────────────────┐                      | dietary
    │ glycogen │                     │                      | CHO
    └──────────┘                     │                      |
                        glucose + insulin                   |
                                 ╱   ╲                      |
                                ╱     ╲                     |
                   ┌──────────────┐  ┌──────────────┐       |
                   │ MUSCLE CELLS │  │  FAT CELLS   │       |
                   │   glycogen   │  │ triglycerides│       |
                   └──────────────┘  └──────────────┘       |
```

Dietary carbohydrate is broken down to glucose which enters the circulation. A proportion is taken up by the liver for storage (glycogen) and the rest passes to the tissues. Glucose that is not required for immediate energy is stored by muscle cells as glycogen and by fat cells as triglycerides, or fat. Insulin is required for the uptake of glucose by the cells.

*An exaggerated insulin response leads to an inappropriate reduction of blood sugar; so high sugar diets may lead to poor blood sugar control.*

Insulin, in addition to its role of facilitating glucose uptake by the cells, also protects the body against sharp rises in blood sugar that may be as equally deleterious to health as low blood sugar levels. Consequently, the amount of insulin secreted by the pancreas will match the glucose load inflicted by the diet. That is to say, when you eat sugar, sweets, biscuits, cakes and chocolate which provide a rapid influx of glucose into the circulation, the surge in blood sugar levels stimulates an exaggerated insulin response from the pancreas. The sugar is then stripped out of the circulation and quickly stored away as fat. Unfortunately, the down-side of this is that you may still feel hungry as the blood sugar has been lowered inappropriately, and the energy you just consumed, far from it being available, is now stored as fat.

**Figure 6.2** Effects on blood sugar with a refined carbohydrate diet

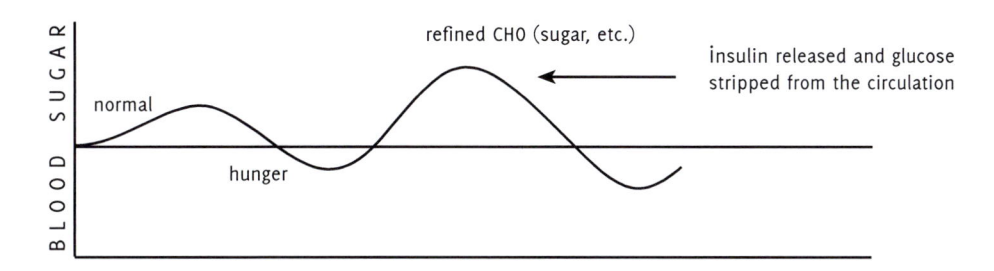

Blood glucose is regulated by insulin. When blood sugar levels falls you feel hungry. Refined carbohydrates result in a sharp rise in blood sugar and an exaggerated insulin response which lowers the blood sugar levels inappropriately giving rise to poor appetite control and cravings.

Perhaps this is easier to understand if you compare the effect of eating six slices of wholemeal bread to one chocolate bar. They both contain the same amount of kilojoules and yet you are more likely to be hungry one hour after eating the chocolate bar than consuming the bread. The kilojoules from the chocolate have already been stored as fat while those from the bread have still yet to be released. The digestion of complex carbohydrate (whole grains, legumes) is a much slower process with the gradual release of glucose. This small but constant elevation of blood sugar does not elicit a strong insulin response and therefore the energy is not stored as fat but made available to the tissues for their activities.

*It is best to take sugar as complex carbohydrates. This will not stimulate an insulin spike and will satisfy your hunger for longer.*

**Figure 6.3** Effects on blood sugar with a complex carbohydrate diet

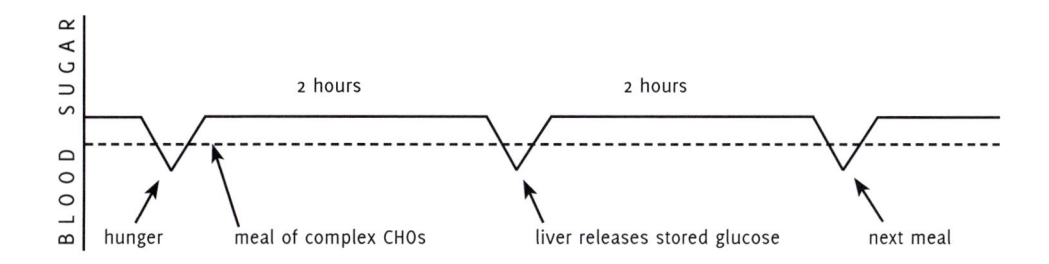

Complex CHOs are digested slowly with a steady release of glucose into the circulation that will not stimulate an exaggerated insulin response. Levels will start to fall approximately 2 hours after your meal when the liver will release its stored glucose. Around 4 - 5 hours later you will be ready for your next meal.

The saying "dieting makes you fat" is not far from the truth. Many weight-loss diets concentrate on calorie reduction, or on how little you must eat in order to lose weight. This invariably undermines effective blood sugar control and gives rise to cravings and bingeing. The types of food we binge on are those which give us a lift - in other words, elevate the blood sugar rapidly - and these foods are immediately converted to fat! Very often it is not the number of kilojoules you consume which is important but their source. Kilojoules derived from foods which have a slower rate of digestion will not turn into fat and are therefore said to be "slimming" while those from refined products are "fattening". For the same reasons the role of fibre, found in complex carbohydrates, also slows the digestive time and therefore indirectly controls blood sugar levels and the appetite.

The other danger with excessive dieting is that you lose muscle bulk as the corticosteroids released during food deprivation actively break down muscle protein for energy. Therefore when you start eating again there is less muscle tissue to take up the dietary carbohydrate to store as glycogen and so fat cells take up the carbohydrate, converting it to fat – and you end up with more fat than muscle.

It is worth mentioning that of the many patients I have treated with eating disorders most had appalling blood sugar control. What begins as a physiological imbalance, where the body tries to maintain its blood sugar through stimulating the hunger centre, rapidly becomes a psychological disturbance where the client feels "out of control". While the body is only dictating for its survival, the thinking process panics, and before long these patterns can become obsessive. Different people react in different ways; some over-eat and become obese while others enter the starvation/bingeing cycle. With a little understanding of how these mechanisms regulate our hunger patterns, we can take control by changing our dietary habits before the situation becomes an entrenched psychological picture.

*Stimulants give an adrenaline-rush which elevates the blood sugar and makes you feel good.*

## The effects of stimulants, such as the caffeine-containing drinks tea, coffee and cola, also raise the blood sugar levels - albeit indirectly. They facilitate the action of adrenaline which stimulates the liver to release glucose. So although they do not provide glucose for energy themselves they promote its release. This is why stimulants are highly addictive and serve as effective energy-boosters. However, they are devitalising and strip valuable nutrients away from the body. People who live on the adrenaline drive become "burnt out" before their time.

*Sex hormones and the corticosteroid hormones inhibit the uptake of sugar by the cell and therefore elevate blood sugar levels. The "drop" in sugar levels around 4pm coincides with the natural fall in cortisone at that time.*

## Sex hormones and the stress hormones also regulate blood sugar levels. The sex hormones, oestrogen and progesterone, are protective of blood sugar levels because they antagonise the action of insulin. This means that they indirectly inhibit cellular uptake of glucose from the circulation and therefore blood sugar levels remain more stable. However, when the levels of these hormones fall prior to menstruation, so too does the blood sugar, and this is when the cravings and erratic moods begin. Remember, hormones may only mask an already existing low blood sugar picture. The true situation is that which arises prior to menstruation and indicates how effectively the liver is able to meet the demands. For those who suffer badly with pre-menstrual symptoms, it is probably wise to start the healing and regenerative process now before you hit the menopause when the sudden loss of oestrogen can have devastating effects. I have treated many women with severe pre-menstrual syndrome that simply "disappears" to the extent that the onset of menstruation comes as a complete surprise.

### Case history 6.1

**Marianne was 30 years old** and an exhausted mother of two. Her elder child, Simon was five years old, overweight and hyperactive while her daughter, Clare was just three. Marianne had no energy or enthusiasm for life, found getting up in the morning difficult, let alone looking after two children. When I asked her about her diet she said that she had been preoccupied with diet since she could remember. She was overweight as a child and adolescent and liked to binge on cake. She also suffered chronic constipation. When she was eighteen she went on a severe diet and lost weight but it soon came back, escalated and spiralled out of control. Marianne tried everything from slimming clubs, slimming pills to hypnotherapy, but the weight kept piling on.

In her early twenties the symptoms of bulimia started and she became emotionally unstable. Over the next few years Marianne felt as though her weight was under control but during her first pregnancy she gained 25 kilos. By semi-starvation she managed to reduce her weight before becoming pregnant for the second time. This time Marianne controlled her eating and managed to stabilise her weight throughout the pregnancy. Currently she was living off strong espresso coffee throughout the day, picking at the children's food around 4.30pm which would satisfy her hunger very often enabling her to miss the evening meal.

We looked back over her case history and discovered that she had a serious chest infection when she was six years old that was treated with antibiotics. It was after this that the asthma started. As there was no medical treatment at that time Marianne attended hospital each week taking classes to improve her breathing. The asthma attacks subsided when she was fourteen years old.

Marianne's menstrual cycle had always been erratic and she had been on and off the pill since she was sixteen. In her 20s she suffered several miscarriages due to a lack of progesterone and had progesterone injections during the first few months of both subsequent pregnancies. Marianne recently decided to stop taking the pill and her periods were practically non-existent.

Marianne was not convinced that if she started eating properly she would not gain weight. It was more important to her, at that stage, that she remained thin than experience greater energy and wellbeing. She hoped that I would give her some mineral supplements that would make her feel better.

Here was a picture of deep congestion (chronic constipation) and poor blood sugar control. Liver congestion is always indicated in low blood sugar conditions and eating disorders. There had been no natural resolution of the chest condition which had subsequently led to asthma. Asthma invariably indicates congestion of the liver, which, in Chinese terms, then rises to obstruct the lungs. As no therapeutic treatment was undertaken at this stage to raise the vitality and resolve the liver disharmony, congestion deepened manifesting in menstrual irregularities (and later difficulties in conception and pregnancy) and a full-blown eating disorder.

There was a deep magnesium and manganese deficiency and I did prescribe magnesium at this stage even though Marianne had suffered asthma in the past. Many of my best patients have been of the obsessive/compulsive type as they find sticking to the diet, once they have resolved to do so, very easy. Marianne decided, two months later, that she would try the diet. She wanted to do the strong detoxification plan and stayed on it for seven months. To her surprise, although she was eating what she considered to be "masses" she did not gain any weight (although her body shape changed and became toned), her energy returned within the first month and her menstrual cycle became regular for the first time ever. Very slight asthmatic symptoms did return so we stopped the magnesium and reduced the vegetable juices until they resolved naturally within a short period of time.

Marianne found that it took at least a month before her stomach felt comfortable with eating breakfast and twice as long for lunch. I had stressed the importance of eating the three meals a day, both for stabilising blood sugar levels and for regeneration. We did a lot of work on the liver with lecithin-based products and by the end of the seven months Marianne was a different person. It was truly a joy to see the transformation. I am still in touch with her today and she tells me that none of the old symptoms have returned and that she still follows the broad guidelines of the diet.

She also decided to bring her son for treatment as she suspected that many of his hyperactive symptoms were due to blood sugar problems. We changed his diet and supplemented with magnesium and zinc and within a few days his concentration was better and his behaviour had improved. He lost a great deal of weight and over the months became a settled, healthy boy.

**Figure 6.4** Antagonism of insulin by the sex hormones at cell level

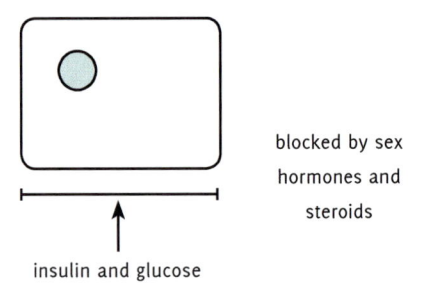

blocked by sex hormones and steroids

insulin and glucose

Increased circulating sex hormones and glucocorticoid steroids (stress hormones) antagonise insulin and inhibit the uptake of glucose by the cells. In stress glucose is spared for the brain and the nerves. During pregnancy this relative insulin resistance supports the laying down of fat reserves and the growth of the baby.

*Replace sugar with complex carbohydrates which contain small amounts of protein and are rich in fibre.*

## What can I do to help stabilise my blood sugar levels?

As a first step, stabilise your blood sugar by changing your diet to include complex carbohydrates and by removing stimulants and sugars. This will ensure that blood sugar levels do not rise and fall inappropriately but maintain a steady concentration. Cravings should abate and it should be possible to go between meals without snacking. In some cases it may be necessary to eat smaller but more frequent meals if the hunger "lows" are very noticeable. This situation indicates that the liver is not capable of maintaining fasting (between meal) blood sugar levels.

Long-term treatment involves regenerating the liver so that we are not dependent on maintaining blood sugar levels from dietary sources alone. In order to achieve this the detoxification plan reduces congestion while re-mineralising the liver. This situation can usually be rectified over a period of a few months, provided that you do not return to bad eating habits.

## Magnesium and B6 play a special role in the control of blood sugar. Magnesium governs the energy cycle. It is involved in the breakdown of dietary carbohydrate to glucose in the gut, the conversion of glucose to glycogen by the liver, the conversion of glycogen back to glucose by the liver between meals, and the utilisation of glucose for energy by the tissue cells.

*Magnesium and B6 are two important nutrients in energy control.*

**Figure 6.5** The role of magnesium in the conversion of glucose to energy

Dietary CHO —Mg→ glucose —Mg→ glycogen —Mg, B6→ glucose —Mg→ energy (cells)
Gut              Liver            Liver                Circulation

You will see that vitamin B6 is also essential for the conversion of stored glucose (glycogen) to glucose. This conversion is essential for the maintenance of fasting blood sugar levels, hence magnesium and B6 are often supplemented together. If you are deficient in magnesium you will suffer from low energy and no matter how much you eat you will never feel as though you derive enough energy from your food. Supplementation with magnesium will make all the difference and remarkably, many find that their cravings disappear once their magnesium status is improved.

## What are the long-term effects of low blood sugar? Quite simply, low blood sugar accelerates the ageing process. The body releases specific hormones (glucocorticoids) which attack and break down our body tissue protein and fat to provide the energy substrates. These substrates are taken to the liver where they are further degraded to glucose and fatty acids. The glucose will be used by the brain and nerves, while most other tissues can use fatty acids. While the body is breaking itself down it cannot regenerate and tissues which have the highest turnover, that is those which need replacing every few days, are the first to suffer. This includes the cells of the immune system, the lining of the small intestine where digestion and absorption take place, and the hair follicles. So the first symptoms likely to appear are an **increased susceptibility to infection, digestive disturbances** and **food allergies, inflammatory conditions of the gut** and **hair loss.** Over prolonged periods of time the bones will be affected and osteoporosis may occur. In short, the regenerative process is inhibited and premature ageing occurs in all the tissues – in other words, your biological age outstrips your chronological age.

# Tips to support your blood sugar levels

- **Don't skip meals**, particularly breakfast; if necessary eat smaller but more frequent meals spread over the day. Do not eat fruit as the main part of the meal as fruit sugar, or fructose, is not converted into glucose and can exacerbate an already poor blood sugar control.

- **Diets rich in complex carbohydrates** take longer to digest and therefore the steady rate of glucose absorption will not encourage wide blood sugar swings. This inhibits an exaggerated insulin response for those predisposed to low blood sugar and, in the case of insulin deficiency (diabetes) or insulin resistance, will not provoke a sudden spike in blood sugar concentration.

- **Small amounts of fat and protein** taken along with complex carbohydrates reduce intestinal motility and slow the transit time in the small intestine. A slower transit time also stabilises blood sugar levels. Legumes eaten with rice are ideal for stabilising blood sugar levels. Protein does not stimulate a strong insulin response and therefore may be useful for those who suffer energy dips following a meal.

- **Dietary fibre**, found in all whole grains and legumes, has a specific role in regulating blood sugar:

    - fibre is bulky therefore it delays entry of food into the small intestine and hence slows digestion and absorption;

    - fibre has a water-holding capacity, forming gels and making the fluid contents of the small intestine viscous. This slows down movement in the small intestine considerably thereby slowing digestion and absorption.

- **Avoid stimulants** - tea, coffee, chocolate and cigarettes.

- **Avoid alcohol** as it causes a sharp rise in insulin with a subsequent fall in blood sugar. In addition it inhibits the release of glucose by the liver so thwarts any attempt by the liver to stabilise blood sugar levels. This is why you may invariably get the "munchies" following alcohol intake.

- **Magnesium and potassium** dominate the energy cycle so choose foods rich in these minerals (vegetables and whole cereals); avoid the use of salt and limit the amount of dairy which tend to negatively influence magnesium and potassium levels. Tea, coffee, alcohol and refined products (sweets, chocolate, cakes etc.) actively deplete the magnesium and potassium status.

- **B vitamins** are essential for glucose metabolism, particularly B1 and B6, so ensure whole foods in the diet. B6 is important in the maintenance of fasting blood sugar levels, while B1 is required in the key steps of sugar metabolism.

- **Zinc** is important for the production of insulin and for maintaining fasting blood sugar levels.

- **Chromium as GTF** (glucose tolerance factor) is important in the binding of insulin to the cell receptor and the subsequent uptake of glucose. The insulin requirement may be reduced in diabetics when GTF is supplemented if the uptake of insulin at the cell membrane is defective.

# The metabolic syndrome

*The stage may be set for this syndrome in early childhood.*

**More recently, metabolic syndrome** (formerly known as Syndrome X or insulin resistance) and the damaging effects of obesity, diabetes and heart disease has been under the spotlight. This syndrome comes about following years of poor dietary habits of too much refined carbohydrate, sugar and fat. These diets increase the risk of insulin resistance, or simply a rejection of insulin by our cells. This syndrome is not always age-related as the background is invariably established at a young age and influenced by early dietary habits.

*Free fatty acids take precedence over glucose as an energy substrate when VAT is high; high circulating fFA levels determine insulin resistance.*

**Why do our cells reject insulin?** Over a prolonged period of time, a sustained excessive consumption of sugars and fats will lead to fatty infiltration of our organs (particularly the liver) and muscles. Organ fat is commonly referred to as VAT (visceral adipose tissue). Fatty organs are inefficient so they will try and clear the fat by continuously breaking it down and releasing it as free fatty acids (fFAs). Circulating free fatty acids will be preferentially chosen over glucose by most tissues, except the brain and the nervous system. This switch from glucose to free fatty acid metabolism is coupled with a reduction of insulin receptor sites on our cell membranes. These receptors function as "doorways"; insulin attaches to these sites which then enable glucose and other nutrients to enter. The average person may have as many as 20,000 insulin receptors per cell, but in insulin resistance these may be down-regulated to a mere 5,000! So if glucose cannot be taken up, then a surplus remains in the circulation which then signals the pancreas to release more insulin to try and lower the glucose load.

*A healthy liver removes both glucose and insulin from the circulation; it converts excess blood glucose to triglycerides and degrades insulin.*

The liver can clear both insulin and glucose from the circulation. So initially, you may not even know that you have insulin resistance as your blood results may not indicate any abnormal changes (high glucose or high insulin). The liver will slowly take up the excess glucose, convert it to fat (triglycerides) and ship it back to the tissues where it will continue to increase the VAT loading. This perpetuates free fatty acid metabolism and the cycle of insulin resistance. As the situation deteriorates, the sustained insulin response "switches on" cholesterol synthesis.

**Prolonged stress** may also induce insulin resistance and obesity. Just as excessive dieting reduces muscle bulk, so too does stress. When under prolonged stress, we release corticosteroid hormones which not only induce the breakdown of body protein, but also oppose the action of insulin. This reduction of muscle bulk means that more of our dietary glucose will be converted to fat instead of muscle glycogen. As our fat tissues and organs become more engorged with fat, then the body switches from glucose to free fatty acid metabolism and the cycle of insulin resistance begins.

**Figure 6.6** The cycle of insulin resistance

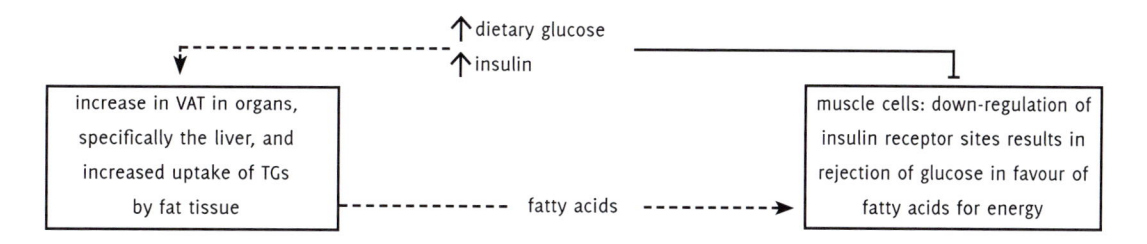

```
                      ↑ dietary glucose
         ┌──────────── ↑ insulin ──────────────────┐
         ↓                                          ┴
┌─────────────────────┐                  ┌─────────────────────────────┐
│ increase in VAT in  │                  │ muscle cells: down-regulation│
│ organs, specifically│                  │ of insulin receptor sites    │
│ the liver, and      │                  │ results in rejection of      │
│ increased uptake of │------ fatty acids ------→│ glucose in favour of   │
│ TGs by fat tissue   │                  │ fatty acids for energy       │
└─────────────────────┘                  └─────────────────────────────┘
```

When glucose is not taken up by the cells, due to the down-regulation of insulin receptors (specifically on muscle cells), blood glucose remains elevated leading to a sustained release of insulin by the pancreas. Glucose is converted to fat by adipose tissue and the liver. The liver ships it out to the tissues as triglycerides (TGs) and lipoproteins for deposition in the organs and muscles.

## The onset of diabetes

occurs when there is insulin resistance at the liver. This means that the liver fails to respond to, and clear insulin. Around this time your blood readings may reflect both high insulin and glucose. You may also start to see your cholesterol levels rising. These are the indications for the onset of type 2 diabetes (non-insulin dependent diabetes mellitus or NIDDM).

*Iodine increases insulin receptor sensitivity and may reverse insulin resistance and type 2 diabetes.*

Under normal conditions insulin acts as a signal alerting the liver that there is sufficient glucose in the blood. When insulin levels fall, the liver will start breaking down glycogen to release glucose into the circulation. In other words, insulin puts the brakes on the release of glucose by the liver. However, if the liver cannot respond to insulin (insulin resistance) then the signalling system fails and the liver will go into glucose releasing overdrive.

**Figure 6.7** Insulin resistance at the liver: the onset of NIDDM (type 2 diabetes)

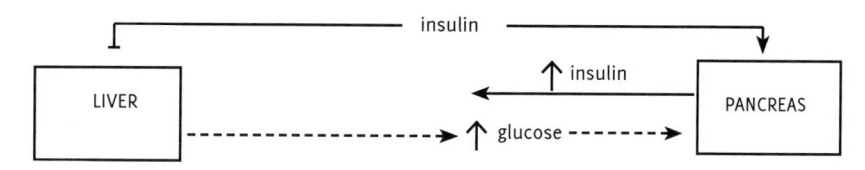

```
           ┌──────────── insulin ─────────────┐
           ┴                                   ↓
      ┌─────────┐        ↑ insulin       ┌──────────┐
      │  LIVER  │ ←──────────────────    │ PANCREAS │
      │         │ ------→ ↑ glucose ---→ │          │
      └─────────┘                        └──────────┘
```

Insulin resistance at the liver leads to uncontrolled glucose output by the liver which elevates blood glucose regardless of dietary input. Elevated glucose stimulates pancreatic release of insulin and a vicious cycle ensues.

We may also see insulin resistance at the pancreas. Normally, insulin signals the pancreas when glucose is in the circulation and this turns on pancreatic production of insulin. Two situations can occur, both of which lead to decreased pancreatic insulin output:
- insulin-resistance at the pancreas where poor signalling capacity fails to stimulate insulin output;
- pancreatic exhaustion due to the deterioration or destruction of the insulin-producing cells of the pancreas.

*Type 1 diabetes (IDDM) may better be described as pancreatic failure to produce insulin.*

The outcome in both scenarios is a relative deficiency of insulin which leads to type 1 diabetes (insulin-dependent diabetes mellitus or IDDM).

**Figure 6.8** Insulin resistance and insulin exhaustion at the pancreas – type 1 diabetes (IDDM)

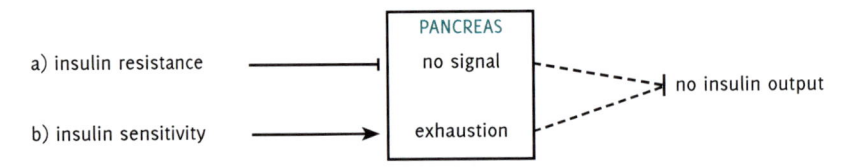

```
                                    PANCREAS
a) insulin resistance    ———————|   no signal    ----
                                                      ---→| no insulin output
b) insulin sensitivity   ———————→   exhaustion   ----
```

Prolonged stimulation of the pancreas by insulin can lead to insulin resistance or exhaustion of the insulin-producing cells of the pancreas. This leads to IDDM, or insulin-dependent diabetes.

**Simply put**, the consequence of either condition, insulin resistance or insulin deficiency, is elevated blood glucose. With insulin resistance the cells fail to respond to insulin and remove glucose, and with insulin deficiency there is no signal for the uptake of glucose.

*Cholesterol and glucose become a problem for the immune system when deposited in the arterial and capillary walls; a perpetual cycle of inflammation and scar tissue production ensues.*

## What are the consequences of diabetes?
The knock-on effect of a poorly controlled insulin metabolism is a rise in blood glucose and cholesterol, both of which oxidise and settle in the blood vessel walls. Oxidised cholesterol elicits an immune response from macrophages (specific immune cells), which take up the cholesterol and in so doing transform to foam cells. These cells resist all continued attempts by the immune system for their removal and are deposited in the arterial wall. Similarly, glucose is oxidised and forms AGEs (advanced glycosylation end products) where it cross-links with proteins in the capillary walls (small blood vessels) and instigates the inflammatory cycle. Local inflammatory reactions try to remove the cause (oxidised products) and heal the damage, but as these products are resistant to removal, a persistent cycle of inflammation ensues which involves free radical activity from the immune cells, the release of growth factors from surrounding healthy tissue, and the formation of scar tissue. (See p57 chapter 4, figure 4.4 *The cycle of inflammation and the healing/disease process*.) This leads to a thickening of the arterial and small blood vessel walls followed by a reduction in blood flow which invariably leads to hypertension, heart disease, stroke, blindness (retinopathy), kidney damage (nephropathy) and, in the case of the nerves, peripheral neuropathy.

*Drugs can offer disease management, but they do not address the cause.*

As is so often the case, we feel confident to ignore the realities of the disease when drugs are offered as a "cure". Conventional treatment either focuses on medications to suppress cholesterol synthesis by the liver (statins), to suppress glucose production by the liver (metformin), or by giving insulin for Type 1 diabetes. None of these treatments are entirely satisfactory, for while they offer a method of managing the disease, they will not resolve the cause nor reverse insulin resistance. These treatments, in themselves produce side effects which carry additional risks, therefore the situation will continue to deteriorate. Although it is necessary in Type 1 diabetes to give insulin, invariably the amount given may be reduced when dietary management forms a major arm of the treatment protocol.

## What can we do?

By changing our own diets and by encouraging better eating habits in our young we protect our bodies from premature ageing and its associated diseases. 60% of diabetics who still have some insulinogenic reserves are able to control their blood sugar levels much better when they adhere to a whole food diet which reduces their medication requirements. These dietary modifications combined with an exercise routine (glucose can be extracted from the circulation without insulin during exercise) also reduces the amount of insulin required and ensures better control. Refraining from picking between meals and encouraging a decent fasting period between meals increases the affinity between insulin and the insulin cell receptors (as does exercise) which helps to lower blood sugar levels.

## Tips to reduce insulin resistance

- Lose weight by reducing general food intake;
- Reduce fats;
- Replace refined bakery products with small portions of whole grain products (barley, rye and brown rice)
- Include small portions of legumes as part of your daily regime;
- If you eat animal protein then take no more than 100g/day for a female or 150g, for a male;
- Eat plenty of vegetables, but omit potatoes, parsnips, beetroot and swede;
- Eat fruit, but omit fruit juices, watermelon and dried fruit;
- Avoid all corn sugar (modified corn syrup) and commercial fructose; these products are common sweeteners and exacerbate insulin resistance;
- Low fat dairy products, such as yoghurt or quark, will complement vegetable protein;
- Avoid caffeine-containing beverages; caffeine switches on fatty acid production;
- Reduce your stress levels; long-term stress increases cortisol production which, in turn leads to insulin resistance; and
- Ensure iodine sufficiency.

## In short, follow the dietary healing program!

If you can stabilise your blood sugar levels through diet, you will lose your cravings and you will guard against obesity, heart disease and diabetes. Remember, there can be no healing or regeneration when blood sugar levels are low or when glucose cannot enter the cells. The detoxification diet not only ensures that the body rids itself of toxins and congestion thereby paving the way for regeneration, but also ensures that the body has the means to regenerate.

It is only through specific dietary changes that cells will be induced to flush out their toxins in exchange for nutrients. Nutritional supplements may aid the process, but very little will be achieved on a long-term basis when taken in isolation of dietary changes.

Both nutrients and toxins pass through the matrix. It becomes more difficult for nutrients to access the cells and for toxins to be cleansed by the lymph when a relative state of dehydration exists.

# 7
# Nutritional supplements - do we need them?

# 7  Nutritional supplements - do we need them?

**Quite often a client will arrive** for their first consultation with a bag filled with nutritional supplements and say, "This is what I've taken over the years and I'm not sure that they've done me any good." When we delve into the bag and pull out the half empty bottles we find everything from bone meal to the latest essential fatty acid, all of which promise a new and younger lease of life. As most of us want to be young and healthy we grab the opportunity to try the latest health fad but ultimately are left with a shelf load of bottles.

In my practice I tend not to over prescribe supplements but work mainly with the diet as a foundation using nutritional aids only when they can benefit the picture. When cells are toxic they cannot take up or retain nutrients so it can be a pointless exercise introducing large quantities of supplements into an already overburdened environment. It will create a greater stress, invariably leading to an aggravation of symptoms.

Although we have covered the rebalancing of sodium and potassium and the reduction of acidity, many people may still remain "stuck" at cell level, as toxins released from the cells may become trapped in the extra-cellular matrix before they reach either the lymphatic system or the blood circulation. So an additional priority is to enable self-cleansing at cell level by opening up or rehydrating the matrix. The matrix is the substance which surrounds all our tissues, through which our nutrients, oxygen, toxins and carbon dioxide have to pass. This "ground substance" is predominantly made from polysaccharide chains which have a high hydration capacity. However, when we lose this matrix, it condenses, shrinks and dehydrates. Under these circumstances there is very little movement of nutrients or toxins and therefore self-cleansing cannot occur. Expansion of the matrix and rehydration then become a top priority.

# Dehydration & detoxification

**Most people are dehydrated.** We consume vast amounts of diuretics which leach fluid from the system (tea, coffee, alcohol and soft, sweetened drinks), large amounts of animal protein (a by-product of protein is urea, which is a diuretic) and the bulk of the diet is made from dry, concentrated foods. In addition, the amount of salt that we consume on a daily basis draws fluid into the cells where it can increase the cells' fluid environment by 20%, and in this high sodium medium toxicity builds up. Dehydration and water logging (fluid retention) are two sides of the same coin: the tissues have lost their capacity to move fluids freely resulting in stagnation and thickening of body fluids. Under these circumstances no cleansing or healing can occur and toxins become trapped both within the cell and in the extra-cellular matrix.

*Both dehydration and over hydration lead to stagnation of body fluids.*

When dealing with the concept of hydration it helps to compare the body to a tree; when it is young it is full of sap and flexible, but as it ages it becomes woody, brittle and breaks easily. The young tree is full of pectin. Pectin plays a decisive role in the water ratio of the plant; the more pectin, the greater the ability to retain water. Pectin is composed of a network of sugar acids, galacturonic acid, joined together forming an electrically charged expanded structure that can attract and trap water. The same is true for cacti that thrive in very dry regions yet still have the capacity to retain water in their leaves. Their hydration capacity is due to the network of sugar acids, mannuronic acid, which, like pectin, also has an expansive hydration capacity.

*Our hydration capacity is determined by our carbohydrate matrix, which, in turn, is determined by the diet.*

## What governs our hydration capacity?

Our carbohydrate matrix is similar to that of the plant; it comprises of a hydrated matrix of carbohydrate chains that permeate the body and has been given the collective name of glycosaminoglycans (GAGs). The specific arrangement of sugar acids (principally glucuronic acid), sugars (galactose, found in dairy, and mannose, found in legumes and aloe vera), sugar amines (glucosamine and galactosamine) and sulphate groups determines the structure and hydration capacity of the tissue. Bones have a more rigidly packed, condensed and relatively insoluble structure. Cartilage is less so, until we come to the tissues that are more flexible in nature and even fluid, such as the lubricating fluid of our joints, the blood plasma and the lymph. So each tissue has a greater or lesser "gelling" capacity. The purpose of this matrix is to fulfil vital lubricative, protective, connective and shock absorbing functions within the body. However, as we age, the level of these polysaccharides (carbohydrate chains) reduces, and hence we become more dehydrated.

*High protein/high fat/low CHO diets are deeply dehydrating as these foods do not supply the sugar acids required for the construction of the matrix.*

*Nutritional supplements - do we need them?*

Equally important are the short sugar side chains (glycoproteins) which coat the cell and protrude like antennae from the membrane. These side chains play crucial biological roles in the recognition of events within the cell's vicinity. These antennae send signals to alert the immune system, receive signals from hormones and neurotransmitters, regulate cell growth and cell-to-cell communication, and by forming an umbrella over potential antigenic sites on the cell membrane, protect it from autoimmune destruction. These glycoproteins even determine our blood type.

*Vegetables, fruits, legumes and grains are high in soluble fire; lemons are very high in pectin. Bone stock is rich in gelatin – an important source of GAGs (glycosaminoglycans).*

When we start losing our matrix we begin to contract; our cells lose their communication capacity and toxins become trapped in the matrix. In order to enable detoxification, we need to open and expand the matrix, increase its hydration capacity, so that toxins can be moved out of the tissues and into the lymph and be detoxified by the liver and kidneys. It's important to understand that the composition of the matrix is determined by what we eat. A high protein, high fat diet will shrink your matrix faster than anything else, as these foods have no hydration capacity; but foods that are rich in the complex carbohydrates that swell with water (such as your beans and whole grains) and are abundant in pectins and soluble fibre, will confer the same hydration properties that they held in the plant to your body. The gelatin found in home-made stocks from bones also contains essential hydration or gelling properties, and I highly recommend this as a base when cooking grains or making soup.

*Increased fluid intake in isolation of dietary changes will not re-hydrate a dehydrated body. Rebuilding the matrix through diet will address dehydration over a period of time.*

You can imagine, as toxicity builds cell activity becomes more and more compromised. Eventually chronic fatigue, recurrent infection and a breakdown of the immune system will start to occur. The degree of toxicity determines the chronicity of the physical illness or in other words, specific disease patterns will manifest at specific levels of toxicity. In addition, the toxins trapped in the matrix become a constant foci of inflammation which will not be resolved until the toxins are removed. The more chronic the problem, the greater the amount of scar tissue, and the matrix becomes more compromised in its capacity to detoxify.

## How can we start the rehydration process?

Firstly, you need to ensure that your fluid intake (water, herb teas, vegetable juices) reaches around 2 litres daily. If you are not used to drinking this amount, and you are dehydrated, you may find that you are forever passing water. The situation is similar to when you water a potted plant that has dried out; it will retain very little, if any, of the water. The dried compost has lost its hydration capacity and it may not be until the compost is renewed that any water will be retained. You will find that as your body rehydrates you will need to pass water less frequently unless, of course, you are still drinking tea, coffee and alcohol!

*Rehydration of the bowel is important. A dry, constipated bowel may be indicative of a dry, stagnant body.*

Secondly, the diet itself needs to contain foods with high water content or the capacity to absorb and retain water in the gut such as the high fibre foods - whole grains (rice and millet), legumes, vegetables (especially raw), fruits (especially apples) and sprouted seeds. This type of diet will hold a vital reservoir of water in the colon that will enhance the rehydration process. If the bowel is very dehydrated (constipation) then the addition of aloe vera juice, psyllium husks (taken with plenty of water) and linseeds will amplify the effect of the diet and prove invaluable in the rehydration process.

Thirdly, the diet must be biased towards vegetables and complex carbohydrates as found in whole grain cereals and legumes. As mentioned previously, these foods deliver the raw materials for the synthesis of the glycosaminoglycans-rich extra-cellular matrix. If you are not vegetarian, then stock made from animal bones is rich in gelatin and will also support the rebuilding of the matrix.

Once the body has started cleansing you may find that you no longer exhibit symptoms of nutrient deficiency. It is very often the case that the body, through its self-cleansing process, is able to re-establish its nutrient status. Nutrients from the diet are better absorbed and then retained by the cells. If you do need extra help, provided that the body is cleansing (you can tell this from the reversal of your symptoms) then nutritional supplementation may be of an advantage.

Never fall into the trap of "symptom" management with supplements. Supplements tend to be marketed for their "symptom relief" capacity. It is true that symptoms do exist in nutrient deficiency states (usually induced by poor diet) but it is the toxicity which then ensues that exacerbates the deficiency state. Under these circumstances, no amount of supplementation will change the overall picture. Transient changes may occur with supplementation, but invariably as soon as the supplement is removed the symptoms return - truly a symptomatic treatment where you are merely treating the symptoms of pollution rather than the pollution itself. This sort of disease management, by default, permits a deepening of the picture and health will continue to spiral downwards.

*Both nutrients and toxins pass through the matrix. It becomes more difficult for nutrients to access the cells and for toxins to be cleansed by the lymph when a relative state of dehydration exists.*

*Make sure when you treat symptoms that you are also treating the cause itself. Very often, by removing the pollution, the symptoms resolve.*

# Valuable nutrients in the detoxification process

**Magnesium and B6** (preferably taken in its active form as pyridoxal-5-phospate) are two of the few nutritional supplements that can be of value in assisting the hydration process. Whether they are introduced at the beginning of treatment or after the first couple of months depends upon the degree of congestion within the body. If you are embarking on a do-it-yourself regime it is probably better to wait a couple of months before introducing magnesium. Magnesium, as you may remember, is important for the distribution of minerals across the cell membrane; it encourages the entry of potassium and the removal of sodium. The cell is then correctly hydrated.

Valuable sources of magnesium  mg/100g

| RDI 350-400mg | |
|---|---|
| Brazil nuts | 410 |
| Cashews | 265 |
| Almonds | 260 |
| Chickpeas | 180 |
| Kidney beans | 202 |
| Butter beans | 185 |
| Haricot beans | 203 |
| Millet | 184 |
| Oats | 120 |
| Brown rice | 100 |
| Wheat germ | 319 |
| Wholemeal flour | 163 |

Valuable sources of calcium  mg/100g

| RDI 400-500mg (for an adult) | |
|---|---|
| Brazil nuts | 180 |
| Almonds | 250 |
| Sunflower seeds | 133 |
| Chickpeas | 167 |
| Kidney beans | 157 |
| Tofu | 504 |
| Haricot beans | 203 |
| Parsley | 330 |
| Watercress | 220 |
| Spinach | 600 |
| Lemon | 110 |
| Orange | 85 |
| Blackberries | 63 |
| Broccoli | 75 |
| Chinese leaves | 155 |
| Leeks | 61 |

Overall calcium balance is dependent upon magnesium status. Therefore diets high in dairy, which induce magnesium deficiencies, do not promote a healthy calcium balance. Legumes, nuts and whole grains all have a good calcium/magnesium ratio.

Many of the nutrient absorption processes are energy dependent, requiring magnesium and B6. When magnesium and B6 deficiencies are made good there will be more efficient absorption of other elements such as iron, zinc, manganese, chromium and selenium, and the body will naturally regain its nutrient status. In addition, don't forget that the absorption and retention of calcium is improved with magnesium supplementation.

**Note:** I do not generally supplement with magnesium in cases of asthma, eczema or high blood pressure as this mineral can initially aggravate the picture, particularly if there is a lot of fluid retention. It is better to work with the high potassium/low sodium diet and then add magnesium later into treatment when the body has sufficiently reduced its excess fluid.

Valuable sources of vitamin D mcg/100g

| RDI 2.5-10.0 mcg/day (100-400 IUs) | |
|---|---|
| Cod liver oil | 213.0 |
| Herrings | 24.7 |
| Salmon | 11.9 |
| Sardines/pilchards | 8.0 |
| Tuna | 6.0 |
| Eggs | 1.75 |
| Butter | 0.75 |
| Liver | 0.4 |
| Cheese | 0.25 |
| Cream | 0.25 |
| Milk | 0.01 |

Vitamin D is essential for the absorption of calcium. 90% of our vitamin D should be metabolised by the skin through the action of sunlight on 7-dehydrocholesterol which forms D3. However, with the growing use of sun barrier creams which inhibit this process, it is likely that we could become vitamin D, and therefore calcium, deficient. As less than 10% of the daily requirement is provided by the diet as D2 (ergocalciferol) or D3, it may be wise to supplement with cod liver oil capsules periodically (never exceed the stated dose, unless under medical supervision). Food sources of vitamin D are not plentiful except in oily fish which accumulate vitamin D from ingesting the surface plankton exposed to the sun. Vegetables, cereals, nuts, legumes and fruit contain no vitamin D, while animal protein and white fish contain comparatively little. Vegans must be particularly careful. Dairy products do not make a substantial contribution unless fortified.

## 7  Nutritional supplements - do we need them?

*During long-term supplementation, balance your w6 series and w3 series in a ratio of 4:1*

**Essential fatty acids** Correct hydration is also dependent upon the type of fats at the cell membrane. As we know fats do not mix with water, they repel it. But when the fatty acid/glycerol units become charged with phosphate and nitrogenous groups to form lecithin (phospholipids), they attract water. The cell membrane, which interfaces with water both on the inside of the cell and the outside, is composed of a phospholipid bi-layer. In addition, the cell membrane depends upon a high proportion of essential fatty acids (found in whole grains, nuts and seeds and the fish oils) in its structure, often referred to as the omega 6 and omega 3 series. However, as most diets are high in saturated fats, cholesterol and damaged fats or trans-fatty acids (formed during the processing of oil and manufacture of margarine) and are low in the essential fatty acids, then these saturated and damaged fats become deposited in the cell membrane making it rigid and compromising its function. Under these circumstances the cell membrane loses its integrity and its capacity to communicate, and toxic waste may gain entry and accumulate within the cell.

*EFAs, with their longer chains and multiple double bonds, are more soluble, and therefore more Yin.*

If we return to the Chinese concept of Yin and Yang, where the Yin is water (or hydration) and the Yang is fire (or inflammation), then the nature of the fatty acids at the cell membrane takes on a new meaning. Essential fatty acids, with their multiple double bonds, carry strong electrical fields which attract water, so are more Yin. You will notice that you can remove flaxseed oil from a container just by using hot water whereas other fats, such as olive oil, may require some detergent. Not only are these oils more water-soluble but they pack more densely in the cell membrane, folding and curling at their double bonds, unlike the rigid, straight packing of saturated fats. So they confer greater integrity, and with their higher electrical potential will readily attract oxygen and essentially bring the cell to life.

*Essential fatty acids may either promote or reduce inflammation. Ensuring adequate intake of the natural oils of both the w6 and the w3 series promotes anti-allergy and anti-inflammatory activity.*

Saturated fats are more Yang; they not only repel water but a predominance of these fats is associated with inflammatory disease. The cell membrane is capable of responding to local conditions, and in any inflammatory condition, whether induced by allergy, infection, trauma or chronic inflammatory disease, these essential fatty acids are released from the cell membrane and converted to local hormones known as prostaglandins. There are different families of prostaglandins depending from which series of fatty acids they derive, but a dominance of omega 3 (derived from fish oils) and omega 6 (derived from nuts, seeds and grains) will generally confer anti-inflammatory and anti-allergic effects, while a predominance of saturated fats will lead to pro-inflammatory activity which may be difficult to quell. If you look at table 5.2 *Saturated and unsaturated fatty acid levels in foods* you will see at a glance which foods deliver high levels of the omega 6 series or linoleic acid.

These cell changes occur on all levels eventually affecting the brain leading to learning, concentration and memory difficulties and mental disorders. Of particular importance for brain cell communication is the long chain fatty acid DHA (docosahexanoic acid) found in fish oils – hence the old saying that eating fish is good for the brain.

When supplementing with the essential fatty acids it is important to balance both the omega 6 and the omega 3 series. Although you may start off with the omega 3 series (**DHA** and **EPA** [eicosapentanoic acid]), particularly if you have an inflammatory condition or suffer from allergies or ADHD, long-term supplementation should include the omega 6 series, usually in the form of

GLA (gammalinolenic acid) as found in **Evening Primrose oil**. Mixing flaxseed oil with sunflower seed oil in a ratio of 2:1 as a salad dressing (do not heat this oil) will give a balanced oil, but hemp seed oil probably provides the best ratio between the omega series. Although flaxseed oil is a high source of the omega 3 series essential fatty acids, only 5%-10% of the oil converts to the more biologically longer chain fatty acids, DHA and EPA.

## Lecithin

There are many people who will find that they don't handle fats or oils very well. Under these circumstances products which assist in the emulsification and removal of fats, such as **phosphatidyl choline, choline bitartrate** and **inositol**, may be used. Commercial lecithins usually contain a high proportion of trans-fatty acids, and therefore should be avoided. Eventually fat handling improves and a stage may be reached when oils pose no problem.

## B vitamins

Vitamin B deficiency arises on diets high in sugar, refined carbohydrates and fat. A diet containing whole grains, nuts and legumes provides adequate amounts of the B vitamins. The refining of grains results in tremendous losses. The example below gives percentage losses of vitamins and minerals incurred in the refining of wholemeal flour to white flour.

| | | | |
|---|---|---|---|
| B1 | 80% | Potassium | 50% |
| B2 | 67% | Magnesium | 75% |
| B3 | 77% | Manganese | 85% |
| B5 | 50% | Iron | 50% |
| B6 | 84% | | |
| Folic acid | 68% | | |
| Vitamin E | 100% | | |

Further losses are sustained during cooking when minerals and the B vitamins are leached into the water. Never throw your cooking water away. All the B vitamins, except B5, are stable to heat and acid. Adding sodium bicarbonate (an alkaline salt) to the cooking water destroys the B vitamins as does cooking in copper or aluminium pans.

## Valuable Sources of B vitamins   mg/100g

|  | B1 | B2 | B3 | B5 | B6 |
|---|---|---|---|---|---|
| RDI | 1.0-1.5mg | 1.2-1.8mg | 13-15mg | 3.0-10mg | 1.7-2.0mg |
| Walnuts | 0.44 | 0.16 | 1.1 | 0.9 | 0.74 |
| Almonds | 0.28 | 0.8 | 4.0 | 0.47 | 0.06 |
| Legumes (average values) | 0.4 | 0.1-0.3 | 1.5-3.0 | 0.3 | 0.5 |
| Lentils | 0.5 | 0.2 | 2.0 | 1.36 | 0.55 |
| Millet | 0.73 | 0.38 | 2.3 |  | 0.75 |
| Whole wheat | 0.4 | 0.1-0.3 | 4-5.5 | 0.8 | 0.5 |
| Brown rice | 2.9 | 0.1-0.3 | 2-4.5 | 0.55 | 0.4 |
| Wheat germ | 2.0 | 0.7 | 3-7 | 1.7 | 0.9 |
| Oats | 0.42 | 0.12 | 0.8 | 1.5 | 0.14 |
| Veg/fruit | 0.02-0.2 | 0.03-0.3 | 0.1-1.5 | 0.1-0.4 | 0.1-5.0 |
| Meat | 0.05-0.15 | 0.15-0.2 | 3.5 | 0.5-1.2 | 0.45 |
| Organ meats | 0.25 | 2.0-4.0 | 7.0-17.0 | 4.0-8.2 | 0.68 |
| Fish | 0.05 | 0.15 | 2.0-7.0 | 0.2-2.0 | 0.4 |
| Dairy | 0.04 | 0.2-0.4 | 0.1-1.2 | 0.3 | — |
| Eggs | 0.08 | 0.47 | 0.1 | 1.6 | 0.12 |

The recommended daily intake for the B vitamin group is estimated according to the kilojoule intake as requirements are dependent upon fuel intake, especially carbohydrates. Therefore for every 4,200 kilojoules:

    0.5mg      B1 is required
    0.6mg      B2 is required
    4.2-6.6mg      B3 is required

**Trace elements** Occasionally I may supplement with specific minerals later on in the case when detoxification is well under way. For example, many people exhibit deep zinc deficiencies which can take a very long time to correct. This is not to say that these people need to be on zinc indefinitely. The zinc status cannot be corrected until fat handling is resolved therefore it is important to work with the lecithins and essential fatty acids first. Vitamin A, a fat-soluble vitamin, and vitamin B6 are both vital in zinc metabolism.

*Make sure that you are taking a therapeutic level of mineral supplementation. Labels may be misleading.*

Many people take a multivitamin/mineral supplement. Usually these products are only significant for their content of B vitamins. When you look at the mineral status there is usually a high ratio of calcium to magnesium (which may adversely affect the magnesium status) and if you look at the elemental weight it may be exceedingly low. For example, you may think that a supplement is giving you 25mg of zinc whereas if you read the label properly you will see that it is providing you with 25mg of zinc sulphate - only 6mg of this is zinc the rest is the sulphate. The orotates also fair badly where the elemental value may be as little as 7.5%; in other words a 100mg of magnesium orotate will only deliver 7.5mg of magnesium.

In addition to the low values found in these supplements, which will have little or no impact on health, the grouping together of nutrients poses yet another problem. Minerals are very competitively absorbed. For example, if iron or calcium is taken alongside zinc, the uptake of zinc is suppressed; if zinc is taken with manganese, the uptake of manganese is suppressed. This also means that if you take a specific mineral for long periods of time you can induce deficiencies in others. For example, a pregnant woman taking iron will suppress her zinc status which endangers the physical and mental development of the unborn child; women at risk from osteoporosis who take large doses of calcium damage their magnesium and zinc status - both critical to the formation of bone.

*When trying to make good mineral deficiencies it may be wise to supplement single minerals rather than a combined formula to ensure uptake.*

It is wise to determine the exact mineral deficiency and supplement with that nutrient until the deficiency is resolved. If you have more than one nutrient deficiency then supplement with each at opposite ends of the day; for example the pregnant woman may require both iron and zinc, the iron could be taken in the morning and the zinc before bed. In addition, certain minerals need other co-factors in order to work properly: zinc requires B6 and manganese requires B1. An experienced practitioner would be able to advise you on your requirements.

Watch out for zinc deficiencies at a dietary level particularly if you have a young adolescent who suddenly decides to become a vegetarian. Meat is an important source of zinc and if suddenly removed from the diet it may be difficult to meet the zinc requirements for a growing teenager. The RDI for zinc is 15mg and you will see from the table below that it is very much a borderline mineral. Nuts, legumes and whole grain cereals provide adequate amounts (if you do not throw away the cooking water) and shellfish, particularly oysters, is high in zinc. However, shellfish is also high in copper which inhibits the absorption of zinc - so perhaps not the best source.

*Switching to a vegetarian diet during adolescence can induce zinc deficiencies – at a time when zinc requirements are high.*

## Valuable sources of zinc  mg/100g

| RDI 15mg | |
|---|---|
| Vegetables (average values) | 0.2-0.3 |
| Fruits (average values) | 0.08 |
| Cheese | 4.0 |
| Egg | 1.5 |
| **Cereals** (average values) | 2.5 |
| Wheat bran | 16.2 |
| Wheat germ | 14.3 |
| **Nuts** | 3.79 |
| **Legumes** | 3.3 |

| Meat | |
|---|---|
| Beef | 5.5 |
| Lamb (lean) | 5.3 |
| Kidney | 2.4 |
| Liver | 3.9 |
| **Fish** | |
| Cod | 0.4 |
| Haddock | 0.3 |
| Salmon | 0.8 |
| Crab | 5.5 |
| Shrimp | 5.3 |
| Oysters | 45-70 |

7   Nutritional supplements - do we need them?

*Anti-oxidant supplements, along with the essential fatty acids, may be of great benefit in inflammatory disease.*

**The anti-oxidants** are a group of nutrients which protect our tissues from damage, hence they are often heralded as anti-ageing factors. They include, vitamins A, C, E, beta-carotene and the mineral selenium. Iron, zinc and manganese also have critical anti-oxidant properties as they are involved in enzyme systems which reduce the damaging oxygen radicals to water. During normal metabolism we produce these free radicals which should be "mopped" up. A good, unrefined diet, low in saturated and damaged fats should provide us with enough anti-oxidants to do the job, but with the additional burden of pollution, which increases the free radical load and introduces carcinogens into the body, our diets may not provide enough.

*Be careful not to overlook the pollution that comes from the diet we eat. A clean diet reduces the burden and provides anti-oxidants.*

The problem with free radicals is that they behave like sparks from a fire which burn holes in the carpet. The anti-oxidants perform the role of a fireguard protecting our cell membranes from being "burned". In addition to this they have anti-cancer properties. For example, vitamin A will suppress malignant cell activity and improve the immune response - both vital responses in the control of cancer. Selenium protects against stomach cancer; vitamin C protects against cervical and stomach cancer (neutralises carcinogens from malt beverages, cured meat and fish products); beta-carotene neutralises carcinogens from smoking and air pollution in the lungs; and most anti-oxidants neutralise the carcinogens formed from chlorine found in drinking water and used as a bleaching product in white flour.

All in all it can be a good idea to take the anti-oxidants as a protective measure, but taken in isolation of dietary changes they may have little impact because toxicity in the cell is by far the greatest determinant of tissue health.

Perhaps conditions that can benefit most from anti-oxidant supplementation are the chronic inflammatory conditions where damaged cells are already producing vast quantities of free radicals. These create more damage by attacking normal, healthy cells and the condition becomes self-perpetuating. Selenium and vitamin E are particularly beneficial in heart disease and thrombosis as they protect against fatty build-up in the arteries and help to reduce stickiness of the blood.

Valuable sources of selenium mcg/100g

| RDI 25mcg (dose should not exceed 300mcg/day) | |
|---|---|
| Organ meats | 40 |
| Fish and shell fish | 32 |
| Muscle meats | 18 |
| Whole grains | 12 |
| Dairy products | 5 |
| Fruit and vegetables | 2 |

Selenium deficiency arises among populations where the soil is selenium-deficient, increasing the risk of cancer. It can be invaluable in liver cleansing and as an immune stimulant. *Note: an average shelled brazil nut contains between 12-25mcg of selenium!*

## Valuable sources of vitamin E mg/100g

| RDI 12-15mg | |
|---|---|
| Almonds | 24.0 |
| Brazil nuts | 6.0 |
| Hazelnuts | 21.0 |
| Sunflower seeds | 49.5 |
| Wheat germ oil | 133.0 |
| Sunflower oil | 55.0 |
| Wheat (whole grain) | 0.99 |
| Wheat germ | 11.0 |

Vitamin E is found in all whole cereals, nuts and seeds.

## Valuable sources of vitamin C mg/100g

| RDI 30-60mg | |
|---|---|
| Broccoli tops | 110 |
| Cabbage | 60 |
| Parsley | 150 |
| Green capsicum | 100 |
| Red capsicum | 204 |
| Watercress | 60 |
| Blackcurrants | 200 |
| Citrus fruits | 40-80 |
| Strawberries | 60 |

Vitamin C is destroyed by heat and exposure to the air. Cooking, bruising and long-term storage reduce the amount of available vitamin C. There is no shortage of vitamin C in diets that contain fresh fruit and vegetables. The RDI is too low in my opinion.

## Valuable sources of vitamin A mcg/100g

| RDI 750-1,000mcg (2,500-3,000 IUs) | |
|---|---|
| Liver | 18,000 |
| Margarine (fortified) | 800 |
| Butter | 750 |
| Cheese | 385 |
| Eggs | 140 |

Vitamin A is only found in animal sources. Dairy produce is often fortified with vitamin A. People on a vegan diet must watch their vitamin A status. The formation of vitamin A from beta-carotene is dependent upon the zinc and iron status. It may be wise to supplement this vitamin in recurrent infection of the digestive, respiratory or genito-urinary tract or in immune deficiency states and cancer. Vitamin A in doses above 3,000 mcg (10,000 IUs) can be toxic especially to the pregnant woman.

Valuable sources of beta-carotene mg/100g

| RDI 5mg | |
|---|---|
| Apricots (fresh) | 1.5 |
| Broccoli | 2.5 |
| Cantaloupe melon | 2.0 |
| Carrot | 12.0 |
| Parsley | 7.0 |
| Prunes | 1.0 |
| Spinach | 6.0 |
| Spring greens | 4.0 |
| Tomatoes | 0.6 |
| Watercress | 3.0 |

*SCFAs not only provide the colonocytes with fuel for growth leading to a healthy bowel mucosal wall, but they also prime a positive immune response.*

**Bowel flora products** have a major part to play in the case when there has been antibiotic abuse, chronic candida, digestive problems, bowel disease (including irritable bowel), autoimmune disease, allergies and leaky gut. Specific resident bowel flora species dictate the integrity and resilience of the gut and have a profound effect on the immune system as a whole. An overgrowth of pathogenic strains may lead to inflammation of the gut mucosa, a loss of integrity and leaky gut. From here, increased levels of food antigens may pass through the intestinal barrier and trigger the allergic response.

By ensuring populations of beneficial bacteria, such as the lactobacillus bifidobacterium, we not only encourage gut integrity, but the by-products of their metabolism (short chain fatty acids - SCFAs) stimulate and enhance positive immune responses against infection (bacterial and viral) and tumour tissue. On the other hand, fungal colonies produce prostaglandin-like molecules that have a negative impact on the immune system, suppressing immune responses against infection and cancer, while stimulating the allergic response.

*Allergy is more prevalent in those who have reduced faecal levels of bifidobacterium.*

Quite simply, the intestinal microflora orchestrate how the immune system expresses itself. By working with the bowel flora, reducing the more pathogenic strains and re-establishing the beneficial species, we may alleviate allergy and simultaneously increase resistance to recurrent infection and cancer. Some authors refer to the gut mucosa as the heart of the immune system, where healthy immune responses are either promoted, altered, switched on or switched off.

The re-establishment of the gut flora can be an expensive process which involves not only taking the specific strains of microflora, but also prebiotics, which feed and establish their growth, and natural "antibiotics" which either compete with pathogenic strains (such as the non-pathogenic saccharomyces boulardii yeast which competes with candida) or directly kill pathogens such as the herbs, Pau d'Arco, golden seal, olive leaf, citrus seed extract and garlic, and inorganic iodine.

However, supplementation of these products and herbs without changing the diet will do little to change the environment which promoted their growth in the first place. A diet which is high in fibre and whole foods while low in animal protein, dairy, tea, coffee and alcohol, creates a habitat which will support the acid-loving bacteria and will maintain the colonies after treatment has finished.

*You cannot expect to have a clean body if your colon is toxic.*

Nor must we forget the toxic by-products produced by the pathogenic strains feeding off stagnating faeces. These by-products re-circulate back into the body from the colon increasing its toxic load with the liver receiving the bulk of these products. If the liver cannot detoxify these they will pass into the systemic circulation and increase the toxic toll.

**Remember, supplements** - as their name implies - should be used to supplement the diet. If you make no dietary changes then you will probably be wasting your time and money. It is not until the body is cleansed that supplements can be of any real value, except those used specifically in the cleansing process - and even these can't fight against an inappropriate diet.

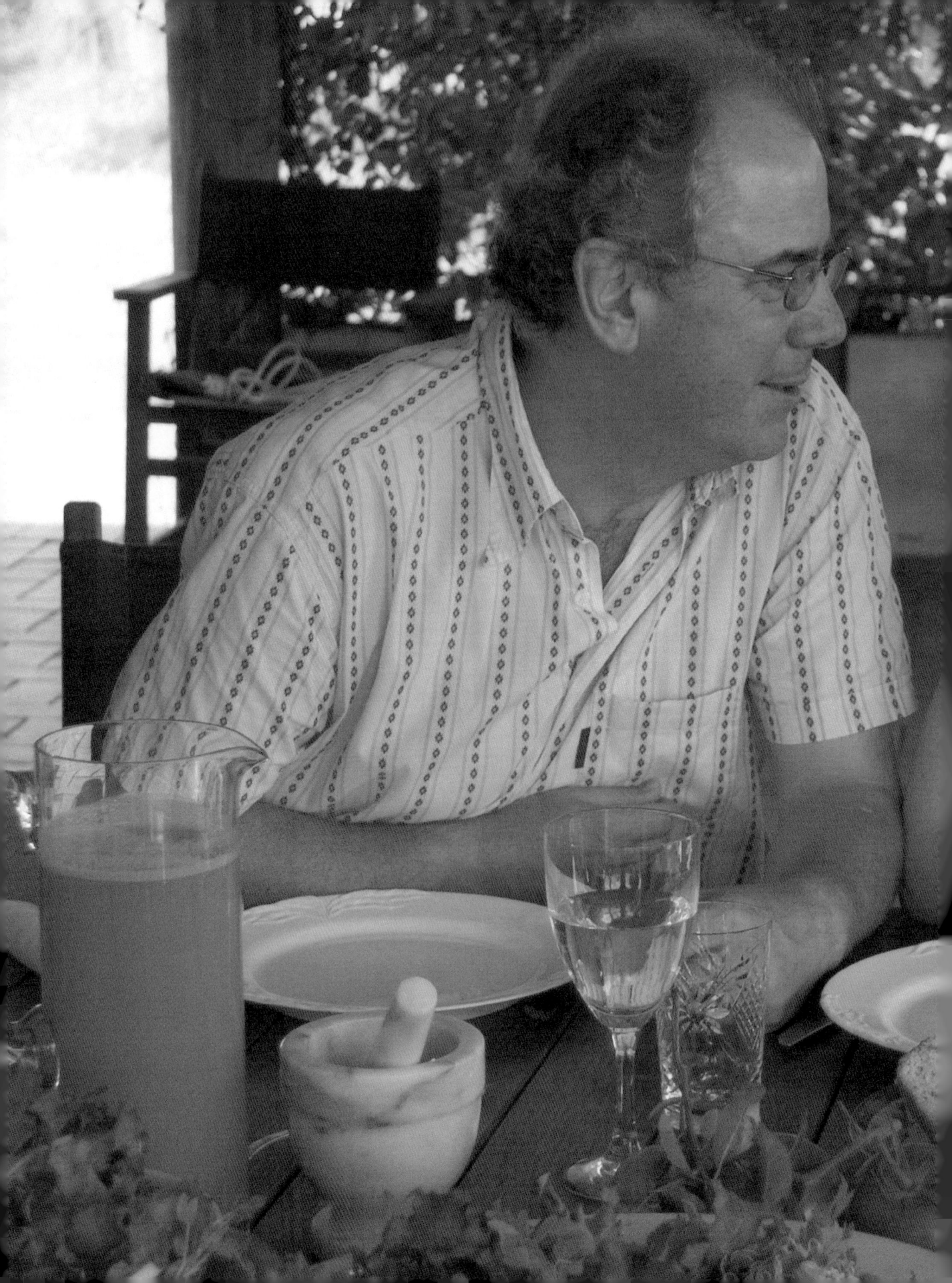

# Part 3

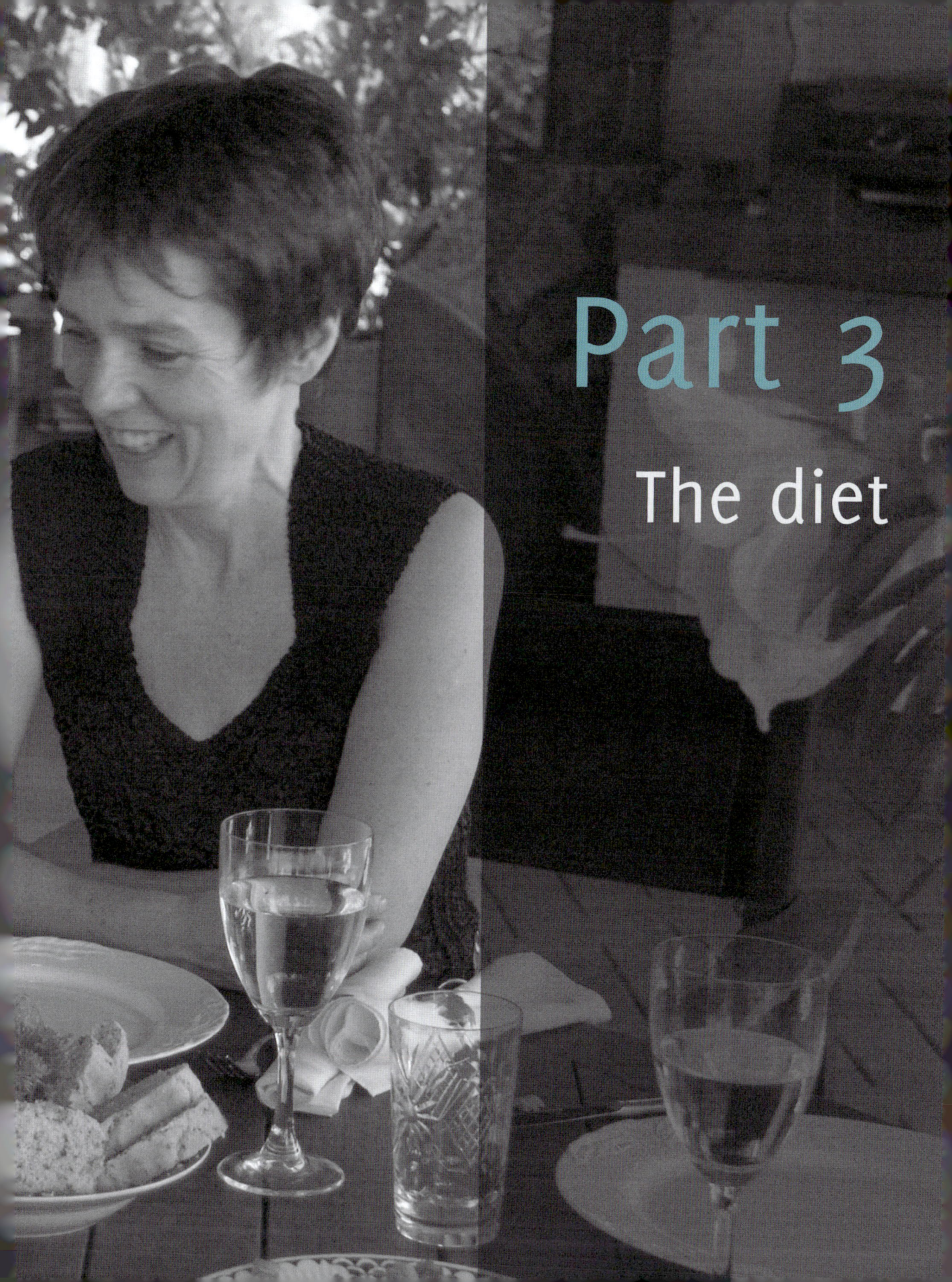

## The diet

Make sure you understand your condition and your inherent level of vitality before you embark on your program. It is best to proceed on a detoxification program where the rate of toxin removal keeps pace with elimination.

Dietary healing is a twofold process: detoxification and regeneration. It takes time to regenerate – so factor this into your timeframe.

# 8

## The diet
## - not for the
## faint-hearted

# 8 The diet - not for the faint-hearted

**By now you will have some idea** of what a basic detoxification plan entails. So you need to decide which detoxification plan would suit you best based upon your total health picture and how readily your body can remove toxins without causing aggravations. In order to help you choose your program I have set a simple questionnaire. From this you can determine whether you follow plan A, B, or C.

**Turn to the vitality questionnaire** and tick the boxes which apply to you. If most of the boxes you tick are in the A category, then you should be able to follow a fairly strict detoxification plan - the A plan. The answers you have given indicate that you can resolve illnesses without resorting to medication, that you have suffered no major health set-backs and that you are emotionally and mentally well. You should be able to detoxify without major aggravations.

If most of the boxes ticked are in the B category, then you should take things more slowly and follow the B plan. Detoxification will occur but at a rate that you can comfortably eliminate to the outside. It should be possible, having followed this plan, to progress to plan A after a couple of months.

If any of the boxes you tick are in the C category then you may initially find detoxification quite difficult. Plan C will enable you to detoxify at a much slower pace - but don't be fooled because detoxification will still occur at this level. Children respond very well to plan C and rarely need to follow anything stronger. I would recommend that you seek professional guidance when embarking upon detoxification if you are suffering from any major illness or mental health problems, if you have suffered cancer, any of the autoimmune diseases such as multiple sclerosis, motor neurone, Crohn's, coeliac, systemic lupus erythematosus [SLE], rheumatoid arthritis etc., or had major surgery. I say this because although it is possible for anyone to go on a detoxification plan it can be quite difficult, if not impossible, to manage your own case.

# Vitality questionnaire

**Into which age group do you fall:**

A. 18-35 years ☐
B. 35-50 years ☐
C. Over 50 ☐

**How would you describe your energy levels:**

A. Good ☐
B. Easily fatigued ☐
C. Permanent low energy ☐

**How do you resolve your illnesses:**

A. Rarely take medication ☐
B. Take medication more than once/year ☐
C. Permanent medication for control of illness ☐

**Have you ever suffered with the following:**

A. Tonsillitis ☐
B. Glandular fever ☐
C. Hepatitis/jaundice/malaria or any other liver disease ☐

**Do you, or have you suffered from:**

A. Boils or abscesses ☐
B. Asthma, eczema, psoriasis ☐
C. Recurrent infection of the lungs or kidneys ☐

**Do you suffer from:**

A. Mild constipation ☐
B. Chronic constipation and/or diarrhoea ☐
C. Irritable bowel syndrome/diverticular disease/colitis ☐

**How would you describe your digestion:**

A. Good ☐
B. Indigestion, bloating, cravings, food allergies ☐
C. Any disease (Crohns, coeliac, ulcer) ☐

**How would you describe your nervous state:**

A. Irritability, dissatisfaction ☐
B. Anxiety or phobias ☐
C. Depression ☐

**How would you describe your mental state:**

A. Inspired and creative ☐
B. Mental lethargy, poor concentration, forgetfulness ☐
C. Obsessive/compulsive disorders, eating disorders, schizophrenia ☐

# The dietary program

**Now for a quick appraisal of the dietary plans,** including the long-term maintenance plan. If you follow the chart *Overview of Dietary Plans* (p176) you will see that all three diets share some basic principles which include:

- fresh, organic (whenever possible) whole foods;
- a high proportion of fresh vegetables and fruits;
- legumes daily;
- whole grains (excepting wheat or rye) taken at each meal;
- nuts (except peanuts);
- sparing use of unrefined oils such as olive, sunflower, safflower and flaxseed oil;
- limited use of animal protein (none if you are vegetarian) and dairy products; and
- the omission of salt

For a fuller understanding of your program you will need to read through *Dietary Recommendations* (p197) which gives specific instructions and an in-depth explanation for each recommendation.

## General principles for each plan

**Plan A** is the strictest detoxification plan. You will need to take note of the margin text throughout the *Dietary Recommendations* section. This program is virtually vegetarian, but for non-vegetarians, fish may be included twice weekly (one serve measures 100g per serve for a female and 150g per serve for a male). You are not permitted dairy, eggs or wheat products (wheat germ is allowed if you are not sensitive to gluten). Vegetable juices are included on this program. The only oils that are included are a mix of flaxseed oil and sunflower seed oil, taken as a dressing.

**Plan B** is a slight modification of Plan A. We may omit the vegetable juices which reduces the pace of detoxification. Follow Plan A but include:

- 2 eggs/week;
- organic skimmed milk yoghurt (100g daily) or quark (50g daily); and
- optional - 1 serve of whole wheat or rye weekly (1 serve = two slices of sour dough wheat or rye bread, or a modest serve of wholemeal pasta).

**Plan C** represents a modification of Plan A and Plan B. It is easier for most people to follow and detoxification will still take place. Follow Plan B but include:

- animal protein at 5 meals of the week (fish twice weekly, organic lean meat three times weekly: 100g per serve for a female and 150g per serve for a male);
- 2 eggs/week – in replacement for one of the meat meals. Keep 2 days animal protein free (other than yoghurt); and
- optional – 2 serves of whole wheat or rye weekly (1 serve = two slices of sour dough wheat or rye bread, or a modest serve of wholemeal pasta).

**The maintenance plan** may be adopted once you've reached your desired state of health. You will now be asking how you can maintain your health without permanently being on some sort of diet. Hopefully, by this time you will have changed many of your eating habits, and the contents of your kitchen cupboards will include organic salt-free, additive-free products and seasonings.

The problem "give an inch - take a mile" exists for all of us and it's really deciding where to draw the line between healthy eating and obsessive dieting. So bear in mind the tips on p213 for long-term healthy eating.

# 8 The diet - not for the faint-hearted

## Overview of dietary plans

| Plan A | Plan B | Plan C | Maintenance |
|---|---|---|---|
| **Beverages:** 2L fluid intake daily is generally adequate. Requirements may increase with exercise. Drinking too much water will increase urinary mineral losses. No tea, coffee, alcohol or soft drinks ||||
| 2 litres of fluid daily; includes vegetable juices, water & herb teas | 2 litres of fluid daily; includes vegetable juices (optional), water & herb teas | 2 litres of fluid daily; this amount includes water & herb teas | 2 litres of fluid daily; this amount includes vegetable juices, water & herb teas |
| **Vegetable Juices:** these should be freshly prepared. Use organic produce only. ||||
| 600ml – 1 litre daily | Optional | Nil | 300ml daily |
| **Vegetables:** you are looking to take at least 2.5kg daily. Juicing increases the volume of vegetables taken. 300g of apple + 300g vegetables = 300ml juice ||||
| Around 2.5kg daily; take raw and cooked, twice daily | As for Plan A | As for Plan A | Take vegetables twice daily; be conscious of keeping up amounts |
| **Fruit:** can be taken as a snack or part of the meal. Do not substitute vegetables for fruit as vegetables have a higher mineral value ||||
| Up to 4 serves daily (excluding those used in juicing) | As for Plan A | As for Plan A | As for Plan A |
| **Cereal Grains:** small amounts at each meal. Brown rice and oats are preferred. If you are sensitive to gluten then exclude wheat, oats, rye and barley. Sour dough breads are preferred to yeast-proved breads. 1 serve of wheat/rye = 2 slices bread or small portion of pasta, or equivalent ||||
| Permitted grains: oats, brown rice, buckwheat, millet, quinoa, barley and sweet corn. | + 1 serve of whole wheat or rye once weekly | + 1 serve of whole wheat or rye twice weekly | + 1 serve of whole wheat/rye daily as the grain portion of a meal |
| **Legumes:** peas, beans and lentils ||||
| Taken once or twice daily with cereal grain | As for Plan A | As for Plan A | As for Plan A |
| **Soy products:** over-consumption is best avoided. Minimal amounts of soy as tofu, soy milk or yoghurt may be taken ||||
| Tofu once weekly (optional) | As for Plan A | As for Plan A | Tofu 1-2 times weekly |
| **Nuts:** these should be taken as part of a meal. Nut butters are not allowed, but a little tahini is permitted on occasion ||||
| Almonds, cashews, hazelnuts, pine nuts; sunflower, pumpkin, sesame and linseeds | As for Plan A | As for Plan A | + small amounts of walnuts, brazil nuts |
| **Oils:** these should be cold-pressed and organic. Keep refrigerated. Never heat flaxseed, sunflower or safflower oils ||||
| Flaxseed 20ml + sunflower seed 10ml as a dressing | + olive oil (minimal use) | + olive oil (minimal use) | + unsalted butter/ghee in moderation |
| **Fish:** best taken fresh or fozen. Canned tuna may contain high levels of mercury. ||||
| Twice weekly (optional) | Twice weekly (optional) | Twice weekly (optional) | Twice weekly (optional) |
| **Meat:** 1 serve = 100g for a female and 150g for a male. Take maximum of one serve daily (meat or fish), if not vegetarian. Aim to have 2 days of the week meat/fish free. De-fatted chicken stock is allowed ||||
| Nil | Nil | 3 serves meat/week; lean chicken, beef or lamb | Daily serve of animal protein |
| **Eggs** ||||
| Nil | 2 eggs/week (optional) | 2 eggs replace 1 serve of meat | 2 eggs/week (optional) |
| **Dairy:** always choose organic dairy products ||||
| Nil | 100g skimmed milk yoghurt or 50g quark daily | As for Plan B | + small serves of cheese on occasion |

# Dietary recommendations

**The dietary guidelines below** will help you devise your diet. The recommendations made may be adopted long-term. If you wish to follow a stronger detoxification plan then take special note of the suggestions made in italic. However, it is advisable to seek professional help to ensure that detoxification does not exceed the rate of elimination and that the treatment is regenerative at all times.

**Animal protein**, such as fish, organic chicken and lean red meat (lamb or beef) may be taken at five meals of the week, but not twice daily. Two days of the week will be vegan (no animal produce) as this speeds up the detoxification process. Fish, especially the oily fish, such as salmon, tuna, mackerel, sardine, herring, cod's roe, should be eaten twice weekly. However, there is concern about the levels of heavy metals and other contaminants found in oily fish, and therefore if you are unsure of your source, then opt for the deep sea white fish. If you are a vegetarian, then meat or fish is not included in the diet but ensure that you complement your protein sources.

*Meat is not included on Plan A but fish is recommended twice weekly. Avoid shellfish.*

- Avoid salted, smoked, cured or processed fish and meat products.
- Shellfish should be avoided on the strict detoxification plan.
- Avoid pork including pork products such as ham and bacon.

**Eggs** are limited to two a week. They may take the place of one of the animal protein meals (chicken, lamb or beef) on Plan C.

*Eggs are excluded on Plan A*

**Dairy products**, such as milk and cheese, are either excluded or limited. Watch for hidden milk products such as casein, whey and lactose. Goat, sheep or organic cow's milk yoghurt may be taken. If you suffer milk protein allergy or lactose intolerance then no dairy products should be included. The inclusion of small amounts of yoghurt for those following a vegetarian diet provides an invaluable source of protein. Although yoghurt is low in protein, it complements grains and legumes thereby increasing the protein value of a diet to that of a first class protein. It is important to ensure that you get protein quality rather than quantity.

*Diets high in dairy aggravate existing mineral imbalances. All dairy is excluded on Plan A for the initial 2 month period.*

**Vegetables** will form around 40% of the diet and therefore should be included at both lunch and dinner. Organic vegetables are recommended whenever possible. It is important to remember

*The diet - not for the faint-hearted*

that potatoes and peas are not vegetables and therefore do not form part of the vegetable component. Peas are legumes and potatoes are storage organs. Potatoes are allowed but not at the expense of the cereal grains (see below).

It is good to take vegetables in the form of soups, salads and cooked whole vegetables. Do not boil your vegetables (unless you intend to use the cooking water in soups) as vitamins and minerals leach into the water. Lightly steaming is acceptable. Cooking vegetables in their own juice helps to retain the nutrients. Do not use aluminium or copper pans, nor add bicarbonate of soda. These factors destroy most of the B vitamins. Never add salt.

*Vegetable juices enhance the detoxification process and can be taken daily. Take no more than 1 litre daily, unless under supervision. When juicing, use organic vegetables and apples only.*

- Leaf, stem and root vegetables are preferred.
- Potatoes, tomatoes, eggplant, capsicums, spinach and the squash family should be used in moderation. Omit if you have reactions to any of these foods particularly tomatoes, eggplant, capsicum and potatoes.
- Mushrooms should be avoided if you suffer recurrent fungal infections.

Vegetable juices are included in Plan A and are optional in Plan B. These should be made from organic vegetables and fruits, and taken freshly prepared. Use an equal quantity of apple to vegetable (carrot, celery, green leafy vegetables). Generally 300g of apple + 300g mixed vegetables will deliver 300ml of juice.

## Legumes include the peas, beans and lentils. They are an excellent source of minerals and vitamins, are low in fat, high in fibre and provide a good source of quality protein when taken with cereal grains. In addition, they help to stabilise blood sugar levels for those people who suffer from low blood sugar or those with diabetes.

When preparing any seed in its whole state (this includes cereal grains, such as rice, and legumes [beans, peas, lentils]) I recommend that you soak the grain or legume in water for 12 hours, and then rinse and drain and place in a bowl covered with a damp cloth for a further 12 hours before cooking as normal. Do not let the seed sprout – just the tip of the shoot should show. This procedure is known as semi-germination which increases its digestibility and its nutrient value. The initial soaking neutralises the anti-nutrient, phytic acid, found in the outer coating of the grain or seed. Unless deactivated, phytic acid will bind with dietary iron, zinc, calcium and magnesium and inhibit their absorption thereby causing nutrient losses. The "standing" for 12 hours under a damp cloth starts the germination process and deactivates the enzyme inhibitors which ordinarily stop the grain/seed from sprouting until suitable conditions prevail. If these enzyme inhibitors are not deactivated before cooking, they will inhibit your own digestive enzymes from digesting the food. Additionally, legumes contain significant amounts of short chain sugars, known as oligosaccharides, which are difficult to digest causing flatulence. The semi-germination process will reduce these sugars by 50% thereby relieving the flatulence factor! If you wish to semi-germinate in bulk, you may do so and then freeze the rice or legumes in small serving sizes.

Remember, you do not have to have a plate full of beans - a small amount will be adequate. In general, the legumes will form the protein part of the meal (if taken with a whole grain cereal or nuts/seeds) when animal protein is not being taken. As with vegetables, do not discard the cooking water - either use the minimum amount required for cooking or drain the excess and use in the recipe. Always use purified water or, better still, stock prepared from bones. Some people who suffer bowel disorders or severe digestive deficiency may not be able to include any high fibre foods in their diet and should seek advice from a professional therapist.

## Grains

are encouraged, except wheat and rye which tend to be acid-forming, and wheat may be difficult to digest often aggravating existing digestive disorders. Wheat intolerance is very common in many individuals and people generally achieve better results if wheat products are removed completely. Watch out for wheat in bread or bakery products (cakes, biscuits, pastry) and pasta. Avoid hidden wheat in packaged products. Bulgur (cracked wheat) and couscous are both wheat products. Organic grains are preferred. Below is a list of the cereal grains allowed.

- Oats
- Rice - short grain, organic brown rice provides the best nutrient value.
- Buckwheat, millet, quinoa, barley and sweet corn may be allowed in addition to the rice.
- Wheat germ is allowed, unless you are gluten-intolerant.

If you are gluten-intolerant then you should not have wheat, rye, oats or barley.

Grains should be taken as the carbohydrate source for energy requirements and should form part of every meal. Whole grains are rich in minerals and vitamins necessary for their metabolism. Many refined carbohydrates are devoid of these nutrients and deplete body resources which leads to nutrient deficiencies, particularly of magnesium and the B vitamins. As with vegetables, do not throw away the cooking water but try to use the amount required. The cooking water from all grains is rich in soluble fibre, vital for cholesterol metabolism and liver cleansing, so should never be discarded. Always use purified/distilled water in cooking.

On a maintenance plan, two slices of wholegrain bread (wheat or rye) are allowed daily. Wheat flour generally has many additives, bleaching agents and preservatives so choose products made with organic flours which contain no bleaching agents. Sour dough fermentation in bread making is preferable to the yeast proving methods. The slow fermentation process ensures that both the phytates and anti-enzyme factors are neutralised in the cereal grain, and the lactobacilli from the natural fermentation process will digest the gluten – making this bread infinitely more nutritious and digestible.

## Nuts & seeds

are generally allowed but used in moderation, forming part of a meal and not used for snacking. Pumpkin, sunflower and sesame seeds may be used and the less oily nuts such as cashews, almonds and hazelnuts are preferred. The soaking of nuts and seeds for 12 hours improves their digestibility.

*The more oily nuts such as walnuts and brazil nuts should be omitted on a detoxification plan. Peanuts are always excluded.*

**Soy products** are generally best limited – this includes the soy bean, tofu and soy milk. Although the phytosterols in soy are regarded as beneficial for oestrogen metabolism, the studies remain conflicting. We do know that these phytosterols have an inhibitory effect on thyroid function (and therefore overall metabolism) and that soy products are particularly high in enzyme inhibitors and phytates (particularly tofu). However, if you wish to eat soy products, such as tofu, then take no more than once weekly on Plan A and B, and twice weekly on Plan C; and if you are looking to replace milk with another "white" product, choose an organic brand with no additives, taking minimal amounts.

**Fruits** are limited to 4 portions/day (this amount does not include the apples used in juicing). Nutritionally they are not as sound as vegetables, nor do they help stabilise blood sugar levels. They can be taken as part of a meal or as a snack between meals although this may be ill-advised if you are suffering from low blood sugar levels, in which case fruit would form part of a meal.

- Oranges and pineapple may be too aggressive and cause aggravations.
- Watermelon is very high in sugar and should be excluded from the diet if you have insulin-resistance.
- Fruit juices are not included on the diet, except for the inclusion of apple in the vegetable juices.
- Organic, unsulphured dried fruit is also allowed, but not for snacking. This should be reconstituted before eating.

*Fats and oils should be reduced to a minimum during a detoxification diet. Use only small amounts of unrefined flaxseed, safflower or sunflower oil as a dressing. Keep these oils refrigerated and never heat these oils.*

**Fats & oils** include the virgin, cold-pressed oils. Olive oil is the only oil that you should heat, therefore it may be used sparingly in cooking. Clarified butter, or ghee, may also be used in cooking. The other oils such as sunflower, safflower and sesame oil should be unrefined, kept in the refrigerator and used for dressings. Olive oil can also be used as a dressing.

- Flaxseed oil is recommended at 20ml/day. It can be mixed with sunflower oil in a 2:1 ratio as a salad dressing.
- Unsalted butter may be used in moderation (maintenance program only).

In order to secure a detoxification it is best to omit fats and oils entirely (except small amounts of flaxseed oil, safflower or sunflower oil) from the diet. Best results are seen when fats are omitted as the liver can truly release under these circumstances. It is possible to "fry" vegetables in a little water. You need to bring them to the heat slowly, keep agitating so that they don't stick while adding small amounts of water (1 tsp at a time) to stop them from sticking. You may need to cover at intervals to allow the vegetables to build up a sweat, so that they don't keep drying out. If they get too watery, then uncover and turn up the heat. As soon as the plant cells burst, sugars are released and the vegetables can gently cook in their own juices. It takes a little longer to cook in this way, but once the vegetables get going, time wise there is little difference. As onions are quite succulent, it is often easier to start with the onions and bring these to a point of cooking in their own juice before you add any of the other vegetables. Don't be tempted to add vegetables in large quantities otherwise you will end up with a mush.

**Beverages** such as tea, coffee and alcohol are omitted, as are carbonated or popular soft drinks (coke, squash etc.). Mineral water (non-carbonated) is permitted as are the various herb teas and rooibosch tea. Watch for prepared brands of coffee substitutes as they are highly processed and contain additives (lactose, wheat derivatives) and may therefore need to be avoided.

## Miscellaneous

- Honey or maple syrup is allowed but restricted to between 2-4 tsp/day;
- Vinegar: organic wine, apple cider or balsamic vinegar is permitted;
- Herbs and mild spices, garlic and ginger are allowed. Be careful with the hot spices if you suffer digestive problems; and
- Corn flour and arrowroot are allowed for thickening.

## Exclusions

- Most frozen and canned products;
- Processed foods;
- Sugar;
- Salt. Salt substitutes based on potassium can be purchased but watch for additives, but potassium chloride is an acid salt and should be avoided;
- Confectionery, ice-cream, chocolate;
- Carbonated beverages and squashes;
- Alcohol;
- Yeast extracts, stock cubes and products using hydrolysed protein. These products have a high sodium content; and
- Soy sauce, Tamari and Miso.

Focus firstly on the vegetable content of the meal, and secondly on the grain and make this your priority.

When planning a meal from this perspective, you will automatically be looking to see what vegetables you have for salads and cooked vegetable dishes, and choosing the legumes or meat as the accompaniment.

# 9

# The nitty gritty - shopping & menu planning

*9   The nitty-gritty - shopping and menu planning*

**The success of any diet** lies in organisation, particularly when you are embarking on a diet with foods you have never cooked before and recipes and methods that are new. In order to make life easier (!) for you I have devised a two-week menu plan, plus shopping lists which will introduce many different recipes, particularly those using legumes. By the end of the two week period you should feel more confident and have picked out recipes that are definite favourites.

The recipes are simple and most of the evening meals from Monday to Friday are easily prepared even after a day of work. That is, of course, provided you have the ingredients to hand which is the value of having a good shopping list.

The prepared menu plans fit both plan A and B - which just means that no meat is included in the recipes. An asterisk (*) in the recipe indicates an optional ingredient, usually one that should be omitted on plan A.

People following plan C will have a much greater variety and should plan their diet using the breakfast and lunch recipes from the menu, two fish recipes and two of the vegan recipes (legume/nut dishes) from the evening meal selection which leaves three meal slots for your chicken or lean red meat. I have not included many meat dishes in the recipe section as it is easy to adapt these from good cookery books.

You can make the diet as simple as you like and follow your own menu. But I would stress that it is vitally important to make a proper menu plan and shop accordingly. For example, many of my clients choose either the Bircher muesli or porridge with dried, stewed fruit for breakfast, and hummus or a bean dip with green salad and rice salad for lunch (or a soup in the winter). Leftovers from the night before can be a blessing, while hummus, bean dips and soups will keep in the refrigerator for several days, and rice for up to two days. The evening meal may consist of grilled fish or chicken, or a legume dish (usually lentil burgers!) with salad and rice.

**What about bread?** Nothing quite replaces bread! The most common request is - when can I have bread and wheat products again on a regular basis? Remember you are only giving it up for two months - try to overcome the withdrawals. It does become apparent how much we rely on bread and wheat products but this period will allow you to explore the use of other foods while retraining your habits so that you do not dive straight back into the bread bin.

**Eating out and entertaining** is always difficult. Choose a restaurant where they will grill your fish or chicken and serve a good salad with just an oil and vinegar dressing (or take your own dressing). When entertaining at home you will find that many of the Asian, Indian and Mexican dishes can be adapted. Blend your own Indian and Thai spices and make liberal use of fresh herbs, chilli, fresh ginger, lemon grass and coriander. I have included some Indian vegetarian recipes and a Mexican meal for your enjoyment. Eating outdoors is always fun and I have included several dips such as hummus, guacamole, fava bean, eggplant and tofu-garlic dips to enjoy with crudites, along with several rice salads and vegetable salads and a tandoori marinade that can be used with fish or chicken.

Carefully read through the Dietary Recommendations so that you understand the principles of the diet.

# Basic rules

- Have three meals a day and try not to pick between meals. Never skip breakfast as blood sugar levels must be kept stable to allow regeneration to take place. Picking inhibits the cleansing process.
- Avoid processed products.
- Use organic products as much as possible.
- No tea, coffee or alcohol.
- No salt - watch out for hidden salt.
- Oils should include only organic, unrefined, cold-pressed oils. Use a mixture of flaxseed oil and sunflower or safflower oil in dressings. It can be beneficial to take a little flaxseed oil daily. If you choose to fry then only use olive oil or ghee (clarified butter).
- Animal protein in the form of fish is included preferably at only two meals of the week. If you are vegetarian then omit the fish. On Plan C and the maintenance program, meat may be included at a further three meals of the week.
- Ensure that you eat plenty of legumes. These, when eaten with grains or nuts/seeds provide an essential contribution to the protein content of the diet. If you miss out on your legumes and are not eating animal protein then you may suffer decline rather than regeneration.

- 40% of the energy content of the diet should comprise vegetables. Ensure that you have salads and/or cooked vegetables twice daily. The inclusion of raw as opposed to cooked vegetables will step up the detoxification process. Plenty of fresh fruit will also be beneficial but remember fruit does not help stabilise blood sugar levels.

- If juicing, ensure you use organic vegetables. If you are following plan A allow 600mls – 1 litre daily. Use equal quantities of organic vegetables (carrot, celery, green vegetables) to apples.

- Eat plenty of brown rice as your main source of carbohydrate. Ideally this should be taken twice daily. Foods high in soluble fibre, like brown rice, are essential for liver cleansing and the removal of toxins to the outside. Many people who have symptoms of toxicity when they start the diet improve when brown rice is increased in the diet. It will also lower your cholesterol levels and keep cravings at bay. It's a good idea to always have a rice salad in the refrigerator.

- Soy products are limited. Generally they should not be taken more than once weekly on a detoxification program, and twice weekly when following the maintenance program. Small amounts of soy milk may be permitted.

- Dairy products are generally omitted at the beginning of the program (Plan A). The rebalancing of the cell minerals will be accelerated if you can omit dairy for a period of time. Dairy is not eliminated from the diet long-term.

- A supplement may be taken although it is wiser to seek advice from a professional.

- Exercise is important as it stimulates the lymph, which is important for the removal of toxins from the tissues.

- Drink at least 2 litres of fluid daily (preferably water, herb teas and vegetable juice).

# The weekly shopping list

### In the cupboard...
*Oil & Vinegar*
Olive oil - virgin, cold-pressed
Flaxseed oil – unrefined, organic
Safflower or sunflower oil – unrefined, organic
Apple cider, wine or balsamic vinegar
Ghee (optional)

*Dried herbs and spices*
Ground coriander, whole coriander, cumin, turmeric, chilli powder, chillies, cayenne, cinnamon, paprika, cumin seeds, ground cumin
Dried oregano, basil and thyme

### Miscellaneous
Honey
Potassium bicarbonate (Low Allergy Baking Powder)

### From the health shop...
*Grains*
Rolled oats
Brown rice (2 kg)
Wheat germ
Brown rice flour
Buckwheat flour
Masa flour
*Barley, wild rice, roasted buckwheat & millet

*Legumes*
Besan flour (chickpea or gram flour)
Chickpeas
Yellow split peas
Red lentils, green lentils or puy lentils
Haricot beans
Black-eyed beans, red kidney beans
Urid dahl

*Nuts*
Cashews, almonds, hazelnuts
Sunflower, sesame and pumpkin seeds
*Pecan nuts and pine nuts

*Miscellaneous*
Tahini paste - optional
Soy milk - optional
Tofu (fresh bean curd from Asian shops) - optional
Yoghurt (goat, sheep or biodynamic cows) - optional
Dried fruit (unsulphured apricots, dates, prunes, sultanas, raisins)
Caffeine-free beverage/herb tea
Pasta – millet, rice or corn

\* not necessary, but good to have in your food cupboard

### From the supermarket/market...
*Vegetables*
4 kg Organic carrots
Dark green leafy vegetables (spinach, chard, silver beet)
Avocado
Broad beans (frozen)
Broccoli, cabbage
Celery, eggplant
Green beans, mushrooms
Onions, potato
Red cabbage, zucchini

*Salad stuff*
Tomatoes, lettuce, avocado, sprouted beans
Capsicums (red and green), sweet corn etc.

If making the green juice then you will need additional cos lettuce, green capsicum, red cabbage + a few dark green leafy vegetables (as described on p58

*Herbs*
Fresh basil, parsley, mint, coriander, chillies, ginger, garlic

*Fruit*
4 kg Organic apples
Lemons (6-8)
Fruit in season: kiwi, melon, peaches, pears, grapes, mango

*Meat/Fish*
Fish portions for two meals (tuna, salmon, white fish)
4 Chicken carcasses (for making stock)

*Miscellaneous*
Sun-dried tomatoes (not in oil)
4-6 x 400g canned tomatoes (salt-free, organic)
Tomato paste (salt-free, organic)

9  The nitty-gritty - shopping and menu planning

# Menu plan – week 1

Sunday - Preparation Day:
- Prepare the muesli base
- Prepare chicken or vegetable stock and freeze
- Prepare some tahini sauce (optional)
- Prepare the hummus having soaked and semi-germinated the previous day
- Prepare one of the brown rice salads
- Prepare the basic vinaigrette
- Prepare the basic tomato sauce

Breakfast: Choose from the breakfasts. If you are on Plan A then it is probably better to go with the porridge or barley with stewed fruit.

On plan A start each day with 300mls of freshly prepared carrot and apple juice. Aim to have another 300mls later in the day. The green juice is a better option for those with insulin resistance or high cholesterol.

|           | Lunch | Dinner |
|-----------|-------|--------|
| Monday    | Spicy Moroccan Lentils  p227<br>Mixed salad with dressing<br>Brown rice salad with nuts & vegetables  p233 | Fish with roasted vegetables  p253<br>Mixed Salad with dressing<br>Steamed vegetables<br>Brown rice |
| Tuesday   | Broad bean soup with mint  p222<br>Mixed salad with dressing<br>Brown rice salad with parsley & pine nuts  p230 | Lentil burgers  p248<br>Vegetables and/or mixed salad<br>Raita / Tomato & coriander salsa  p244<br>Brown rice with tomato sauce  p238 |
| Wednesday | Hummus  p228<br>Mixed salad with dressing<br>Brown rice salad with parsley & pine nuts  p230 | Bean goulash  p248<br>Steamed vegetables<br>Spinach & red capsicum salad  p233<br>Brown rice |
| Thursday  | Dahl soup  p222 or minestrone soup  p223<br>Mixed salad with dressing<br>Brown rice salad with nuts & vegetables  p233 | Hazelnut zucchini loaf  p261<br>Spicy tomato sauce  p238<br>Red cabbage & apple  p262<br>Brown rice |
| Friday    | Falafel  p227 with tahini dip (optional)  p243<br>Avocado & kiwi fruit salsa  p244<br>Mixed salad with dressing<br>Brown rice salad with parsley & pine nuts  p230 | Salad nicoise  p234 or<br>Grilled tuna/salmon and salad<br>Steamed vegetables<br>Brown rice |
| Saturday  | Chickpea flour pancakes  p228<br>Avocado & kiwi salsa  p244 or ratatoullie  p261<br>Mixed salad with dressing<br>Wild rice salad with orange & mint  p230 | Eggplant lasagna  p262<br>Mixed salad with dressing<br>Steamed vegetables<br>Brown rice |
| Sunday    | Bean & nut roast  p249<br>Tomato & red capsicum sauce  p238<br>Cooked salad  p234<br>Beetroot salad (optional)  p233<br>Brown rice | Simple pasta with tomato sauce<br>Mixed salad with dressing |

# Menu plan – week 2

Sunday - Preparation Day:
- Prepare the muesli base
- Prepare chicken or vegetable stock and freeze
- Prepare some tahini sauce (optional)
- Prepare the hummus having soaked and semi-germinated the previous day
- Prepare one of the brown rice salads
- Prepare the basic vinaigrette
- Prepare the basic tomato sauce

Breakfast: Choose from the breakfasts. If you are on Plan A then it is probably better to go with the porridge or barley with stewed fruit.

On plan A start each day with 300mls of freshly prepared carrot and apple juice. Aim to have another 300mls later in the day. The green juice is a better option for those with insulin resistance or high cholesterol.

|  | Lunch | Dinner |
|---|---|---|
| Monday | Hummus *p228*<br>Mixed salad with dressing<br>Brown rice salad with parsley & pine nuts *p230* | Tuna fish risotto *p256*<br>Spinach & red capsicum salad *p233* |
| Tuesday | Minestrone soup *p223*<br>Mixed salad with dressing | Chickpea flour pancakes *p228*<br>Avocado & Kiwi fruit salsa *p244*<br>Mixed salad with dressing<br>Wild rice salad with orange & mint *p230* |
| Wednesday | Fava bean dip *p240*/eggplant dip *p243*<br>Mixed salad with dressing<br>Beetroot salad (optional) *p233*<br>Brown rice salad with parsley & pine nuts *p230* | Curried tofu *p251*<br>Spicy eggplant *p243*<br>Mixed salad<br>Pilau rice *p262* |
| Thursday | Dahl soup *p222*<br>Mixed salad with dressing<br>Brown rice with nuts & vegetables *p233* | Chickpea burgers *p249*<br>Spicy mushroom sauce *p238*<br>Steamed vegetables/mixed salad<br>Brown rice |
| Friday | Spicy Moroccan lentils *p227*<br>Wild rice salad with orange & mint *p230*<br>Mixed salad with dressing | Wheat free pasta with creamy lentil sauce *p250*<br>Spinach & red capsicum salad *p233* |
| Saturday | Indian dosas with potato stuffing *p252*<br>Raita (optional) *p244*<br>Spicy eggplant *p243*<br>Pilau rice *p262* | Fish with tandoori marinade *p255*<br>Raita / tomato & coriander salsa *p244*<br>Wild rice salad with orange & mint *p230* |
| Sunday | Falafel *p227* with tahini dip (optional) *p243*<br>Avocado & kiwi fruit salsa *p244*<br>Mixed salad with dressing<br>Brown rice salad with parsley & pine nuts *p230* | Mexican chilli with corn tortillas *p251*<br>Guacamole *p243*<br>Mixed salad with dressing<br>Brown rice |

**To recap** - each recipe is coded by the letters A, B or C. Those following the C plan can enjoy all the recipes; those on the B plan can have both the A and B coded recipes, while those on the A plan must stay with those that have the A code.

Most of the recipes have been adapted to omit any oil used in the cooking. The difficulty with detoxification programs is whether you can make your meals tasty enough without cooking in oil or adding salt. It can be hard to come to grips with oil-free cooking as the ingredients can easily begin to lose their individual taste when you are cooking them together, and end up as a watery mush on the plate. However, if you can master the art of "water frying" then you will be surprised that not only is it possible to cook in this way, but that you can also make the food taste good. The art in this type of cooking is not to have the heat too high so that the food sticks and burns, and not to have it too low that it just sweats and stews. This means that you need to supervise it!

# Water frying

When "frying" vegetables in water do not try to do large volumes at once, and add only one type of vegetable at a time. The plant juices are full of sugar, and by gently heating the vegetables, the vegetable cells swell and burst, releasing this sugar. By cooking and evaporating the excess moisture, the sugar will start to caramelise and bring out the sweet flavour of the vegetable. It is easier to start with onions as they are quite succulent. Heat them to the point where they release their own sugars and start gently caramelising before you add any of the other vegetables. Alternatively, you can cook each vegetable separately in this manner and then assemble together when all are cooked.

## Method

Place the onions in the frying pan and bring them to the heat slowly. Keep agitating to prevent them from sticking, if necessary adding small amounts of water or good strong stock (1 tsp at a time) to prevent them sticking. You may need to cover at intervals to allow the vegetables to build up a little moisture so that they have sufficient juice to "fry" in, but keep an eye on this because if they get too watery they will merely stew. Be ready to turn up the heat to evaporate any excess moisture. It's a bit of an art but you will get the hang of it eventually.

There are a number of reasons why we do not fry our foods on a healing program. As a main priority is to reduce of the burden on the liver I often give the analogy - why would one wash a greasy floor with greasy water? But there are other reasons. The structure of all foods, proteins, carbohydrates and fats, changes when high temperatures or high pressures are applied. When we fry food, its temperature can rise to 230°C; when we cook food with water or in its own juice, the temperature does not exceed boiling point, 100°C. Carbohydrates, such as rice or potato, when fried or puffed, may plasticise and their chemical structure changes to form acrylamides. Acrylic is a good description for rice cakes and puffed cereal grains! The chemical structure of protein also changes when fried or barbecued, and fats, as we know, are converted to their trans-fatty acid state. In short, these compounds then become "non-foods"; they are more difficult to digest and they are toxic to the system, while some may act as carcinogens.

The dilemma when preparing recipes for this book was how to make food tasty so that one could enjoy and stay with the program. The truth is that once you become used to eating without salt, the taste buds become alive and you can actually start tasting the subtle flavours of the food. On the occasion when you do take salt, say in a restaurant – it actually burns the mouth. Incidentally, when you reduce the amount of fried foods, then these too become unpleasant to the palate. Some recipes are not possible to use without a little oil, such as in the preparation of curry pastes, or smearing a pan with a little ghee or butter when making omelettes or pancakes, or brushing burgers with oil before grilling – and if this becomes the sticking point (literally) of whether you stay with the diet or not – then a few teaspoons of oil a week may be a small price to pay and surely worth it. If you simply can't get to grips with no-oil cooking, then use a minimum of oil and cook at low temperatures - no fast and furious frying! Additionally, you will see that some recipes use a little tahini – again if you opt to be really strict, particularly in the first two months, then this is not advised.

## A word of advice...

I have noticed that for many clients it's easy to lose the overall perspective by becoming too focused on what we normally consider to be the main part of the meal: to a Western perspective this is the animal protein or the legumes (beans); to an Eastern perspective it is the vegetables and rice. We need to focus firstly on the vegetable content, and secondly on the rice content of the diet and make this our priority. When planning a meal from this standpoint, you will automatically be looking to see what vegetables you have for the salad and cooked vegetable dishes, and then choosing the legume or meat accompaniment. There are many wonderful combinations for salads (combining crispy salad vegetables, bean sprouts, a little avocado and topped with some toasted pumpkin seeds) and cooked vegetables, and it is these that you need to collate so that you have a thick repertoire of vegetable cuisine.

So your starting point is the vegetable part of the meal, and then you focus on the carbohydrate and the protein portions. Adding a small amount of beans to complement the rice will give you good quality protein and after two months, if you are following Plan A, you will be able to include some yoghurt which will increase the protein quality further. Remember, we are aiming for protein quality, not quantity.

If you are not a menu planner then simply create a daily eating plan based on the outline on p212. You can work quite successfully from this point and create your own program. You can gradually start to add some of the recipes from this book, or adapt recipes from other cookery books to increase your repertoire.

When you think "detoxification" - think of giving your body a holiday or rest probably for the first time ever so that it can regenerate and heal!

## Your basic daily diet

### Breakfast

- Oat porridge or other grain such as rice, quinoa or barley with stewed fruit (dried or fresh) and a few soaked nuts and seeds. Add a dollop of yoghurt (Plan B & C)
- *Or* the Bircher muesli

### Lunch

- Mixed salad and/or cooked vegetables
- Brown rice salad (preferred grain)
- + legume dish (soup, burger, spicy Moroccan salad, humus)
- + yoghurt (Plan B & C)

### Evening meal

- Mixed salad and/or cooked vegetables
- Brown rice or other grain
- For those on Plan A or B the evening meal will be similar to lunch, but you may include fish on two nights of the week, and for those on Plan B you may include 2 eggs weekly.
- On Plan C include an additional two meals of meat. Grill, steam, casserole or bake your fish or meat.
- A tasty sauce or salsa will enhance the meal.

## Tips for maintaining your health

- Make sure that you always drink around 2 litres of fluid daily (water, vegetable juices, herb teas);
- Always ensure high fibre foods such as legumes and brown rice;
- Go easy on the wheat products - don't let them creep back in;
- Remove salt as much as possible. Make a rule not to use salt in home cooking. Try not to reintroduce stock cubes, soy sauce or yeast extracts. You can then afford to eat out occasionally without worrying too much about prepared food;
- Generally avoid alcohol except on special occasions. Cooking with wine once in a while is acceptable;
- Don't go back to the tea, coffee, or caffeine drinks such as cola;
- Limit the amount of dairy – i.e. don't let this become a staple part of the diet. Taking some yoghurt or salt-free quark daily is acceptable, but limit cheese to the odd occasion;
- Choose unsalted organic butter as the healthy option to margarines, but aim to keep your saturated fats down;
- Coconut milk in cooking can be used on occasion;
- Keep two days of the week animal protein-free, except for dairy (yoghurt, quark);
- Try to have fish twice weekly, unless you are vegetarian;
- Choose seasonings wisely. Prepared sauces, seasonings, mustards and stock powders generally contain sodium. Be vigilant about not letting those sodium levels creep back up.

NUT MOUSSAKA  *p263*

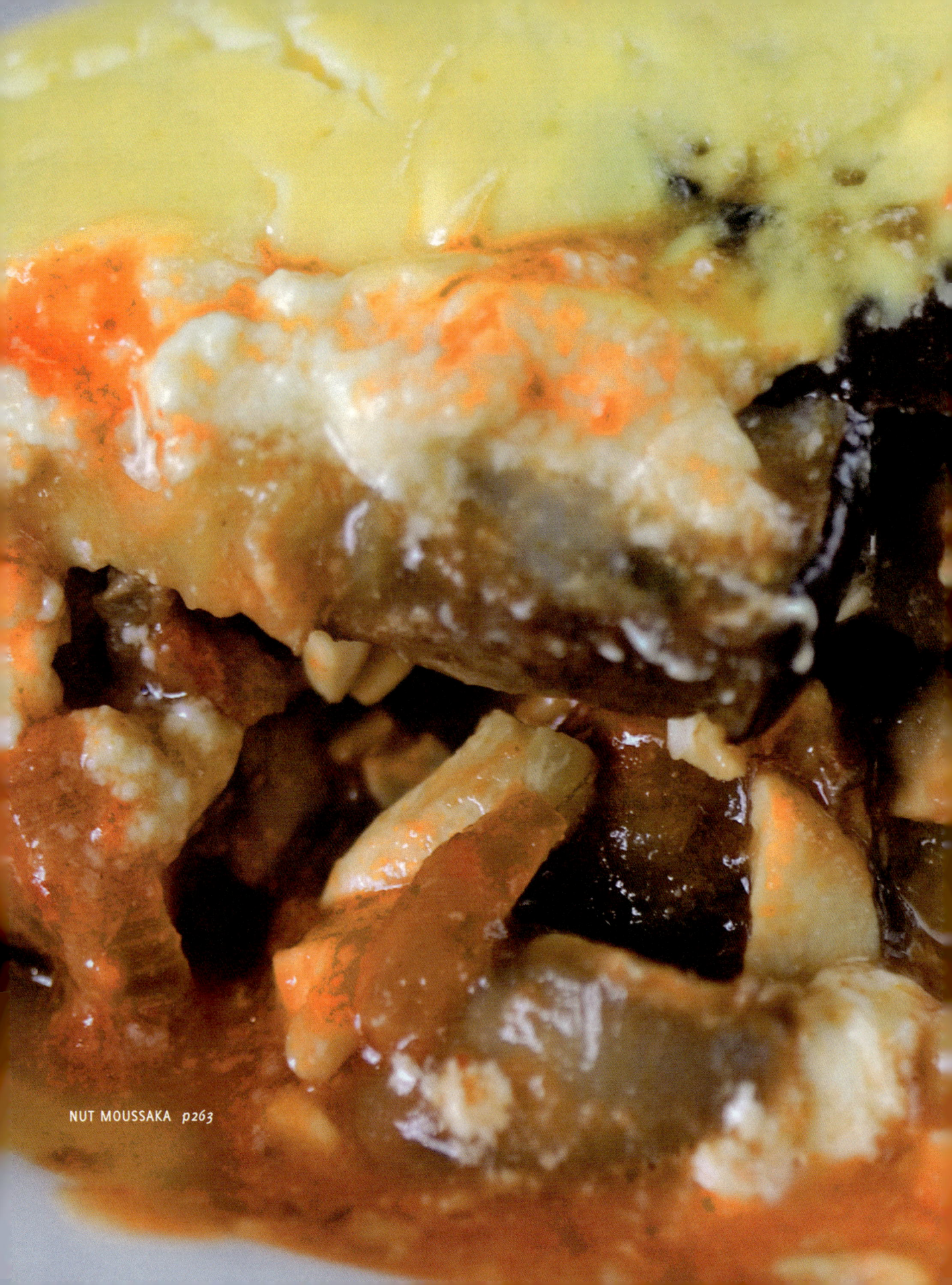

# Part 4

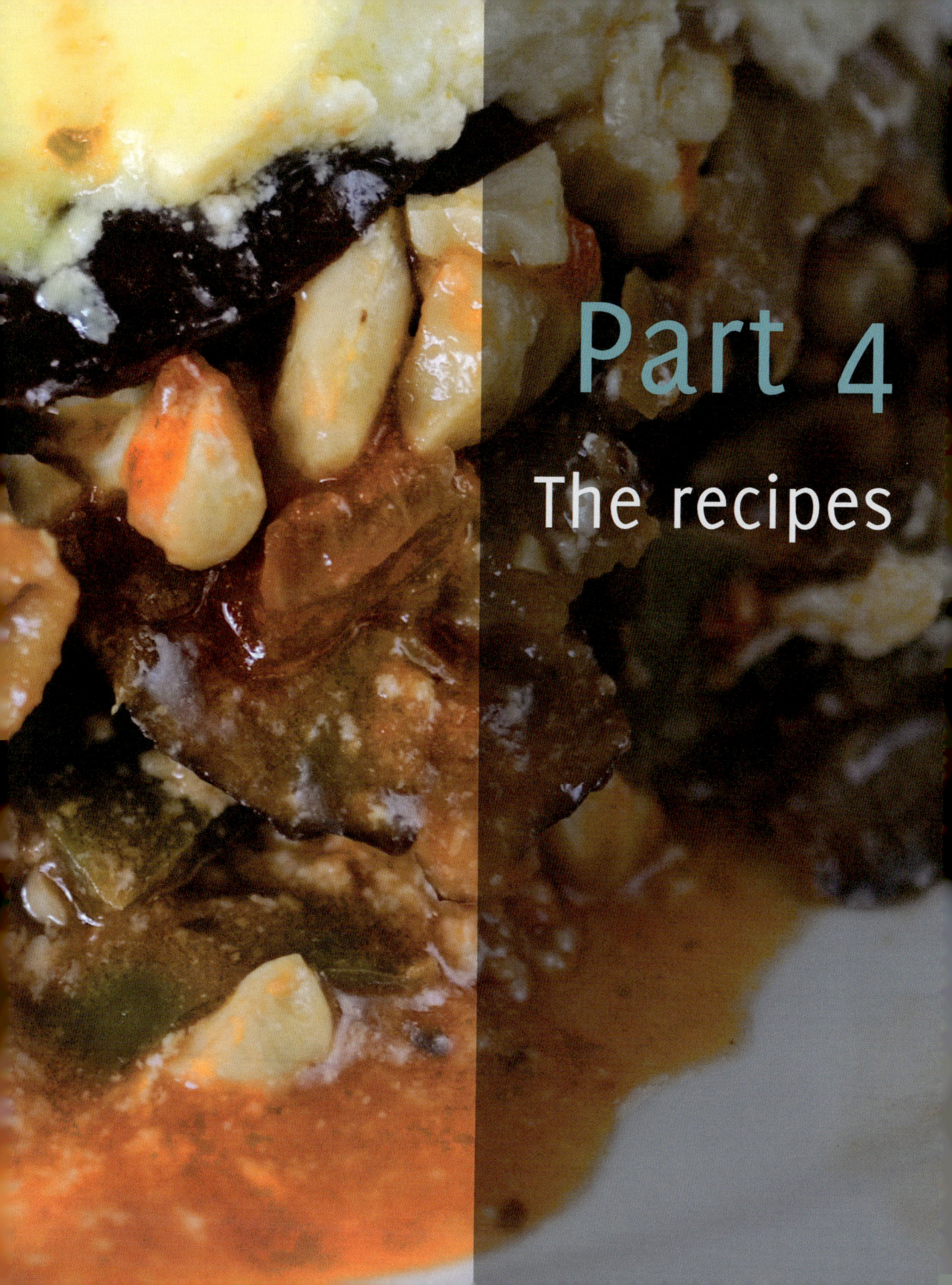

## The recipes

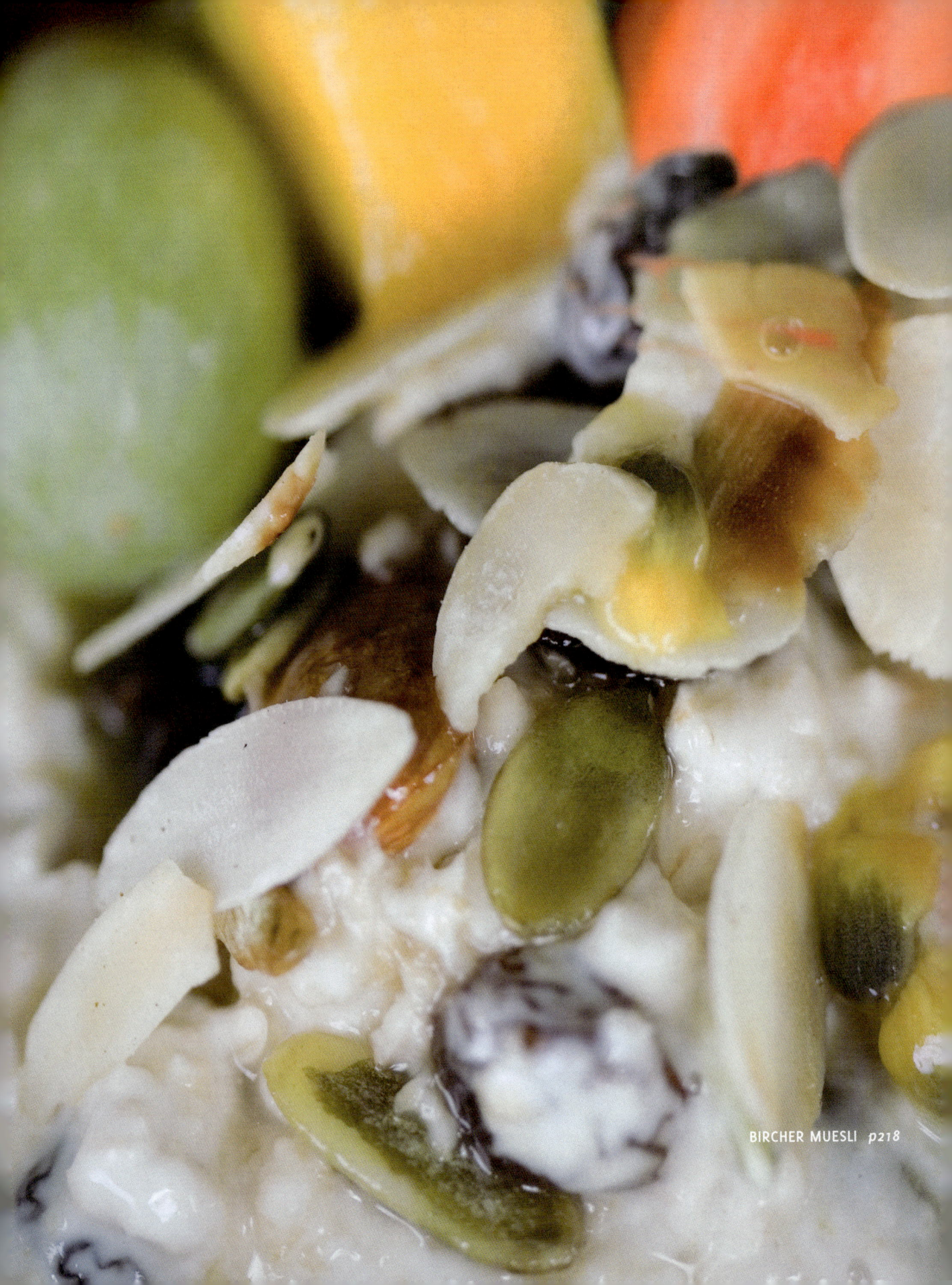

BIRCHER MUESLI *p218*

# Breakfasts

Barley with dried fruit compote  *219*
Bircher muesli  *218*
Fresh fruit salad with wheat germ, yoghurt & pine nuts  *219*
Granola  *219*
Muesli  *218*
Porridge  *218*
Soaked muesli with fresh fruit  *218*
Yoghurt fruit salad dressing  *219*

Recipes

## Porridge  A B C

**SERVES 1**

½ cup of rolled oats
1 tbsp soaked wheat germ (optional)
1 cup of purified or spring water

Soak the oats and wheat germ separately overnight in water. Cook oats on a very low heat in a covered saucepan, adding more water if necessary. Add wheat germ before serving, if desired. Serve with stewed fruit compote or fresh fruit, a little honey, and add a dollop of yoghurt (plan B & C). You will find that the juice from fruit compote will more than adequately suffice any requirement for milk.

## Muesli  A B C

6 cups rolled oats
2 cups dried fruit (sultanas, raisins, dates, unsulphured apricots)
2 cups chopped nuts - almonds, cashews and hazelnuts only (toasted)
1 cup sunflower seeds (toasted)
Add 2 dsp wheat germ per serving (optional)

Combine the first four ingredients and store in an airtight container. Add the wheat germ to each serving. Serve with fresh fruit juice and add chopped fresh fruit if desired (melon, peaches, nectarines, apple, banana etc.).

## Bircher muesli  B C

**SERVES 2**

1½ cups of the muesli base
or
1 cup rolled oats and ½ cup almonds and pumpkin seeds, mixed
2 large dollops of yoghurt
1 apple, grated
Water, distilled or purified

Mix all the ingredients together with enough water to make a runny consistency. Place in the refrigerator overnight. Serve with fresh or stewed fruit.

## Soaked muesli  A B C
### with fresh fruit

**SERVES 1**

Soak ½ cup of oats in ¼ cup spring water overnight. Add a dessertspoon of wheat germ, chopped nuts, fresh fruit of your choice, either grated or chopped. Top with yoghurt.

*Breakfasts*

## Granola     C

- 6 cups rolled oats
- 1 cup wheat germ
- 1 cup sunflower seeds
- 1 cup pumpkin seeds
- 1 cup sesame seeds
- ½ cup olive oil
- ½ cup honey
- 1 cup dried fruit

This recipe makes a more nutritious granola than you would find in the shops. Technically it should just be for those on a maintenance program. However, other family members will love it. Preheat the oven to 190°C. Melt the honey and oil together. Stir evenly into the oats, wheat germ and seed mixture. Place a thin layer on three baking trays and put in the oven for 12-15 minutes until lightly browned. Remove and stir in the dried fruit. Store in an airtight tin - delicious!

## Barley     A B C
### with dried fruit compote

**SERVES 2**

- Equal quantities of figs, prunes and unsulphured apricots (say 6 of each)
- 1 cup of barley
- 1 ½ cups of boiling spring water
- A dollop of yoghurt* or yoghurt fruit salad dressing

This recipe needs preparing the night before. Place the cup of barley into a wide-necked flask, which has been warmed with boiling water and immediately add the 1½ cups of boiling water. Screw on the lid and leave overnight. The barley will be "cooked" by morning. At the same time wash your dried fruit and cover with water, bringing to the boil. Simmer for a minute, turn off the heat and leave covered until morning. This fruit compote will store well in the refrigerator. To serve, place some barley in a dish and add the fruit compote and yoghurt*. The compote is tasty served warm over the barley.

## Fresh fruit salad     B C
### with wheat germ, yoghurt & pine nuts

**SERVES 1**

Make a fruit salad from melon, kiwi fruit, a few grapes or any other soft fruit. Add a tablespoon of pine nuts. Mix a good dollop of yoghurt (or yoghurt fruit salad dressing) with 2 dessertspoons of wheat germ and spoon over the top.

## Yoghurt fruit salad dressing     B C

- 200g yoghurt
- Honey to taste
- ¼ tsp cinnamon
- ¼ tsp vanilla essence

Blend together until smooth and creamy. This makes a delicious substitute for cream by adding the honey, vanilla and cinnamon – just enough to taste.

*Recipes*

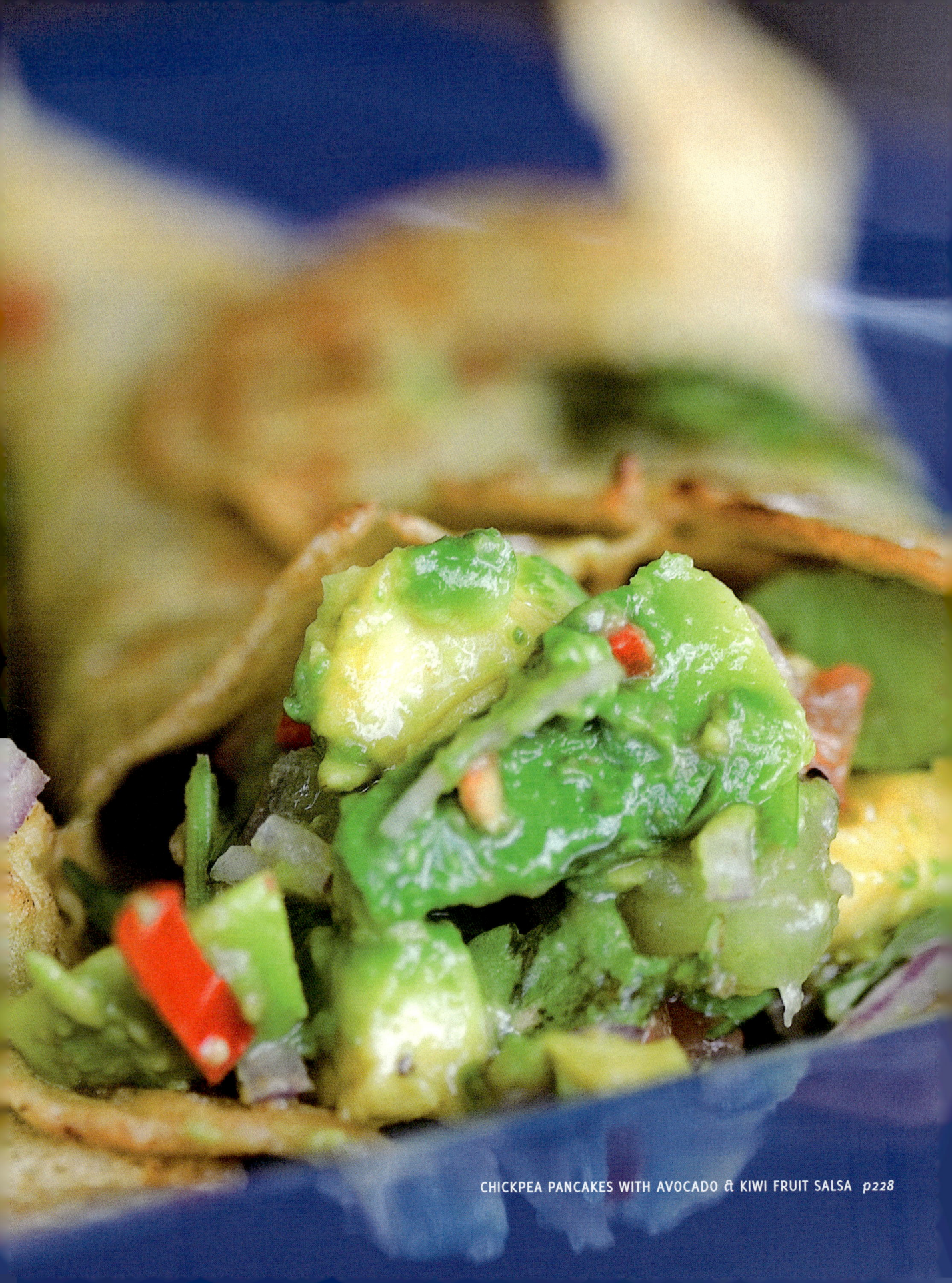

CHICKPEA PANCAKES WITH AVOCADO & KIWI FRUIT SALSA  *p228*

# Lunches

### Soups
Broad bean soup with mint  *222*
Dahl soup  *222*
Gazpacho  *223*
Minestrone soup  *223*

### Light lunches
Bean salad with tuna  *229*
Cashews & zucchini with buckwheat  *229*
Chickpea flour pancakes with 3 fillings  *228*
Eggplant omelette  *224*
Falafel  *227*
Hummus  *228*
Spanish omelette  *224*
Spicy Moroccan lentils  *227*

### Salads
Beetroot salad  *233*
Brown rice salad with nuts & vegetables  *233*
Brown rice salad with parsley & pine nuts  *230*
Coleslaw with savoury tofu dressing  *233*
Cooked salad  *234*
Potato salad  *234*
Salad Nicoise  *234*
Spinach & roasted red capsicum salad  *233*
Wild rice salad with orange & mint  *230*

### Salad dressings
Vinaigrette  *235*
Savoury tofu dressing  *235*

# Soups

## Dahl soup  A B C

SERVES 4

- 2 cups of yellow split peas (mung dahl)
- 1 litre of spring water
- 2 onions, sliced and diced
- 6 cloves of garlic, finely sliced
- 2 tsp each of ground cumin and coriander
- 1 tsp of ground turmeric
- Pinch of chilli powder
- Bunch of fresh coriander, chopped

Soak the split peas in water overnight. Rinse and drain. Add the peas to the water in a pan and simmer for 30-45 minutes until soft, and then blend. If the mixture is too thick for a soup then add more water to achieve the desired consistency. This soup should be fairly thick. Water fry the onion and garlic adding water, a teaspoon at a time to stop sticking, until the vegetables start to brown in their own juice. Then add the spices to the mix and stir in. Stir through the soup mixture and let stand while the flavour develops. Add the fresh coriander immediately before serving. The basic soup mixture may be divided into four containers and frozen, while freshly preparing the vegetables and spices to taste when required.

## Broad bean soup with mint  A B C

SERVES 6

- 500g broad beans or lima beans (fresh or frozen)
- 2 medium potatoes, peeled and thinly sliced
- 1 large onion, chopped
- 1 clove of garlic, crushed
- 1.25 litres chicken or vegetable stock
- 3 tablespoons of fresh mint, finely chopped

Water fry the onion until soft and then add the garlic. Add the fresh or defrosted beans along with the stock and potatoes and simmer for around 30 minutes or until the potatoes are cooked. Strain the soup and blend the vegetables. Return the pureed vegetables to the liquid and heat through before serving, adding chopped mint as a garnish.

Another version of this soup may be made with fresh coriander rather than mint. Omit the garlic, and instead of "frying" the vegetables just combine the onion, potatoes and beans with 1 litre of light chicken stock and simmer for 20 minutes. Strain the vegetables and blend before adding back to the liquid. Before serving, add 2 tablespoons of chopped, fresh coriander.

Soups

## Gazpachio  B C

**SERVES 4**

- 750g ripe tomatoes, skinned and chopped
- 2 red capsicums, skinned and chopped
- 1 large onion, chopped
- 2 cloves of garlic, crushed
- 1 small cucumber, diced
- 3 slices of day-old wholemeal bread, crusts removed.
- 2 tbsp of cider vinegar
- 6 tbsp of sunflower or safflower oil
- 1 litre of spring or distilled water

**Garnish:**
- Croutons from 2 slices of one day old wholemeal bread
- 1 small cucumber, chopped
- 4 tomatoes, chopped
- Onion rings

Grill the red capsicums, turning them allowing the skin to char uniformly. Peel and chop when cool enough to handle. Meanwhile, remove the crusts from the bread and place in a bowl with the garlic, vinegar and oil. Add the tomato flesh, the chopped capsicums, diced cucumber and water. Mix thoroughly and blend in an electric food mixer. Chill before serving.

The garnishes are prepared and served in separate bowls to be added according to individual taste. If you are on the detox program then technically you should omit the croutons; however, if you are on the maintenance plan – then these are fine once in a while. Croutons are prepared by dicing the bread and tossing in a mixture of olive oil with a little crushed garlic. Then place the croutons in a pre-heated oven (180°C) for 25 minutes, turning at intervals to make sure that they do not burn. Croutons made in this way can be stored in an airtight container for up to a day.

## Minestrone soup  A B C

**SERVES 8**

- 1 cup haricot beans
- 2 litres of chicken or vegetable stock
- 1 large onion, diced
- 2 cloves garlic, crushed
- 2 carrots, sliced
- 2 sticks of celery, diced
- 2 tomatoes, diced
- 1 cup sliced green beans
- ¼ cup shredded cabbage
- ½ cup pasta (wheat-free)
- ¼ cup chopped parsley
- Freshly ground black pepper

Prepare the beans by the soaking and semi-germinating method. Water fry the onion and garlic until softened. Add to the beans along with the stock, carrots and celery and simmer for 1 - 1½ hours until beans are tender. Add the cabbage, green beans, tomato and wheat-free pasta and cook for a further 10 minutes. Add the parsley and black pepper before serving.

*Recipes*

# Light lunches

## Spanish omelette  B C

SERVES 4

- 300g potatoes, thinly sliced
- 400g onions, thinly sliced
- 1 cup peas, fresh or frozen
- 1 cup diced red capsicum (roasted and peeled)
- 2 tablespoons olive oil
- 5 large eggs
- Freshly ground black pepper
- Pinch of cayenne pepper (optional)

Water fry the onions until tender and translucent. Add the peas, red pepper, ground black pepper and the pinch of cayenne pepper (optional) to the onions and heat through. Drop the potato slices into boiling water and cook until they soften, but not until they disintegrate! Drain immediately. Gently stir the potato into the vegetable mix. Lightly beat the eggs and add the vegetable mixture to the eggs. Let it stand for 15 minutes. You won't be able to get away without using some oil with this next stage – so wipe out the frying pan and add 1 tablespoon of olive oil to cover the base of the pan. Heat this and pour the omelette mixture into the pan, spreading it evenly. Cook over a moderate heat, shaking the pan from time to time to prevent sticking. When the omelette is browned on the underside, place a plate over the pan and carefully invert so that the omelette falls onto the plate. Add the remaining 1 tablespoon of oil (if required) and slide the omelette back into the pan, browned side up, and continue to cook until the underside is also browned. Transfer to a warmed plate and serve warm for a filling lunch.

## Eggplant omelette  B C

SERVES 4

- 2 ½ cups eggplant, diced into 1cm pieces
- ½ large onion, chopped
- 1 large clove of garlic, crushed
- 5 large eggs
- Freshly ground black pepper
- A squeeze of fresh lemon juice

This is similar to the Spanish potato omelette but using eggplant instead of potato. Steam the eggplant until just tender, but not watery. Meanwhile water fry the onion and garlic until soft and transparent. Add the cooked eggplant and season with black pepper and lemon juice. Pour in the beaten eggs and stir together. Cook the omelette as for the Spanish omelette, cooking each side until browned taking care that the omelette does not stick to the pan.

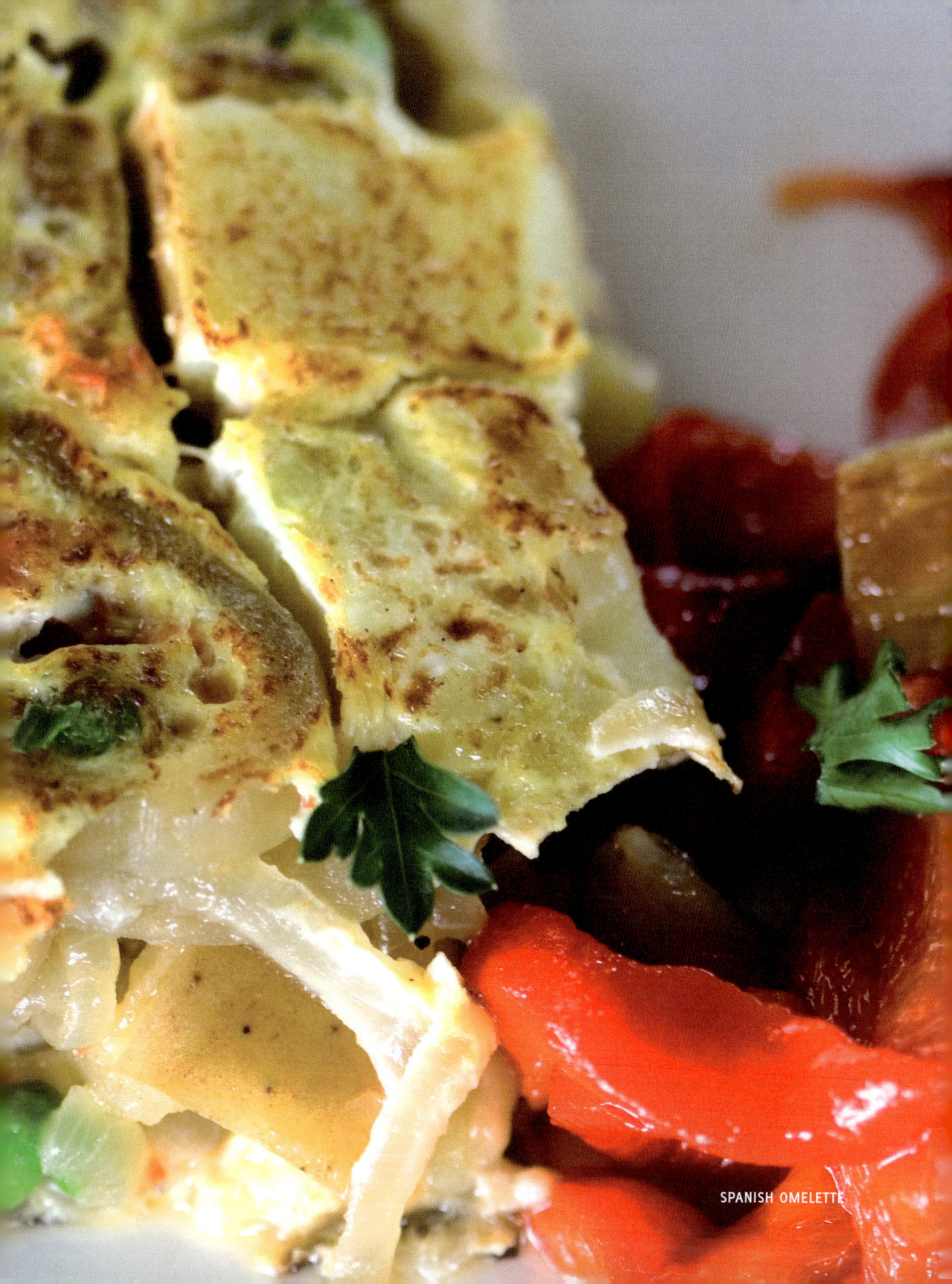

SPANISH OMELETTE

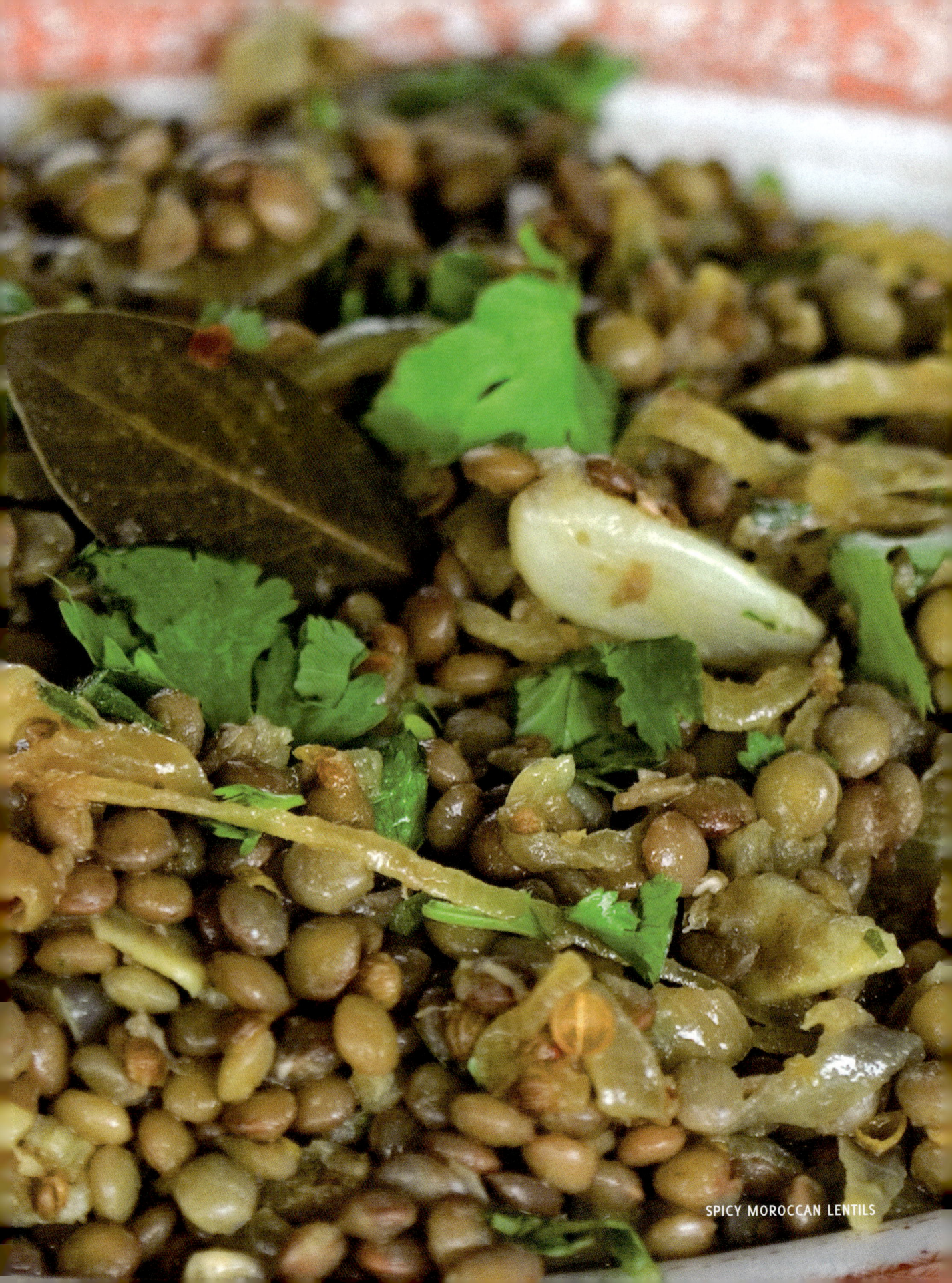

SPICY MOROCCAN LENTILS

*Light lunches*

## Spicy Moroccan lentils     A B C

SERVES 4 - 6

- 1 cup green (or Puy) lentils
- 2 bay leaves
- 2 cloves of garlic
- 1 onion
- 1 level dessertspoon coriander seeds, crushed in mortar and pestle
- 1 tsp dried chilli
- Juice of 1 lemon
- Flaxseed or olive oil
- Bunch of fresh coriander or parsley, chopped

The lentils do not need prior soaking for this dish. Bring the lentils to a boil, then drain. Place them back in the saucepan, cover with hot water and add the bay leaves and garlic. Cook for 30 minutes. Drain, reserving a little of the cooking liquid. Chop the onions and sweat them (without oil) until they are gently caramelised. Add the crushed coriander seeds and dried chilli and stir. Pour in the lentils and mix well. If the mixture is too dry add a little of the cooking water (this shouldn't really be necessary). Add the chopped coriander, lemon juice and flaxseed or olive oil before serving. This dish is best served slightly warm or at room temperature. You can easily turn any leftovers into a soup by adding stock and chopped tomatoes. Add the freshly chopped coriander before serving and put a dollop of yoghurt in the centre. This is one of my personal favourites!

## Falafel     A B C

SERVES 4 (MAKES 16)

- 1 cup dried chickpeas
- 5 cups purified or distilled water
- 1 tsp each of ground cumin and ground coriander (lightly toasted in a frying pan)
- ½ cup of minced onion
- 2 cloves of pressed garlic
- 2 tbsp of chopped parsley
- 1 tbsp lemon juice
- Pinch of cayenne pepper
- Freshly ground black pepper
- 3 tbsp gram flour (chickpea)
- Cold-pressed olive oil, for brushing

Prepare the chickpeas by soaking and semi-germinating and then cook until tender (approximately one hour). Drain, reserving a little of the liquid, and blend the chickpeas in a food processor until the mixture resembles coarse bread crumbs. Turn into a bowl and add all the other ingredients and mix well. Make small patties from the mixture. It should just about hold together without requiring firm handling but if the mixture is too crumbly add a little of the reserved water. Brush the patties with oil and place under the grill, turning once. Serve hot with the *tahini dip (p243) or salsa and salad. This combination may also be used as a filling for pita bread.

* omit on Plan A

## Chickpea flour pancakes  A B C
### with a choice of 3 fillings

SERVES 4

For the batter (makes 8 pancakes):

- 170g chickpea flour (besan or gram flour)
- 1 tsp ground cumin (toasted)
- Freshly ground black pepper
- 450mls of warm spring water
- 2 tablespoons cold-pressed olive oil
- Ghee* or olive oil

This recipe is for a treat. Again it will not be suitable if you are doing the strict plan A or B as it contains oil. However, it makes a wonderful lunch and is worth the effort if you have guests. The best filling is the avocado and kiwi salsa. Whisk together 450mls of warm water, the chickpea flour, pepper and ground cumin. This pancake batter can be used immediately. Add the 2 tbsp of oil to the batter before cooking. Lightly smear a 17cm frying pan with a knob of ghee or oil. When the pan is hot, pour in 3-4 tbsp of batter making sure that batter covers base. Cook 2-3 minutes before turning (don't attempt to turn before the underside is cooked otherwise the pancake will disintegrate!). Cook the other side, remove and keep warm. Regrease the pan before you make each pancake.

Choose from these fillings: avocado and kiwi salsa – favourite choice (p244 ); ratatouille (p261) or mixed salad (fresh bean sprouts, diced or grated apple, carrot, celery and any other crunchy salad vegetable you have to hand) topped with tahini dip (p243 ).

* omit on plan A

## Hummus  A B C

- 250g dried chickpeas
- ¼ cup lemon juice
- 2 cloves of garlic
- ¼ - ½ cup of cooking water

Prepare the chickpeas by soaking and semi-germinating and then cook until tender (approximately one hour). Place in a food processor along with the lemon juice, garlic and ¼ cup of cooking liquid. Blend, adding more cooking liquid until the desired consistency is achieved. Store in the refrigerator. Hummus can be served in wholemeal pita bread* with salad. For those on the maintenance plan, you may add ¼ cup tahini to this recipe and reduce the amount of water by the same.

* omit on Plan A

# Cashews & zucchini A B C
## with buckwheat

SERVES 4

50g buckwheat (roasted)
500g zucchini
125g onions, finely sliced
2 cloves of garlic, crushed
125g mushrooms, sliced
1 tsp chopped fresh basil
400g can of tomatoes (salt-free), chopped or passed through a food mill
50g of cashew nuts
150ml of yoghurt*
Freshly ground black pepper

Water fry the onions and garlic until soft and translucent. Halve the zucchini lengthwise and scoop out the seeds; slice into thin 6 cm strips. Add the zucchini and mushrooms to the onions and cook for around 5 minutes. If the mixture becomes too watery, then turn up the heat to evaporate the excess. Stir in the basil, tomatoes, buckwheat and cashew nuts. Cover and cook for a further 10 minutes. Serve with a dollop of yoghurt.

* omit on plan A

# Bean salad with tuna A B C

SERVES 4

250g dried cannelloni beans
1 tablespoon virgin olive oil
1 tablespoon each of chopped fresh mint and parsley
1 green capsicum, diced
1 red onion, finely sliced
1 green chilli, finely diced
400g tuna, cooked and thinly sliced
Juice of one lemon
½ cup yoghurt*

Prepare the cannelloni beans by soaking and semi-germinating. Cover the beans with purified water by 2 cm and cook for around 40 minutes until tender. Drain, and while still warm toss in the oil and the herbs. Add the tuna to the beans along with the onion and chilli. Mix the lemon juice with the yoghurt* and spoon over the bean mixture gently combining the ingredients.

*If you are on plan A then omit the yoghurt and add enough lemon juice to taste.

Recipes

# Salads

## Wild rice salad  A B C
### with orange & mint

SERVES 4 - 6

¾ cup of wild rice
¼ cup of long grain brown rice
2 cups of purified or distilled water
1 cup of pecan nuts
¾ cup of sultanas
Grated rind from one orange
1/3 cup of fresh orange juice
¼ cup of cold-pressed olive oil
¼ cup finely chopped mint
4 spring onions, finely chopped (green stems included)
Freshly ground black pepper

Cook both the wild rice and the brown rice together in a covered pan with the water for around 40 minutes. The water should be completely absorbed. While the rice is warm add the oil, orange juice, grated orange rind, sultanas, nuts, spring onions and mint and let the flavours develop fully. Add some freshly ground black pepper to the salad.

## Brown rice salad  A B C
### with parsley & pine nuts

SERVES 4 - 6

1 cup brown rice
2 cups of purified or distilled water
3 tablespoons of pine nuts (toasted)
Large bunch of parsley, chopped
4 spring onions, finely chopped (green stems included)
Juice from one lemon
2 tablespoons each of cold-pressed olive oil & safflower oil

Cook the rice in a covered pan with the water. The water will be absorbed when the rice is done (40-45 minutes). While rice is still hot add the lemon, oil and pine nuts. When cooled, add the other ingredients and black pepper if desired. This salad will keep for a couple of days in the refrigerator. Toasted almonds can be used instead of pine nuts.

WILD RICE SALAD WITH ORANGE & MINT

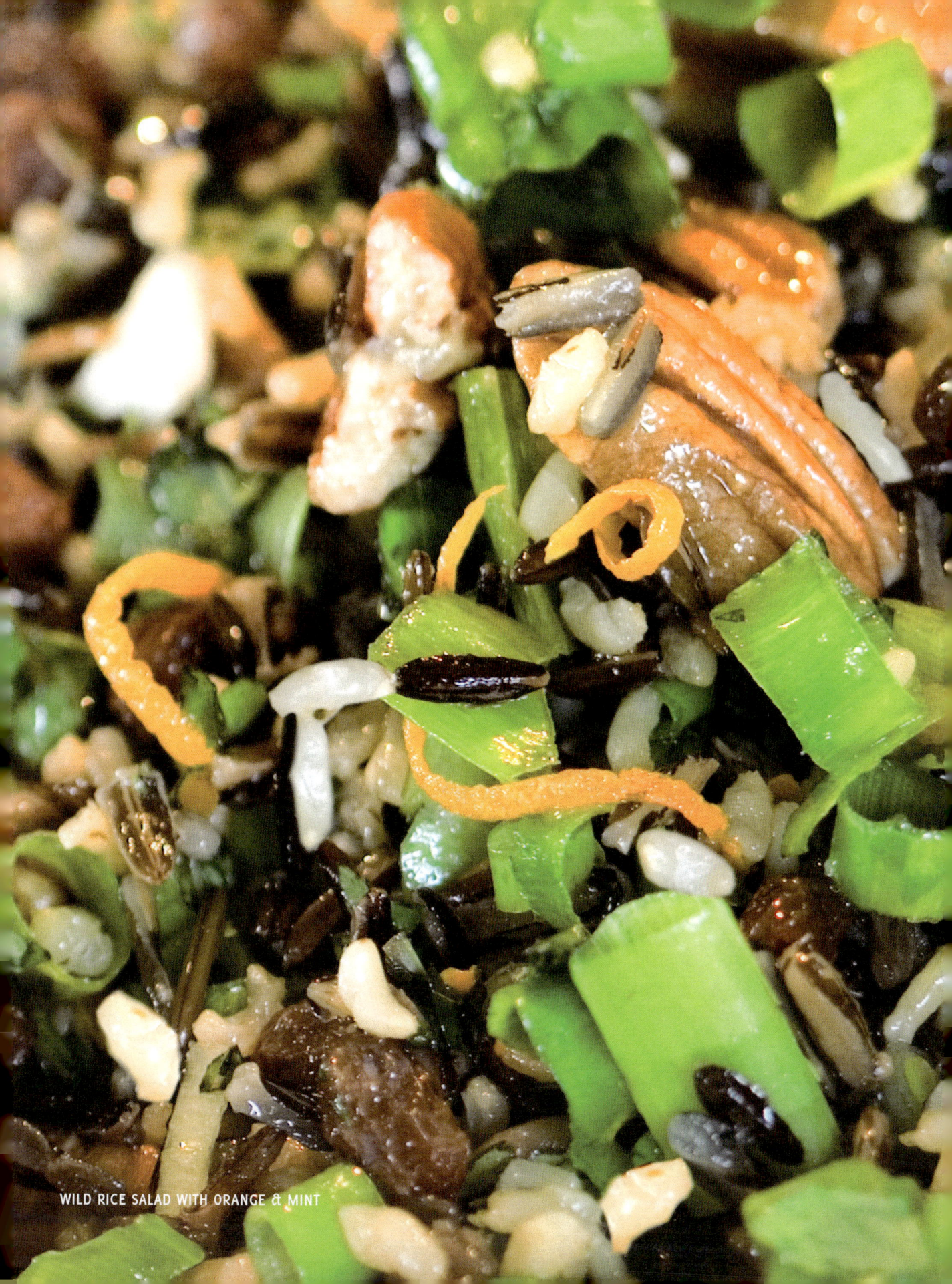

BEETROOT SALAD

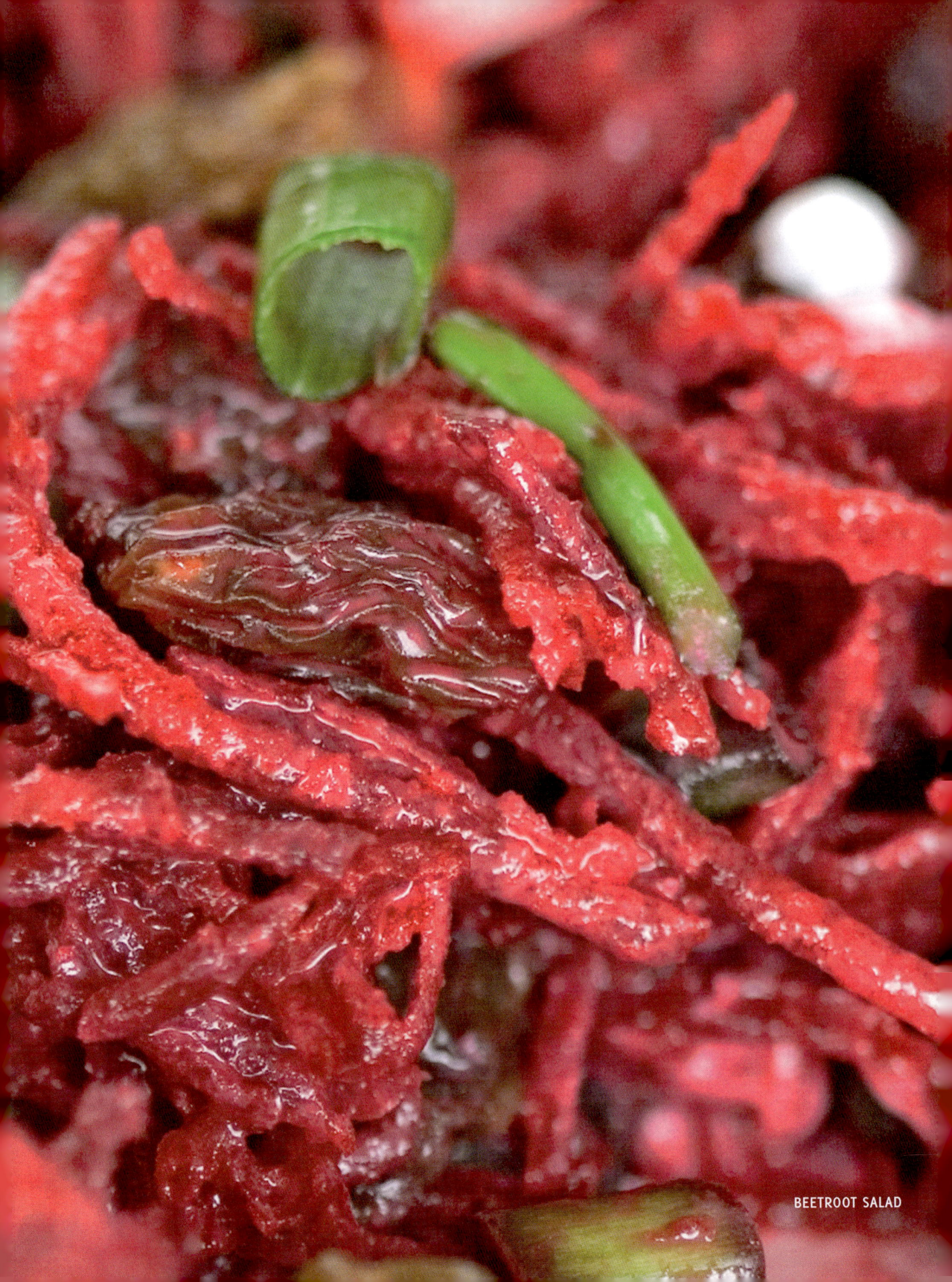

Salads

## Brown rice salad   A B C
### with nuts & vegetables

SERVES 4 - 6

- 1 cup of brown rice
- 2 cups of purified or distilled water
- A mixture of chopped carrots, celery, radish, cucumber, Spring onions, red and green pepper
- ½ cup of coarsely chopped and toasted hazelnuts
- Juice from one lemon juice
- 4 tablespoons safflower oil (unrefined, cold-pressed)
- Chopped fresh herbs - mint, parsley and basil
- Freshly ground black pepper

This rice salad makes use of whatever salad vegetables you may have to hand. You can use leftover cooked rice although the lemon juice and oil dressing is best added to the rice while still warm. Cook the rice in 2 cups of purified water in a covered pan on low heat for 45 minutes. Meanwhile chop up the vegetables and fresh herbs until the mass of vegetables roughly equals the mass of rice. Mix the vegetables, herbs, nuts and rice with the oil and lemon juice dressing. If you desire a more lively taste then just increase the amount of lemon juice and spring onions.

## Beetroot salad   B C

SERVES 4

- 1 medium beetroot, uncooked, peeled and grated
- Small handful of sultanas
- 5 spring onions, finely sliced
- Low fat yoghurt to mix
- 1 tablespoon flaxseed oil

Mix all the ingredients adding enough yoghurt to taste.

## Coleslaw   A B C
### with savoury tofu dressing

SERVES 4 - 6

- 250g of white cabbage, shredded
- 3 celery sticks, diced
- 3 red-skinned apples, diced
- 4 spring onions, sliced (with green tops)
- 3 tablespoons chopped parsley
- 50g of cashew nuts, toasted
- 150mls savoury tofu dressing (p235)

Combine the chopped vegetables, apple and nuts in a bowl and add the savoury tofu dressing.

## Spinach & red capsicum   A B C
### salad

SERVES 4

- 500g of young spinach, shredded
- 2 large red capsicums
- 2 large yellow capsicums
- 125g button mushrooms, sliced (optional)
- 4 tsp chopped fresh basil
- Freshly ground black pepper
- Vinaigrette (p235)

Place the capsicums under a hot grill, turning when the skin becomes charred. Place them in a plastic bag until cool enough to handle, then peel away the skin, remove the stalks, seeds and watery contents. Slice into thin strips. Place the spinach on a serving platter and top with the mushrooms and peppers. Sprinkle with the chopped basil and pour over vinaigrette. Toss before serving.

## Cooked salad  A B C

**SERVES 4**

- Cauliflower broken into small florets
- Raisins/sultanas
- Onion, diced
- Red capsicum
- Sweet corn
- Snow peas
- Fresh marjoram
- Tomatoes
- Lemon juice and flaxseed oil dressing

Lightly steam the cauliflower and snow peas. Roast the red capsicum in the oven or char under the grill. Place it in a plastic bag until cool enough to handle, then peel away the skin, remove the stalks, any seeds and watery contents before slicing and dicing. Water fry the onion over a low heat. Assemble the cauliflower, snow peas, red capsicum and onion and add the sultanas, sweet corn, tomatoes and fresh marjoram to the salad along with a lemon juice and flaxseed oil dressing. You may add crushed, fresh garlic for additional taste.

## Potato salad  B C

**SERVES 4**

- 4 potatoes, boiled in jackets on slow heat
- ¼ cup celery, diced
- ¼ cup green capsicum, diced
- 5 spring onions, finely sliced
- Chives, diced
- Parsley, finely chopped
- Yoghurt
- 1 tablespoon flaxseed oil

Dice the potatoes and mix with all the other ingredients. Add the yoghurt and flaxseed oil to taste.

## Salad Nicoise  A B C

**SERVES 4**

- 1 large lettuce (not iceberg)
- 1 x 425g can of tuna fish in spring water or equivalent of cooked fresh tuna
- 2 tablespoons olive oil
- 1 large red capsicum, seeded and sliced
- 6 large cloves of garlic, unpeeled
- 400g green beans, cut into 5cm lengths.
- 3 hard-boiled eggs, quartered*
- 3 tomatoes, diced
- 1 avocado, diced
- Vinaigrette (p235)

Place the capsicums in the oven with the unpeeled cloves of garlic. Remove the garlic when soft, and peel. Turn the capsicums to ensure they do not burn, and when the skin is loosened, remove from the oven and place in a plastic bag until cool enough to handle. Peel away the skin, remove the stalks, any seeds and watery contents. Slice into thin strips. Lightly steam the green beans. Wash and coarsely shred the lettuce. Place in the serving dish and top with the capsicum, garlic, green beans, tomatoes, avocado, egg and tuna. Add sufficient basic vinaigrette as a dressing.

* omit on plan A

# Salad dressings

## Vinaigrette  A B C

1 part organic apple cider or balsamic vinegar
1 ½ parts organic virgin olive oil (cold-pressed)
1 ½ parts organic unrefined safflower oil or sunflower oil (cold-pressed)
Raw garlic, pressed (optional)

Combine all the ingredients in a glass bottle and shake vigorously. Always store in the refrigerator. You may use lemon juice or orange juice instead of the vinegar. Fresh herbs may be added to this mixture. A little organic sugar is also permissible if you prefer a sweeter dressing.

## Savoury tofu dressing  A B C

250g tofu
¼ cup of safflower or olive oil (cold-pressed)
1 tablespoon fresh lemon juice
1 tsp honey

Blend all the ingredients.

AVOCADO & KIWI FRUIT SALSA p244

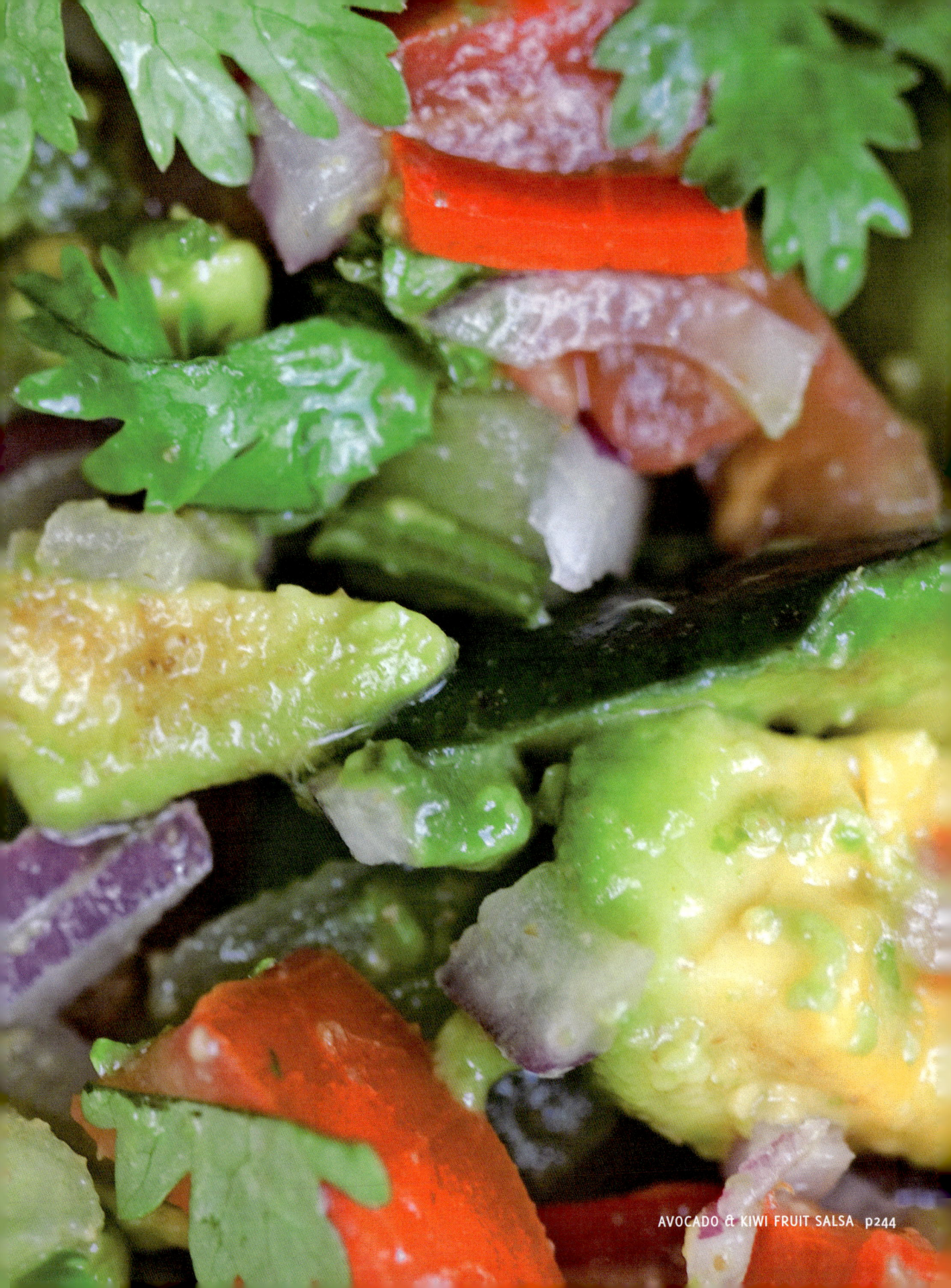

# Sauces, stocks, dips & pastes

**Sauces**
  Basic tomato sauce  238
  Spicy mushroom sauce  238
  Tomato & red capsicum sauce  238

**Stocks**
  Chicken stock  239
  Vegetable stock  239
  Gravy  239

**Dips & pastes**
  Avocado & kiwi fruit salsa  244
  Eggplant dip  243
  Fava bean dip  240
  Guacamole  243
  Indian curry paste  245
  Raita  244
  Spicy eggplant  243
  Sun-dried tomato & chilli pesto  240
  Sun-dried tomato, lemon & garlic pesto  240
  Tahini dip  243
  Thai green curry paste  245
  Thai red curry paste  245
  Tofu garlic dip  240
  Tomato & coriander salsa  244

# Sauces

## Basic tomato sauce     A B C

Makes around 5 cups

- 2 x 400g cans of tomatoes (salt-free), chopped or put through a food mill
- 3 tablespoons of tomato puree
- ½ cup of purified water
- 1 large onion, chopped
- 2 sticks of celery, finely sliced
- 4 - 6 large cloves of garlic, crushed
- Fresh or dried basil and oregano
- 1 tablespoon of apple cider vinegar

Gently water fry the onions and then add the garlic and celery. Add the canned tomatoes and tomato puree mixed with the water. Add the herbs and vinegar and simmer for around 30 minutes. If the sauce is too thick, then more water may be added. You may also add extra tomato puree if the sauce is not strong enough. For a smooth sauce, puree in a blender.

It is a good idea to make this sauce up in batches as it can be used as a base for many dishes. For example, you may add tuna or other seafood along with peas to make a good pasta sauce. Alternatively, you may omit the herbs, adding chilli for a spicy tomato sauce or the base for a chilli bean casserole. When buying pasta choose the rice, millet or corn pasta, which is wheat-free and salt-free.

This sauce may also be used to accompany bean burgers, nut loaves or bean bakes. Poured over rice with a few extra steamed vegetables makes an easy lunch.

## Tomato & red capsicum sauce     A B C

- 150g onion, diced
- 125g celery sticks, diced
- 3 large cloves of garlic, crushed
- A few fresh basil leaves
- ¼ cup fresh parsley, chopped
- A sprig of thyme
- 350g red capsicum, charred under the grill, skins and seeds removed, and diced
- 125g very ripe tomatoes, skinned and chopped
- 300mls chicken or vegetable stock
- 2 tablespoons salt-free tomato puree
- 10mls cider vinegar
- 2 tablespoons lemon juice
- Freshly ground black pepper

Water fry the onion, then add the celery, 2 garlic cloves and herbs (except parsley) until softened. Add the tomatoes, capsicum, stock, tomato puree and black pepper, and simmer in a covered saucepan for 20 minutes. Liquidise and then push through a fine sieve for a smoother consistency. Add the parsley, remaining garlic clove, lemon juice and cider vinegar. Serve with burgers, bakes or on steamed vegetables.

## Spicy mushroom sauce     A B C

- 2 cups of basic tomato sauce without added herbs
- 1 fresh red chilli, deseeded and finely chopped
- 125g mushrooms, sliced
- 2 tsp paprika
- 2 tsp chopped fresh thyme
- Freshly ground black pepper

Water fry the mushrooms and as soon as some moisture is generated, stir in the chilli, thyme and paprika. Add the basic tomato sauce. You may add additional tomato puree to taste.

# Stocks

## Chicken stock  A B C

4 chicken carcasses (+ 8 chicken feet if you can obtain these)
2.5 litres of purified water
2 onions, chopped
2 celery sticks, chopped
1 leek, chopped
3 cloves garlic, chopped
Juice from 1/2 lemon
Bay leaf
Sprig of thyme
Black peppercorns

Place all the ingredients in a large pan, add the water and bring to a boil. Simmer, covered for 2-3 hrs. Strain and if you manage to get the chicken feet, then try to squeeze as much of the gelatin from the feet into the stock. Discard all the carcasses and vegetables and pour the stock into glass jars and freeze until required. Use in savoury dishes, and for cooking rice and legumes.

## Vegetable stock  A B C

20 whole black peppercorns
2 medium onions, sliced
2 medium carrots, sliced
1 stalk celery, chopped into chunks
Handful of parsley sprigs
A few celery leaves
1 bay leaf
2 litres purified water
2-3 cloves of crushed garlic (optional)

Place all the ingredients in a large saucepan with the water and bring to the boil. Cover and simmer for 40 minutes and then strain. Pour the stock into glass jars and freeze until required.

## Gravy  C

The wonderful brown colour of a good gravy comes from caramelised vegetables and the meat juices. To make a gravy, without stock cubes or colouring agents, place the roasting joint on a bed of finely chopped vegetables (onions, carrots, mushrooms) and whole garlic cloves and let these roast and slowly darken with the meat. When the meat is cooked, remove it and allow to rest, while returning the vegetables to the oven to allow them to brown further.

Before removing the vegetables and meat juices make a roux by melting 15g of unsalted butter with 15g of wholemeal flour. Cook until biscuit coloured. Add the juices and vegetables from the pan stirring so that no lumps form. Add additional vegetable water (or stock) and a little wine for special occasions. If the gravy seems a bit bland (it shouldn't be if the vegetables were caramelised well) then you can add some unsalted tomato puree.

Recipes

# Dips

## Sun-dried tomato & chilli pesto — A B C

280g red capsicum - charred under the grill and peeled
75g (8) sun-dried tomatoes - soaked in boiling water and squeezed
½ cup finely chopped basil
2 red chillies, finely chopped
3 tablespoons pine nuts

Combine all the ingredients in a food processor and process until relatively smooth. Store in an airtight container or freeze in small quantities. This pesto can be added to sauces, soups, pasta etc.

## Sun-dried tomato, lemon & garlic pesto — A B C

280g red capsicum, charred under the grill and peeled
75g (8) sun-dried tomatoes
½ cup finely chopped basil
4 cloves garlic
3 tablespoons pine nuts
Lemon juice to taste

Prepare as for the preceding recipe.

## Fava bean dip — A B C

1 ½ cups of broad beans (fresh or frozen)
½ onion, finely diced
¼ cup lemon juice, freshly squeezed
2 tbsp virgin olive oil
1/3 cup yoghurt* (optional)
1 clove garlic
Pinch of cayenne pepper to taste
1 tablespoon finely chopped parsley

Cook the broad beans until tender (5-10 minutes). Drain and place in a blender with the lemon juice, 1 tablespoon of oil, the garlic, yoghurt and the cayenne pepper. Blend, and then stir in the onion and parsley. If the mixture is too stiff you may add some water. Drizzle the remaining oil over the dip before serving.

* omit on plan A

## Tofu garlic Dip — A B C

500g tofu
¼ cup safflower oil
2 tablespoons fresh lemon juice
4 cloves garlic
1 tablespoon honey
Pinch of cayenne pepper

Blend all the ingredients together and chill.

SUN-DRIED TOMATO, LEMON & GARLIC PESTO

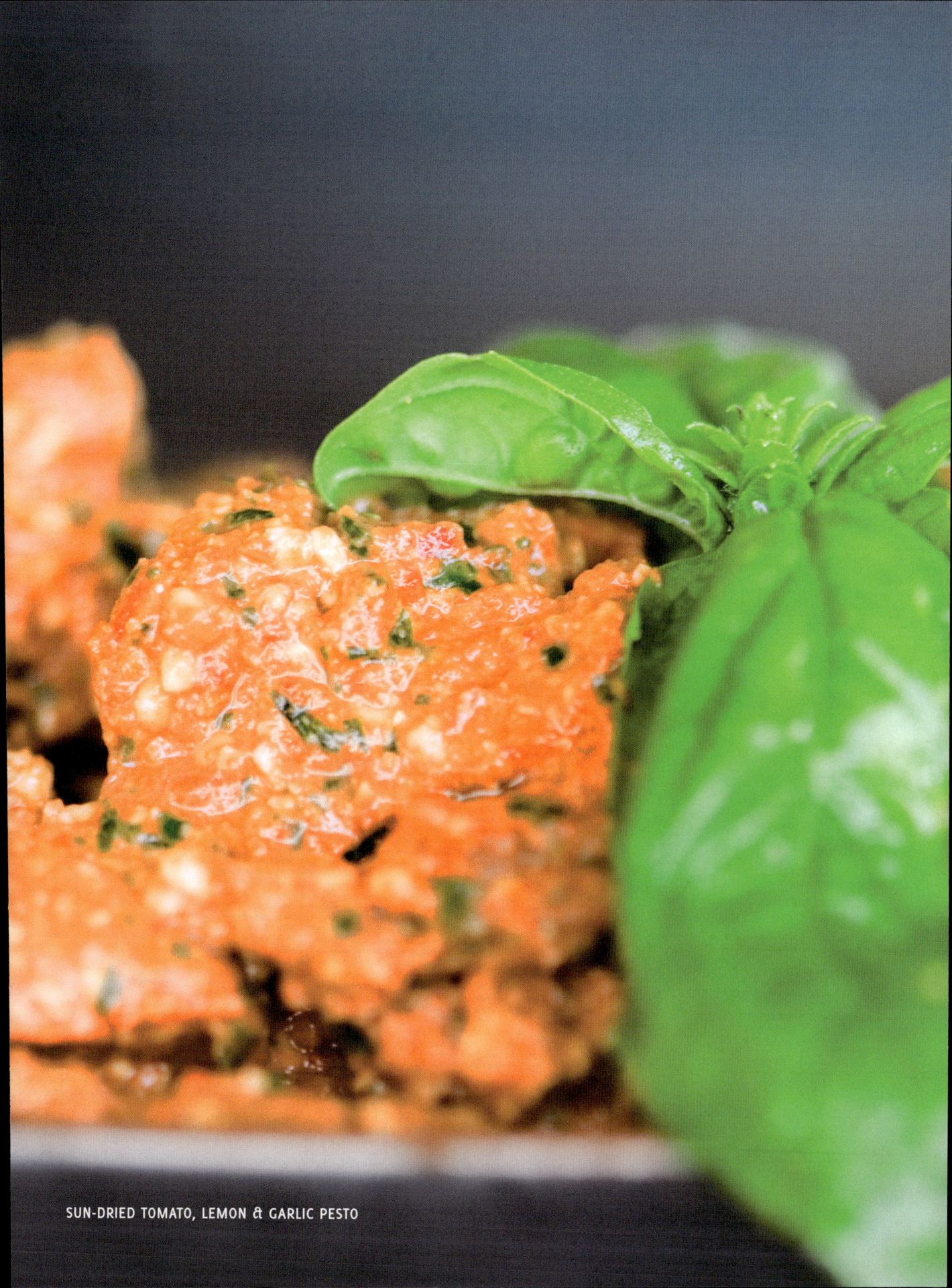

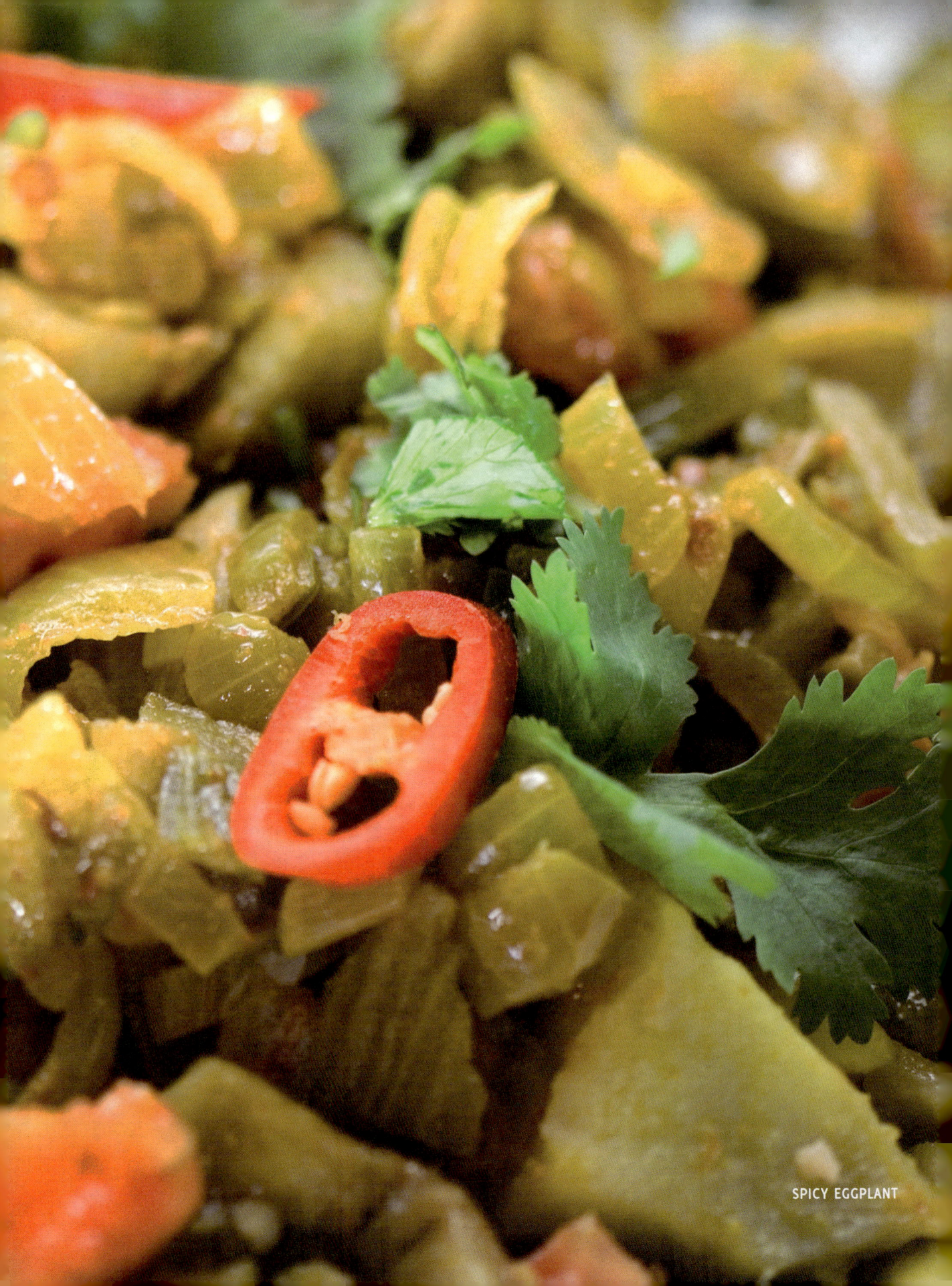

SPICY EGGPLANT

Dips

## Eggplant dip  A B C

- 500g eggplant
- ½ tsp chilli powder
- 2 tablespoon tahini or ½ cup walnuts finely chopped
- 2 cloves garlic
- ¼ cup lemon juice, freshly squeezed
- ½ tsp freshly ground black pepper
- 2 tablespoons parsley, finely chopped (optional)

Char the eggplant under the grill, turning so that all sides are done. Remove, and when cool peel the outer skin. Place in a blender with the chilli powder, tahini (if using), garlic and lemon juice. Place the dip in a serving bowl and stir in the parsley and walnuts (if using).

## Spicy eggplant  A B C

SERVES 4

- 500g eggplant
- 1 large onion, chopped
- 3 tomatoes, skinned and chopped
- 2 green chillies, finely chopped
- ½ tsp each ground turmeric, chilli powder
- ¾ tsp ground coriander
- 2 tablespoons coriander leaves, chopped

Char the eggplant under a grill, turning frequently. Peel when the flesh becomes soft and dice into small cubes. Water fry the onions until soft, then add the tomatoes, coriander leaves and chillies. Cook for a further 3 minutes. Add the eggplant, turmeric, chilli and coriander stirring thoroughly.

## Guacamole  A B C

- 2 cups of chopped avocado
- 1/3 cup of chopped coriander
- 3 tomatoes, chopped
- 1 green chilli, finely sliced and chopped
- ½ onion, finely chopped
- ¼ cup lemon juice, freshly squeezed

Blend the avocado. Add the rest of the ingredients and combine evenly. Cover with greaseproof paper until ready to serve.

## Tahini dip  B C

- ¼ cup tahini
- 4 tablespoons lemon juice
- 2 cloves of crushed garlic
- 3 tablespoons cold water

Place all the ingredients in a blender. This sauce can be kept in the refrigerator in a sealed container and is used to accompany many Middle Eastern dishes, or may simply be used to top a vegetable salad.

## Avocado & kiwi fruit salsa    A B C

Salsa:
- 2 avocados, peeled and diced
- ½ red onion, finely diced
- 2 tomatoes, seeded and diced
- 2 kiwi fruit, peeled and diced
- 1 small fresh red chilli, deseeded and finely diced
- 3 tablespoons fresh coriander, finely chopped

Dressing:
- 2½ tablespoons sunflower oil/safflower oil
- Juice and grated zest of ½ lime
- 1 tsp ground cumin, toasted
- Freshly ground black pepper

Mix salsa ingredients and make the dressing. Combine. Serve salsa either with the chickpea pancakes (p228) or as a side dish to enliven any meal. You may use mango in place of kiwi fruit for a sweeter combination.

## Raita    A B C

- 500g yoghurt* or soy yoghurt
- ½ tsp roasted cumin
- 1 tablespoon of chopped mint or coriander

Mix all ingredients and serve as a side dish.

* omit on plan A

## Tomato & coriander salsa    A B C

- 4 tomatoes, seeded and diced
- ½ onion, finely sliced
- 2 tablespoons fresh coriander leaves, chopped

Mix all ingredients and serve as a side dish.

# Pastes

## Thai red curry paste  A B C

- 10 red chillies
- 2 large onions
- 1 tsp black pepper, ground
- 1 tablespoon ground cumin
- 2 tablespoons ground coriander
- 2 tsp ground turmeric
- 1 tablespoon paprika
- 1 cup fresh coriander, chopped
- 4 tablespoons lemon grass, finely sliced
- 4 tablespoons galangal, chopped (or 2 tsp powder)
- 2 tablespoons garlic, chopped
- 3 tablespoons olive oil

Soak the chillies in a small amount of boiling water for 15 minutes. Remove the stems and seeds and place in an electric blender with all the other ingredients and a little of the soaking water to make a smooth paste. Freeze in small pots until required.

## Indian curry paste  A B C

- 1 cup ground coriander
- ½ cup ground cumin
- 1 tablespoon black pepper, ground
- 1 tablespoon black mustard seeds
- 2 tsp chilli powder
- 2 tablespoons crushed garlic
- 2 tablespoons grated ginger
- a little apple cider vinegar
- ¾ cup olive oil

Combine all the ingredients (except the oil) with enough vinegar to make a thick paste. Heat the oil in a heavy based pan. When hot add the paste, reducing the heat and stirring until the aroma from the spices is released and until the oil has separated around the mixture. Cool and store in a jar in the refrigerator.

## Thai green curry paste  A B C

- 10 fresh green chillies
- 2 cups fresh coriander, chopped
- 1 tsp black peppercorns
- 2 onions, chopped
- 2 stems lemon grass, finely sliced
- 1 tablespoon ground coriander
- 2 tsp cumin
- 1 tablespoon galangal, chopped (or 1 tsp powder)
- 1 tsp ground turmeric
- 2 tablespoons oil

Soak the chillies in a small amount of boiling water for 15 minutes. Remove the stems and seeds and place in an electric blender with all the other ingredients and a little of the soaking water to make a smooth paste. Freeze in small pots until required.

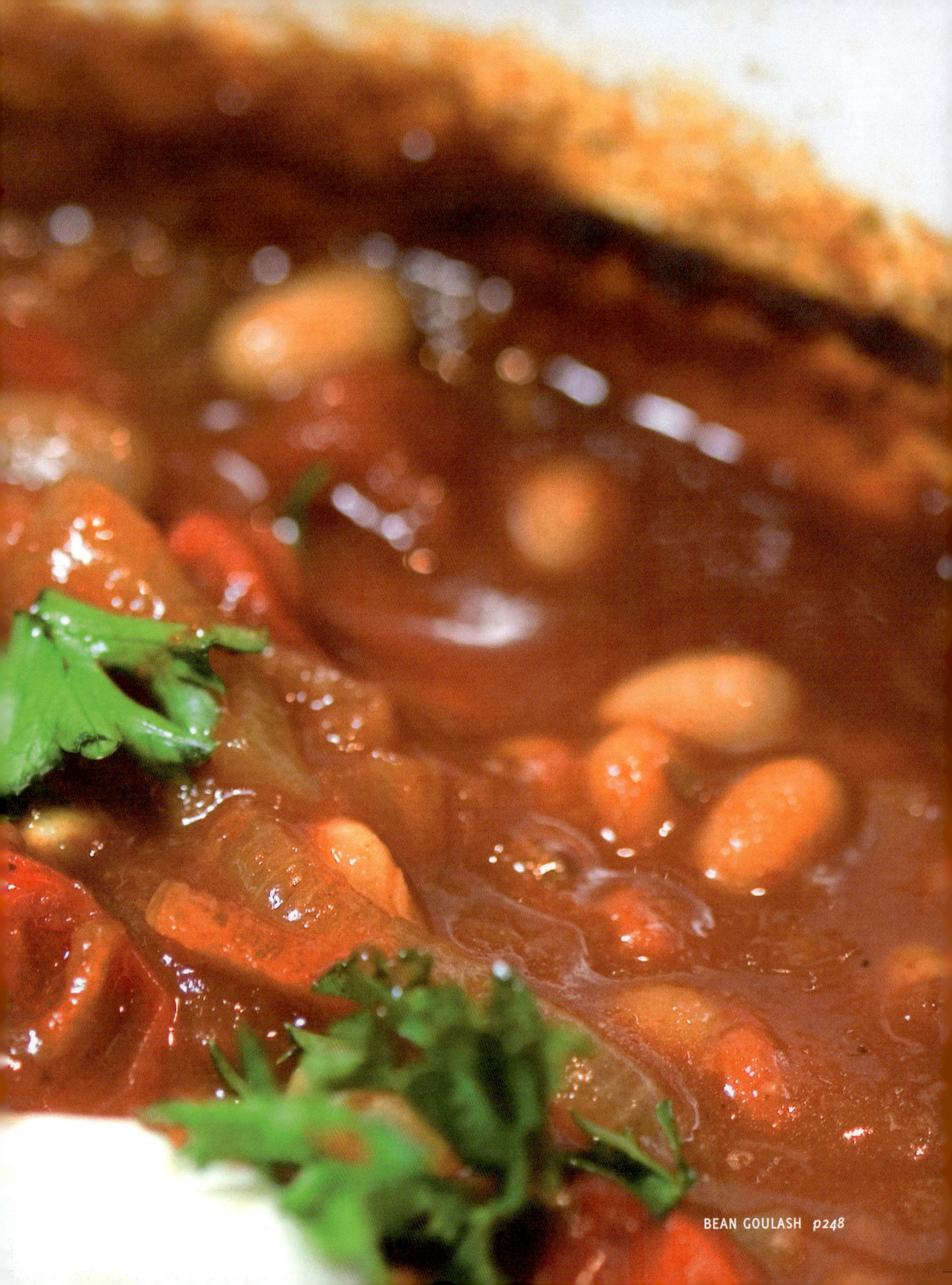

BEAN GOULASH  *p248*

# Dinners

**Beans**
Bean & nut roast  249
Bean goulash  248
Chickpea burgers  249
Curried chickpeas  250
Curried tofu  251
Indian dosas  251
Lentil burgers  248
Lentil curry  250
Mexican chilli with corn tortillas & guacamole  251
Pasta with creamy lentil sauce  250

**Meat & fish**
Cassoulet  253
Fish with roasted vegetables  253
Fish with tandoori marinade  255
Laksa  256
Paella  254
Pasta with tomato & tuna sauce  254
Seviche with Mediterranean salsa  255
Thai chicken green curry  257
Thai fish red curry  257
Thai fish salad  256
Thai-style yellow curry with fish  258
Tuna risotto  256

**Vegetable dishes**
Cabbage & red capsicum  263
Eggplant lasagne  262
Hazelnut zucchini loaf  261
Nut moussaka  263
Pilau rice  262
Ratatouille  261
Red cabbage & apple  262

# Beans

## Bean goulash  A B C

**SERVES 4-6**

- 1 cup dried haricot beans, soaked and semi-germinated
- 400g can of tomatoes (salt-free)
- 3 tablespoons of tomato puree (salt-free)
- 2 dsp of paprika
- 1 tsp cumin seeds
- 2 medium onions, sliced
- 2 red capsicums, deseeded and sliced
- 2 cloves of garlic, crushed
- 300mls chicken or vegetable stock
- *Plain yoghurt or soy yoghurt

Begin by cooking the haricot beans for 20 minutes. Meanwhile water fry the onions, garlic and red capsicums. When moist enough add the paprika and cumin seeds, stir in and continue cooking for a few minutes. Add the canned tomatoes (chopped or passed through a food mill) and the tomato puree along with the chicken or vegetable stock. Bring to the boil and add the haricot beans. Place all the ingredients in a covered casserole and bake in the oven at 150°C for 1½ hrs. Serve with a dollop of yoghurt, brown rice and a green salad. This is good the next day for lunch!

* omit on plan A

## Lentil burgers  A B C

- 1½ cup red lentils (250g)
- 2¼ cups water
- 1½ large onions, chopped
- 1 tablespoon olive oil
- 2 cloves of garlic, chopped
- 2 tsp ground coriander
- 2 tsp ground cumin
- 2 tsp ground turmeric
- 4 tablespoons of chopped fresh coriander leaves

Bring the lentils to boil in the water, turn the heat off and let soak for at least 30 minutes. Cook in a covered saucepan over a very low heat for around 20 minutes being careful that the lentils don't burn. Leave to rest until required. This part of the recipe can be done in the morning while you are getting breakfast etc. and then left in the pan until the evening. When the mixture has cooled it will form a stiff paste. Water fry the onions and garlic and then add the spices. When the vegetables are cooked, stir into the lentil mixture. Add the fresh coriander leaves. Form into burgers (you should be able to make about 10). These freeze well provided that they are separated by greaseproof paper. You can make any quantity in batches so that you have quick easy meals - especially at lunchtime. To cook, brush with a little oil and brown under the grill, turning once. Serve with brown rice, yoghurt and vegetables with a spicy tomato or red capsicum sauce.

## Bean & nut roast      A B C

SERVES 4

    1 cup dried black-eyed beans, soaked and semi-germinated
    ½ cup of hazelnuts, coarsely chopped
    ¼ cup of pumpkin seeds
    ¼ cup of sunflower seeds
    ¼ cup of fresh lemon juice
    Zest from one lemon
    2 tablespoons olive oil
    ½ cup chopped celery
    1 large onion, chopped
    1 large red capsicum, peeled
    12 sun-dried tomatoes
    ½ cup of finely chopped basil
    200g of canned tomatoes (unsalted), chopped

Bring the beans to the boil and simmer until cooked (1-1½ hours). While cooking, place the sun-dried tomatoes in boiling water and leave for 30 minutes. Char the red capsicum under the grill and place in a plastic bag until cool enough to handle, by which time the skin should peel away easily. Squeeze out the tomatoes and combine with the capsicum and basil in the blender to make a paste. Dry roast the nuts and seeds in a pan, agitating until lightly browned. Water fry the onion and celery until soft and translucent. When the beans are cooked, drain and mash gently. Add the onions, celery, nuts, the paste from the blender, lemon juice and zest, and tomatoes. Combine thoroughly and turn into a loaf tin lined with greaseproof paper that has been lightly greased with oil and place in a shallow tray of hot water. Cover and bake at 180°C for an hour. Remove the cover 30 minutes before the end of cooking. Let the loaf stand in the tin for 10 minutes before easing out. Serve with a tomato and capsicum sauce (p238), brown rice and vegetables.

## Chickpea burgers      A B C

SERVES 4

    1½ cups (375g) chickpeas, soaked and semi-germinated
    ½ cup parsley, finely chopped
    Lemon zest from one lemon
    4 cloves of garlic, finely chopped
    A pinch of cayenne pepper

Cover the chickpeas with water and simmer covered for one hour. Drain the beans (there should not be much cooking fluid left) and place in the food processor. If the mixture is too dry then add a little of the cooking water but it should resemble a stiff paste.

Combine the chopped parsley, lemon zest and garlic and chop the ingredients together so that they are well mixed. Add this to the chickpea mixture and form into burgers. These can be lightly brushed with oil and grilled. Serve with a tomato or tahini sauce, rice and salad.

Recipes

## Pasta & creamy lentil sauce  A B C

SERVES 4

- 1 cup brown lentils
- 4 cups chicken or vegetable stock
- 2 onions, diced
- 2 cloves garlic, crushed
- 1 tsp each of ground cumin and coriander
- ½ tsp ground chilli
- 2 tablespoons tomato paste
- 4 tomatoes, diced
- ¼ cup each of chopped parsley and coriander
- Black pepper
- 4 tablespoons yoghurt* or soy yoghurt

Simmer the brown lentils in the stock for 20 mins. Drain, reserving the liquid. Meanwhile, water fry the onions and garlic until translucent and stir through the spices. Add the lentils, tomato paste and enough stock to make a creamy sauce. Heat through. Before serving, stir in the fresh herbs and black pepper. Serve with a wheat-free pasta with chopped tomatoes and a tablespoon of yoghurt on each serving.

* omit on plan A

## Curried chickpeas  A B C

SERVES 4

- 2 heaped tablespoons curry paste (p245)
- 1 cup chickpeas, soaked and semi-germinated
- 1 potato, cubed
- A few fresh curry leaves (if available)
- 1 cup of frozen peas or 4 cups of fresh spinach, chopped

Cook the chickpeas in water for 30 minutes. Mix the curry paste with ½ cup of water and heat in a pan until bubbling. Add the chickpeas, along with their cooking water and curry leaves. Add water to cover by 2 cm. Simmer for 15 minutes, add the spinach or frozen peas. Serve with pilau rice (p262) and a tomato and cucumber salad, or raita (p244).

## Lentil curry  A B C

SERVES 3-4

- 1 heaped tablespoon curry paste (p245)
- ¾ cup brown lentils
- A few fresh curry leaves (if available)
- ¾ cup frozen peas

Place the lentils in a pan with the curry paste and gradually mix with water until covered. Simmer with the curry leaves for 20-30 minutes, being careful not to let the mixture dry out. Five minutes before the end of cooking add the peas. Serve with pilau rice (p262) and raita (p244), or tomato salad.

## Mexican chilli     A B C
### with corn tortillas & guacamole

**SERVES 4**

For the chilli
- 1 cup red kidney beans, soaked and semi-germinated
- 1 large onion, finely chopped
- 1 small green capsicum, chopped
- 1 cup of corn kernels
- 6 button mushrooms, sliced (optional)
- 1 tsp cumin seeds
- 10 sun-dried tomatoes
- 2 hot red chilli peppers, finely chopped
- 1 tsp chilli powder (to taste)
- 200g chopped tomatoes
- Salt-free tomato paste to taste

Cover the kidney beans with water and bring to the boil and simmer until tender (1 – 1½ hours). Soak the sun-dried tomatoes in boiling water for around 30 minutes. Drain, squeeze out the liquid and reserve. Meanwhile water fry the onion and when translucent add the cumin seeds, green capsicum, chilli peppers and mushrooms and cook until tender. Add the corn kernels to this mixture and heat through. When the beans are cooked, mash lightly and add to the vegetable mixture along with the sun-dried tomatoes (chopped) and their liquid, and chopped tomatoes. Add chilli powder and tomato paste to taste. Cover the pot and heat through until the flavours mingle. Add more water if required to prevent drying out.

For the tortillas:
- 2 cups of masa flour
- 1 cup warm water

Stir the water into the flour and mix until it forms a ball. Divide into 12 balls and roll into thin rounds between greaseproof paper. If you own a tortilla press, then these take just a few minutes to prepare. Heat a frying pan (no oil needed) and cook your tortillas, turning once. They do not take long to cook - make sure that they do not burn. Keep warm under the grill or in the oven until all are cooked.

Top the tortillas with the Mexican chilli and guacamole (p243) and serve with a salad.

## Curried tofu     A B C

**SERVES 4**
- 500g tofu, crumbled or cut into bits
- 1 chilli
- 2 onions, chopped
- 2 cloves garlic, crushed
- 2 tsp turmeric
- ¼ tsp ground cumin
- 3 tomatoes
- 6 mushrooms, sliced
- ¼ cup chopped coriander leaves

Water fry the onions, garlic and chilli until translucent. Add the turmeric and cumin and cook for two minutes. Add the mushrooms, then the tomatoes and lastly, the tofu. Heat through for one minute and add the coriander just before serving.

# Indian dosas A B C

**SERVES 4 (8 PANCAKES)**

    1/3 cup urid dahl
    1 cup brown rice flour
    ½ cup finely chopped onion
    1 tsp each of ground cumin and coriander, toasted
    4 tablespoons chopped fresh coriander
    2 tablespoons plain yoghurt* (optional)
    pinch of chilli
    a knob of ghee

**Filling:**

    450g potatoes, peeled and cubed (0.5cm)
    4 tablespoons olive oil
    ½ tsp mustard seeds
    2 green chillies, finely sliced
    1 tablespoon channa dahl
    ¼ tsp asafetida
    3 tablespoons chopped cashew nuts
    2 cm ginger, grated
    1 large onion, finely chopped
    ½ tsp ground turmeric

You will need to start this recipe 36 hours before your planned meal. Grind the urid dahl in a coffee grinder and mix with the rice flour. (If you do not have a grinder then soak the dahl for 8 hours in water and then strain reserving the liquid. Blend in a food processor until you have a coarse paste and add to the brown rice flour). Place in a bowl along with the brown rice flour and add 2 cups of purified water. Mix thoroughly until you have a smooth batter. Let it rest at room temperature for 36 hours.

Before cooking, stir the yoghurt, onion, spices and chopped coriander into the mixture. Heat a small frying pan (approximately 15 cm diameter) and coat with just enough ghee to prevent the pancakes sticking. When hot, pour in ½ cup of the batter. Allow to cook for about 4 minutes before attempting to turn. The pancake needs to develop a good coating on the underside before you turn or else it will tear. Turn and cook the other side for a minute. Keep warm in the oven until you have cooked all the pancakes.

* omit on plan A

Cook the potatoes until tender. Drain and set aside. Heat the oil and add the mustard seeds, asafetida, chillies, nuts, dahl and ginger. Fry for 10 seconds and then add the onion. Cook until tender. Add the potatoes and turmeric along with 100mls of water and heat through, making sure that it doesn't stick. Fill the pancakes with this mixture and serve with a yoghurt and mint raita (p244), fresh tomato and coriander salsa (p244), and spicy eggplant (p243).

# Meat & fish

## Cassoulet     C

SERVES 4-6

- 250g haricot beans
- 2 carrots
- 5 large cloves of garlic
- 1 tsp mixed herbs
- Bay leaf
- 1 boned shoulder of lamb (fat removed) or 750g of diced lamb
- 2 onions
- 400g tin chopped tomatoes (salt-free)
- 2 tablespoons salt-free tomato puree
- Bunch of parsley chopped
- 1 glass of white wine (optional)

Prepare the beans by the soaking and semi-germinating method. Water fry the onion and garlic until softened. Cook the haricot beans in enough water to cover by 3cm with the lamb bone, garlic, chopped carrots, herbs and bay leaf for 1¼ hours. Watch that it doesn't dry out. The beans should absorb most of the water but there should be some left. Meanwhile dice the lamb place in the bottom of a casserole. Add the onions to the lamb. Next pour a can of chopped tomatoes over the lamb and stir adding the parsley. Drain the beans reserving their cooking liquid and remove the bone. Place the beans over the lamb and vegetable mixture. Mix the tomato puree with a little cooking liquid and add to the remainder of the cooking liquid. Pour over the meat (do not stir) ensuring that the liquid rises to the level of the beans. Cover with a lid and place in an oven (220°C) for 20 minutes until bubbling and then reduce the temperature to 160°C for around 2 hrs. Serve with brown rice and a salad.

## Fish & roasted vegetables     A B C

SERVES 4

- 750g of firm-fleshed white fish, cut into chunks
- 1 eggplant
- 2 zucchini
- 2 red capsicums
- 1 onion
- 1 fennel bulb
- 4-8 cloves of garlic, left whole
- 4 tomatoes, diced
- 400g can of chopped tomatoes (salt-free)
- Mixed herbs of your choice

Water fry the onion until translucent. Stir in the diced, fresh tomatoes. Place the rest of the prepared vegetables and herbs in a bowl and stir through the onions and tomatoes until all the vegetables are moistened. Place in a roasting pan making sure that you have a fairly shallow layer of vegetables. Roast for one hour at around 190°C - 200°C turning at intervals. Make sure that the vegetables don't burn. If they look as if they are drying out, then add just enough of the canned chopped tomatoes to keep moist. When the vegetables are roasted add the remainder of the chopped tomatoes and stir through. Allow to heat for a further 5 minutes and then add the raw fish diced into chunks. Stir in but do not stir again after this. Cook in the oven for a further 10 minutes until the fish is done and serve. This is also delicious served cold for lunch.

Recipes

## Paella  C

**SERVES 4**

- 2 large chicken breasts and 4 chicken wings
- 8 raw king prawns, unshelled
- 125ml olive oil
- 4 large cloves of garlic, thinly sliced
- 1 large onion, thinly sliced
- 1 large red capsicum, skinned, seeded and sliced into wedges
- 2 tomatoes, peeled and chopped
- 250g fresh green beans
- 100g fresh (or frozen) baby broad beans or lima beans
- 1 tablespoon paprika
- 1/8th tsp of crushed saffron threads
- 1¼ litres (5 cups) of chicken stock
- 2 cups of organic brown rice
- 3 tablespoons chopped parsley, plus extra for garnish

Place the red capsicum under the grill and char the skin on all sides. Remove and peel when cool enough to handle. Prick the tomatoes with a sharp knife and immerse in a bowl of boiling water. Peel and chop the flesh. Cut the chicken breasts into a total of eight pieces and season with black pepper.

Heat the olive oil and saute the chicken, lightly browning and sealing on all sides. Remove from the pan. Saute the king prawns for no longer than 3 minutes and remove. Saute the onion and garlic until soft. Add the tomatoes, green beans, broad beans and cook for one minute. Remove the pan from the heat and add the paprika, parsley and saffron.

Pour in the stock and add the chicken pieces and cook until the chicken is tender (about 15 minutes). Lift out the solids from the pan and measure the stock. (There should be around 1 litre (4 cups), if not then make up the quantity with either more stock or water). Add the stock to the rice, bring to the boil and cook covered on the lowest heat. As brown rice takes much longer than the traditional white rice, I cook the rice for around 30 minutes (covered) before transferring it to a large paella pan. At this stage add all the other ingredients (including the red capsicum) except the king prawns, burying the chicken in the rice.

Continue cooking (covered) for a further 5-10 minutes until the rice is done being careful not to let the dish dry out. If there is a danger of this then add more stock or water. The dish needs to rest for 10 minutes before serving and at this stage add the king prawns. Keep the dish covered to allow the heat to bring out all the flavours. Serve with a green salad.

## Pasta  A B C
### with tomato and tuna sauce

**SERVES 4**

- 3 cups of basic tomato sauce (p218)
- 200g fresh tuna (preferred) or canned tuna
- 125g peas
- 125g button mushrooms
- 1 leek, finely chopped
- 3 tablespoons olive oil
- 2 cloves garlic, finely sliced
- 1 onion, finely sliced
- Pinch of chilli powder

Water fry the garlic and onion with the pinch of chilli until translucent. Add the leeks and then the mushrooms and cook for a further 5 minutes. Add the tomato sauce and cook for 10 minutes. Add the peas and diced fresh tuna and continue to cook until just done. If using canned tuna, add just before serving. Add more tomato puree if the sauce is too bland. Serve with rice and millet or corn pasta which can be purchased from most health shops.

## Seviche   A B C
### with Mediterranean salsa

SERVES 4

    500g firm white fish, skinned and boned

For the marinade:

    75mls fresh lime juice (lemon will substitute but lime is better).

    2 tsp grated ginger

    1 tablespoon fresh coriander, finely chopped

    2 tsp lemon grass, thinly sliced

For the salsa:

    1 small eggplant

    2 tablespoons olive oil

    3 tomatoes, skinned with flesh diced

    1 green capsicum, diced

    1 fresh green chilli, finely diced

    ½ red onion, thinly sliced

    1 tsp fresh mint, chopped

    1 tsp fresh tarragon, chopped

    Freshly ground black pepper

    Fresh lime juice and olive oil as a dressing

Mix the ingredients of the marinade and place the diced fish in a bowl with the marinade. Leave in the refrigerator for several hours, turning at intervals until it has become firm and milky white.

Slice the eggplant into 1 cm rounds and brush with the oil. Place under a hot grill, turning once until cooked. When cool dice into 1 cm cubes and mix with the rest of the prepared ingredients, adding some lime juice and a little olive oil as a dressing.

Drain the fish and place on a serving dish, spooning the salsa over the fish. Pour the remaining marinade over the top with a liberal grinding of black pepper. Chopped coriander may be used instead of the mint and tarragon.

## Fish with tandoori marinade   A B C

SERVES 4

    4 firm fleshed fish fillets, steaks or whole fish

    Juice of a large lemon

    1 tsp chilli powder

Tandoori paste:

    150mls yoghurt*/soy yoghurt

    6 cloves garlic, crushed

    1 tablespoon fresh ginger, grated

    1 tsp garam masala

    ½ tsp ground cumin

    1 tsp paprika

This dish is excellent cooked on the barbecue. Marinate the fish in the lemon juice and chilli powder for one hour. If you're using whole fish make several slashes down to the bone and rub the marinade well into the flesh.

Prepare the tandoori paste and add to the marinade, leaving for a further hour. Cook the fish on the barbecue or under the grill, taking care not to burn the marinade. It should take between 10-12 minutes to cook through.

Serve with raita mixed with chopped cucumber and the tomato and coriander salsa (p244).

* omit on plan A

## Tuna risotto    A B C

**SERVES 4**

- 600g fresh tuna, cubed, or canned tuna
- 1½ cups short grain brown rice
- 2 large onions, chopped
- 4 cloves garlic, crushed
- Oregano and basil to taste
- Cracked black pepper
- 2-3 tablespoons salt-free tomato paste
- 400g canned tomatoes, salt-free
- 1 bay leaf
- Vegetable stock

Preheat oven to 190°C. Water fry the onion and garlic until translucent. Add the oregano and basil along with the tomato paste and cook for a few minutes. Add the tuna, continue to cook and after 2-3 minutes stir in the rice. Add the canned tomatoes and continue to simmer. Add enough vegetable stock or water to cover the ingredients by 3-4cms. Bring to the boil and simmer for 3 minutes. Pour the ingredients into a covered casserole and place into the preheated oven for around 40 minutes or until the rice is cooked. The dish should be moist but not wet. Serve with a garnish of fresh basil or parsley and black pepper.

## Thai fish salad    A B C

**SERVES 2**

- 1 salmon cutlet, boned and cubed
- 2-3 tablespoons Thai green curry paste (p225)
- 1 tablespoon olive oil
- 1½ cups cooked wild rice
- 1 red capsicum, cut into strips
- 15 snow peas, topped and sliced
- 2 cups bean shoots
- Coriander leaves, chopped
- A sprinkling of sesame seeds, lightly toasted

Heat the oil in a wok and when hot add the green curry paste. Add the fish and cook for a few minutes until done. Add the wild rice, capsicums, snow peas and bean shoots and toss through for a few minutes. Serve topped with the chopped coriander leaves and sesame seeds.

## Laksa    C

**SERVES 2**

- 100ml coconut milk
- 1 heaped tablespoon of Hogan's Laksa paste
- 1 tablespoon olive oil
- 1 chicken breast, cut into strips
- 400ml chicken stock
- 100g rice vermicelli
- 15 snow peas, cut into large pieces
- 1 cup bean shoots
- 100g tofu, cubed (optional)

Mix the laksa paste with the coconut milk and the stock. Bring to simmer and then add the chicken and cook for 5 minutes until done. Add the snow peas and tofu and continue to cook for a further 2 minutes. Meanwhile, soak the rice vermicelli in hot water according to instructions on the packet. Drain the vermicelli and place in a serving bowl. Top with the bean sprouts and pour over the hot soup. Garnish with shaved carrots, cucumber and freshly chopped coriander.

Meat & Fish

## Thai chicken green curry  C

SERVES 4

- 3 chicken breasts, cubed
- 6-8 tablespoons green curry paste (p245)
- Juice from 2 limes
- 4 fresh lime leaves, coarsely chopped
- 1½ cups frozen peas
- 2 medium eggplant, diced in chunks
- 2 onions, diced
- 1 stem of lemon grass, cut into 4 cm lengths
- ½ cup coconut milk
- 1 tablespoon olive oil
- A bunch of fresh coriander, chopped

Steam the diced eggplant until softened. Place to one side. Soak the lime leaves in 200ml boiling water for 15 minutes. In a wok heat 1 tablespoon of oil over a hot flame. Add the paste and cook for 2-3 minutes until the aromas are released. Add the chicken with the onions and the lemon grass. Cook for 3-4 minutes and add the coconut milk with the strained lime leaf juice, eggplant and peas. Cook for a further 3-4 minutes. Add plenty of chopped coriander and stir through before serving. Serve with brown rice.

## Thai fish red curry  A B C

SERVES 4

- 800g firm fleshed white fish
- 2 leeks, cut into 1 cm slices
- Small bunch of fresh basil
- 3 baby bok choy, cut into 3 cm lengths
- Juice of 2 limes
- 3 lime leaves, coarsely chopped
- 6 tablespoons Thai red curry paste (p245)
- 2 tablespoons olive oil

Mix 1 tsp Thai red curry paste with the lime juice and a dessertspoon of the oil. Dice the fish into large chunks and add to the marinade. Leave for 1 hour. Infuse the lime leaves in 100ml of boiling water for 15 minutes. Heat the remaining oil in a wok over a hot flame. Pour in the curry paste and cook for 2-3 minutes until the aromas are released. Add the fish and the leeks. Stir until almost cooked. Add the bok choy. Strain the lime leaves and discard adding the lime water to the pan. Cook for a few minutes stirring in the chopped basil before serving. Serve with brown rice.

## Thai-style yellow curry
### with fish

B C

SERVES 4

- 600g of salmon steak, cut into bite sized chunks
- 1 piece of fresh turmeric, 10 to 15cm long
- 2 to 4 tablespoons of coconut milk
- 1 stalk of lemon grass, cut diagonally into 4cm lengths
- 4 lime leaves (fresh if possible), finely sliced
- I tsp of dried chilli
- 8 cherry tomatoes, sliced in half
- 3 shallots, sliced lengthwise into 1/8th sections
- 1 large red chilli, de-seeded and sliced diagonally into 1 cm pieces
- ½ tsp of palm sugar (optional)
- 1 bok choy or equal amount of spinach, coarsely chopped
- 1 handful of white oyster mushrooms, sliced into 1½ cm strips
- 1 handful of chopped coriander

Peel and dice the fresh turmeric, then using a mortar and pestle, pound into a creamy paste. Add the coconut milk to 250ml of water and slowly bring to gentle simmer in a broad based pot. Add the turmeric, lemon grass, fresh lime leaves and dried chillies to the pot. Add the cherry tomatoes, shallots, red chilli and palm sugar (if using) to the simmering pot. Simmer for 5 to 10 minutes until the shallots soften. Add the bok choy (or spinach) and sliced mushrooms to the pot and simmer for a further 2 minutes. Finally add the salmon chunks and simmer for a few minutes until the middle of the fish starts to turn colour. Add the fresh coriander to the pot and cook for 2 minutes. Serve with brown rice.

THAI-STYLE YELLOW CURRY WITH FISH

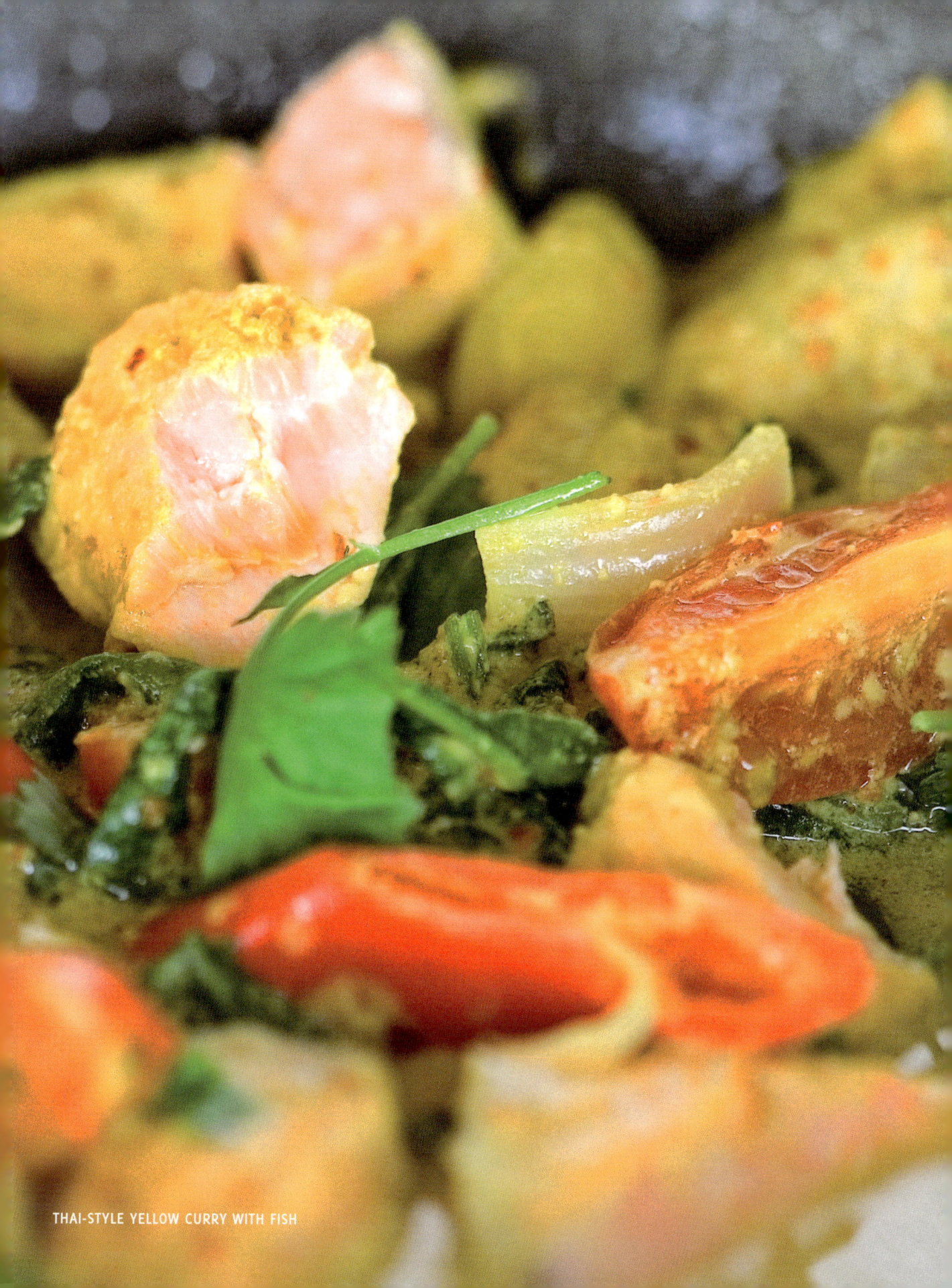

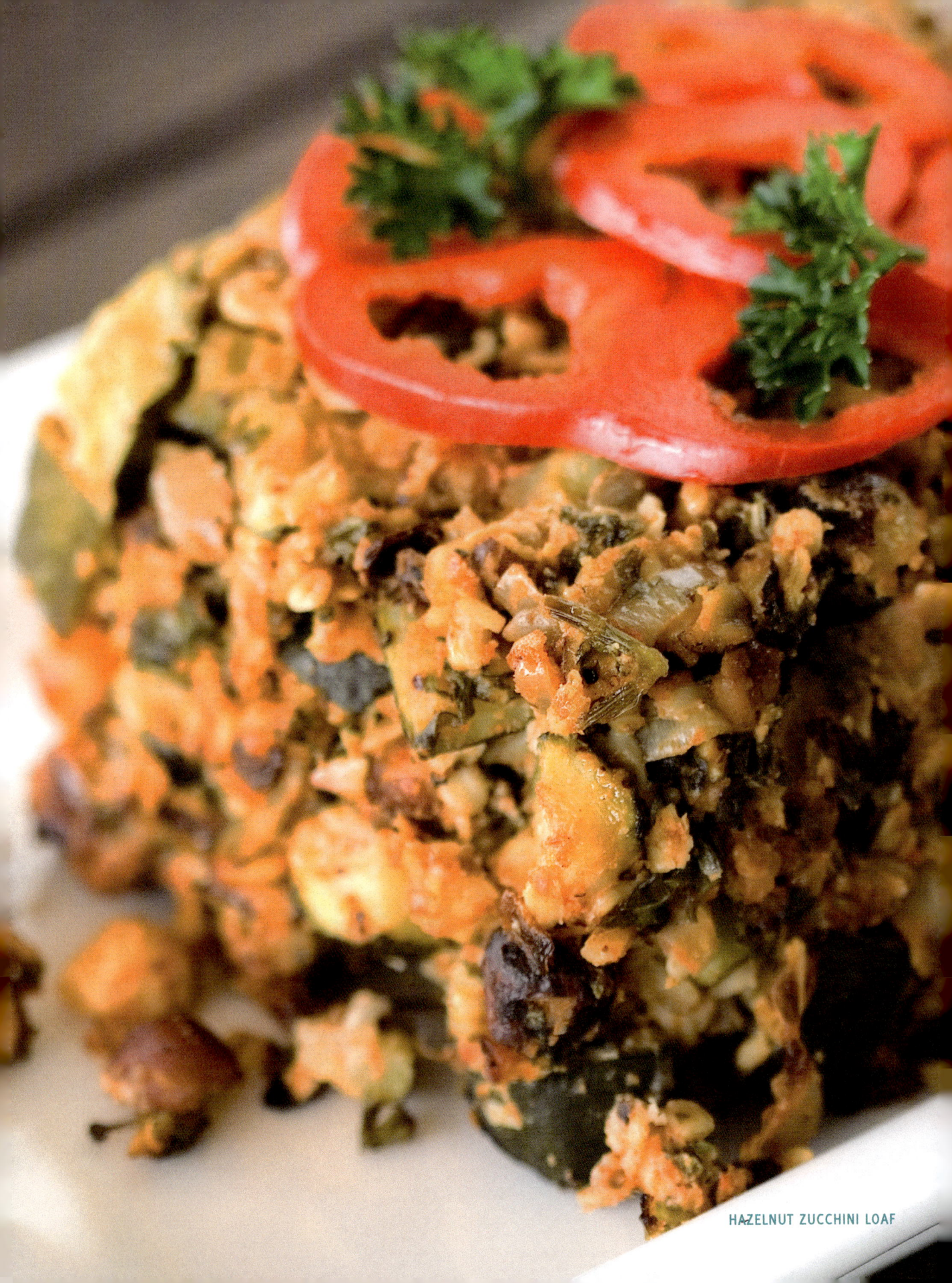

HAZELNUT ZUCCHINI LOAF

# Vegetables

## Ratatouille  A B C

- 1 medium eggplant
- 2 medium zucchini
- 2 red capsicums
- 10 cloves of garlic
- 2 medium onions
- 6 tomatoes

Place the capsicums under the grill and turn frequently until they are evenly charred. Set to one side until they are cool enough to handle; peel and slice lengthwise into 4cm strips. Meanwhile pierce the skin of the tomatoes, dunk in boiling water for a few minutes until the skin splits, then drain, peel and chop the flesh, discarding the seeds. Set aside. Halve the zucchini lengthwise and scoop out the seeds; then slice lengthwise into 4cm strips. Prepare the eggplant by slicing lengthwise into 4 cm thin strips. Thinly slice the onions and water fry, adding the garlic. As soon as they begin to turn translucent, add the eggplant and continue cooking until it softens, then add the zucchini and the capsicum and give a good stir. Pour in the chopped tomatoes, stir briefly and place on a very low heat, cover and cook until the zucchini is just cooked. Do not stir but make sure the mix doesn't stick to the pan. Leave to cool before serving.

## Hazelnut zucchini loaf  A B C
### SERVES 4

- 150g hazelnuts, coarsely chopped
- 50g sunflower seeds
- 50g of ground almonds
- 500g of zucchini
- 1 onion, chopped
- 4 cloves of garlic, crushed
- 6 tablespoons lemon juice
- Grated zest from 1 lemon
- ¾ cup parsley, finely chopped
- 200g canned tomato (salt-free), chopped or milled
- 75g rolled oats
- Freshly ground black pepper

Water fry the onion and garlic until translucent. Halve the zucchini and scoop out the seeds, then dice. Add to the onion mix and cook for a further 5 minutes until soft. Meanwhile dry roast the hazelnuts and sunflower seeds in a frying pan, agitating so that they do not burn. In a large bowl mix the nuts, ground almonds, vegetable mixture, lemon juice and rind, parsley, oats and tomato. Grind some black pepper into the mixture. Turn into a loaf tin lined with greaseproof paper that has been lightly greased with oil, placing the tin in a shallow tray of hot water. Cover and bake at 180°C for an hour. Remove the cover 30 minutes before the end of cooking. Serve with brown rice, green beans and the basic tomato sauce (p238).

## Eggplant lasagne A B C

**SERVES 4**

- 750g eggplant, sliced lengthwise into 1 cm slices
- 275g red capsicum, charred and skinned
- 6 tablespoons olive oil
- 2 large cloves garlic, crushed
- 2 tsp dried oregano
- 15 sun-dried tomatoes, soaked in boiling water for 30 minutes

For the creamed tofu:
- 400g tofu
- 1 tablespoon fresh basil, finely chopped
- 1 clove of garlic, crushed
- 3 tablespoons lemon juice
- 1 tablespoon olive oil
- 1 cup of basic tomato sauce (p238)

Mix the 6 tablespoons of olive oil with the garlic and oregano. Lightly brush the slices of eggplant with the olive oil mixture and place in a single layer under the grill, turning to brown each side. Meanwhile, blend the ingredients for the creamed tofu together. Squeeze the excess water from the sun-dried tomatoes. Slice the roasted capsicum. Spread     cup of the tomato sauce over the base of a baking dish. Cover with a layer of eggplant and spread half the creamed tofu over the eggplant. Place half the sun-dried tomatoes and capsicum over the tofu and repeat this layering ending with a layer of eggplant. Pour the tomato sauce over the dish and bake in a preheated oven at 180°C for around 30 minutes.

## Pilau rice A B C

**SERVES 4**

- 2 cloves garlic
- 1 medium onion
- 3 cloves
- 3 bay leaves
- 1 cinnamon stick
- 2-3 cardamom pods
- A pinch of garam masala
- 4 cups of chicken or vegetable stock
- 2 cups of short grain brown rice

Water fry the onion and garlic until softened. Add all spices and continue to cook. Add rice and stir thoroughly. Pour in the stock and bring the mixture to the boil. Lower the heat and cover, simmering for 35-40 minutes or until all the liquid is absorbed.

## Red cabbage & apple A B C

**SERVES 2**

- ¼ red cabbage, finely sliced
- 1 onion, finely sliced
- 1 green apple, peeled and thinly sliced
- Small handful of raisins

Water fry the onion over a low heat in a little water until it starts to release its own juices. Add the apple, raisins and later the red cabbage. Cover with a tight fitting lid and cook for 45-60mins on a very low heat, checking occasionally to make sure that it doesn't stick or burn.

*Vegetables*

## Nut moussaka        B C

SERVES 4

- 1 kg eggplant sliced into ½ cm thick rounds
- 6-8 tablespoons olive oil
- 3 large cloves garlic, crushed
- 1 tsp dried oregano

For the sauce:

- 2 tablespoons olive oil
- 1 onion, chopped
- 1 clove of garlic crushed
- 125g mushrooms, sliced
- 100g cashew nuts, coarsely chopped
- 3 tablespoons tomato puree
- 150mls spring water
- 1 green pepper de-seeded and sliced
- 2 tsp chopped fresh basil

For the topping:

- 500g plain yoghurt
- 4 eggs

Mix the olive oil with the garlic and oregano in a large bowl and lightly brush the eggplant with the oil. Grill the eggplant in a single layer turning until both sides are lightly browned and the eggplant is soft. Place to one side.

To make the sauce, water fry the onions and garlic until translucent and then add the mushrooms and pepper for a further 10 minutes. Stir in the cashew nuts, basil, tomato puree and water to make a thick sauce.

Place half the sauce in a baking dish measuring approximately 22cm x 32cm. Next place a layer of eggplant followed by the remaining sauce. Cover with the remaining eggplant slices. Beat the yoghurt and eggs together and top the moussaka with the yoghurt mixture. Bake at 190ºC until the top is set (approximately 15 -20 minutes).

## Cabbage & red capsicum        A B C

SERVES 2

- ¼ white cabbage, shredded
- 1 red capsicum, sliced thinly
- 1 onion, thinly sliced
- 2 medium tomatoes, chopped

Water fry the onion over a low heat in a little water until it starts to release its own juices. Add the capsicum and later the tomato. Finally, add the shredded cabbage and cover with a lid. Cook over a very low heat until done.

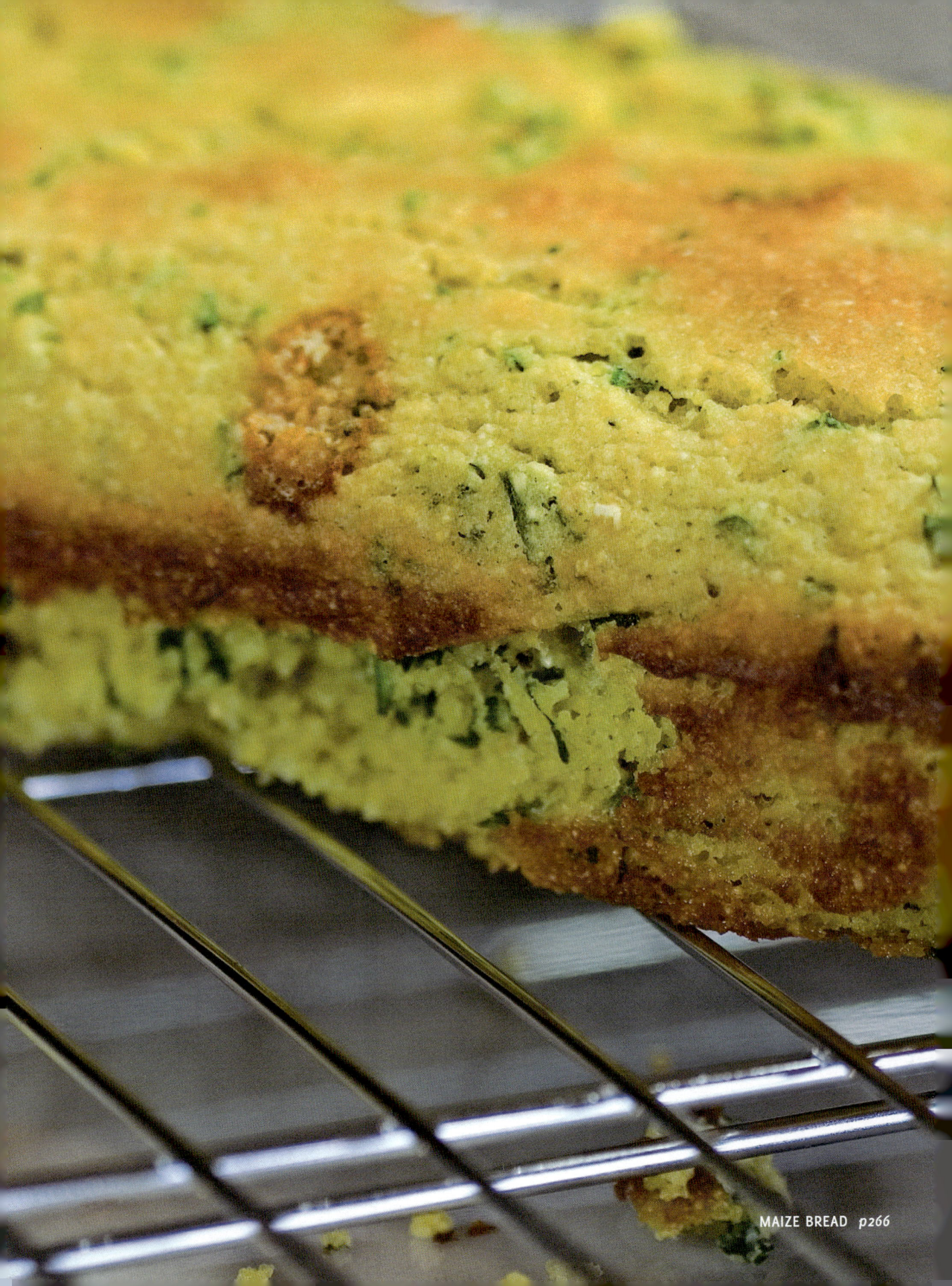

MAIZE BREAD  p266

# Extras

Fruit scones  *266*
Granola biscuits  *266*
Honey cheesecake  *266*
Maize bread  *266*

Recipes

## Fruit scones  B C

MAKES 8

- 50g buckwheat flour
- 125g brown rice flour
- 2 tsp Low Allergy Baking Powder
- 50g unsalted butter
- 50g dried fruit
- 100g grated apple with skin
- 6 tablespoons milk or soy milk

Preheat oven to 230°C. Sift flours and baking powder together and rub in butter. Add dried fruit and apple and mix to a soft dough with the milk. Drop mixture with a spoon onto a greased baking sheet. Bake in oven for 15-20 minutes and cool on a wire tray.

## Maize bread  B C

- 175g maize meal (cornmeal)
- 1½ tsp Low Allergy Baking Powder
- 1 egg
- 150mls yoghurt or soy yoghurt
- 1 tablespoon chopped chives
- 1 tablespoon chopped parsley
- 2 tsp honey
- 2 tablespoons olive oil

Preheat the oven to 200°C. Mix the cornmeal with the baking powder, add the beaten egg, yoghurt, honey and oil. Pour into a greased tin and bake for 15-20 mins. Turn out to cool. You can make a sweet loaf by exchanging the herbs for 75g of raisins and 50g chopped walnuts.

## Granola biscuits  B C

- 50g unsalted butter or ¼ cup olive oil
- 2 tablespoons honey
- 100g oatmeal
- 100g granola (homemade as per recipe p199)
- 75g chopped nuts
- 50g rice flour
- ½ tsp Low Allergy Baking Powder

Preheat the oven to 200°C. Melt the butter or oil with the honey and stir into all the dry ingredients mixing well. Grease a shallow rectangular tin or a round cake tins and press the mixture in firmly. Bake for 15-20 minutes. Cut when cool.

## Honey cheesecake  B C

- 1 kg tofu
- ½ cup safflower oil
- 1 cup honey
- 3½ tablespoons lemon juice
- 1 tablespoon vanilla essence
- ¼ mixture for granola biscuit, baked as a base

Heat the oven to 180°C. Blend all the ingredients for the cheesecake and pour onto the baked biscuit base. Bake for one hour. Serve chilled with fresh fruit.

CHEEKY!

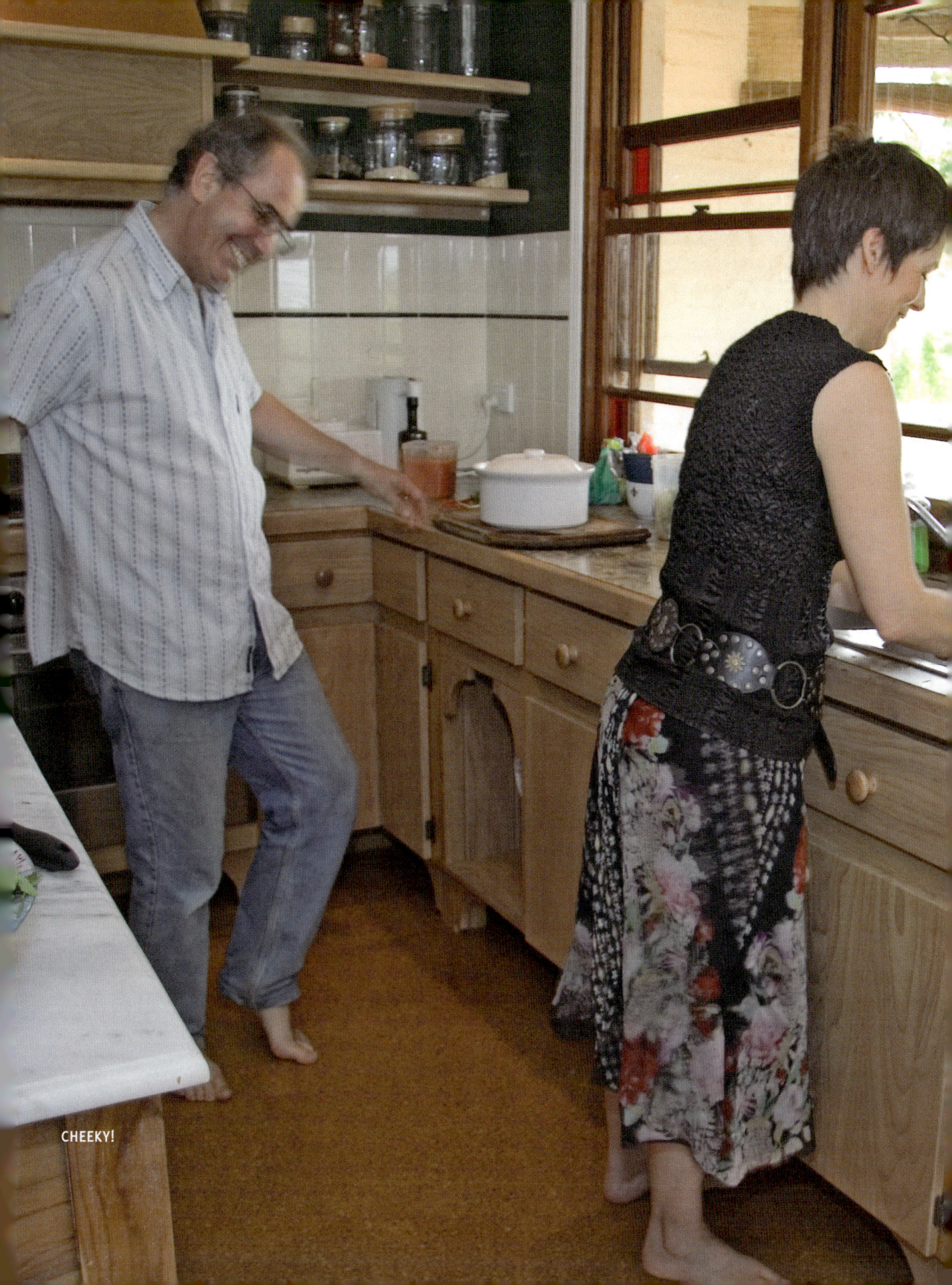

# Glossary

**A**

**adenosine triphosphate (ATP):** the chemical energy of the body.

**acetylation:** the transfer of an acetyl group to a compound during conjugation reactions in the liver.

**acylation:** the transfer of an amino-acid, such as glycine or taurine, during conjugation reactions in the liver as in the conversion of bile acids to bile salts.

**ADHD (Attention Deficit Hyperactive Disorder):** a condition where the brain is physiologically less active (less reactive brain waves), leading to a poor concentration span, while the body is more physically active (hyperactive).

**adrenaline:** a hormone secreted by the adrenal glands in response to stress and low blood sugar. It stimulates the liver to convert glycogen to glucose to raise blood glucose levels. The release of adrenaline can cause hot and cold sweats, shaking, heart palpitations and panic attacks.

**Advanced Glycosylation End-products (AGEs):** formed by the cross linking of glucose and proteins along capillary walls. They are usually formed when there is poor management of glucose, as in diabetes and insulin resistance. Long-term inflammatory reactions at these sites lead to neuropathy, retinopathy and nephropathy.

**alpha lipoic acid:** an anti-oxidant that protects against oxidative damage in both water and fat phases. It is particularly beneficial against oxidative damage in the capillaries in diabetes and insulin resistance. It contains a thiol group (sulphur) and can chelate heavy metals.

**amino acids:** the building blocks of protein.

**anaemia:** relates to any condition that reduces the capacity of the red blood cells to transport oxygen to the tissues.

**anovulation:** failure to ovulate during the menstrual cycle.

**anti-oxidants:** a group of nutrients which protect our tissues from oxidative damage, often termed anti-ageing factors. They include the vitamins A, C, E, beta-carotene, and the mineral selenium.

**apoproteins:** small water soluble peptide units (from proteins) produced by the liver to aid in the processing, packaging and transport of fats. The liver requires a good source of protein, magnesium and vitamin B6 to synthesise apoproteins.

**arteriosclerosis:** hardening of the arteries caused by calcium and fat deposits within the arterial wall.

**ASD (Autistic Spectrum Disorders):** an umbrella group of disorders including autism, Asperger's syndrome, Rett's Disorder, Pervasive Developmental Disorder (PDD) and Child Disintegrative Disorder (CDD).

**atheroma:** an abnormal mass of fat or lipids deposited in an arterial wall. Literally means "porridge".

**B**

**beta-glucuronidase:** an enzyme produced by intestinal bacteria that cleaves the oestrogen-glucuronide bond allowing free oestrogen to be reabsorbed from the intestinal tract into the systemic circulation. Calcium D-glucarate may be taken as a supplement to inhibit this enzyme and facilitate the elimination of oestrogen.

**bile acids:** synthesised from cholesterol in the liver and is the pathway for cholesterol degradation and elimination from the body. They are essential for the solubility of bile (acts as an emulsifier) and the prevention of gall stones; and aids in the emulsification and digestion of dietary fats.

**bile:** the main secretory product of the liver, stored in the gall bladder and aids the digestion of fats. It contains water, bile acids, lecithin and cholesterol and is the medium for the elimination of toxins. It is also the body's natural laxative.

**bilirubin:** a breakdown product of haemoglobin from worn out red blood cells and cleared by the liver. Failure to clear bilirubin, which occurs in blockage of the bile ducts (as in gall stones) or cholestasis, causes jaundice.

## C

**calcium (Ca):** a major mineral found mainly outside the cells which governs muscle contraction, blood coagulation and integrity of membranes. 90% of calcium is stored in the bones. RDI: 600mg - 1,000mg. Amounts greater than 1,000mg serve no useful purpose.

**calcium d-glucarate:** a phytonutrient found in oranges, grapefruit and broccoli; important for the elimination of oestrogen.

**carbohydrate (CHO):** a dietary nutrient broken down to glucose to provide our main source of energy

**cardiac asthma:** impaired breathing due to heart failure.

**catalyse:** to speed up chemical reactions

**chelation:** the use of a chemical substance to bind with a metal or mineral to facilitate its removal from the body.

**cholestasis:** a stoppage or slowing of the flow of bile in the biliary ducts of the liver, usually due to gall stones or liver damage.

**cholesterol:** a sterol related to fat compounds. Found exclusively in foods of animal origin. The liver synthesises its own cholesterol therefore a dietary source is unnecessary. High fat, high sugar diets promote the formation of excess cholesterol. Elimination occurs through its conversion to bile acids by the liver. Inhibition of this pathway (nutrient deficiencies, contraceptive pill, sex hormone replacement therapy) may exacerbate gall stones, atheroma and heart disease.

**choline:** one of the raw ingredients of lecithin; essential for the metabolism of fats.

**co-factor:** a mineral or a vitamin required by an enzyme system for function. For example, iron is a co-factor for haemoglobin and enables the uptake of oxygen.

**conjugation:** the transfer and binding of a naturally available substance to a foreign or potentially toxic substance rendering it water-soluble for detoxification.

**cysteine:** a sulphur-containing amino acid required for the detoxification of a range of toxins including heavy metals.

**cytochrome p450 oxidases:** a group of 50-100 enzymes responsible for oxidation-reduction reactions in Phase 1 liver detoxification. These enzyme systems are also active within the cells.

## D

**diabetes mellitus:** reduced or absent insulin production by the pancreas leading to high blood glucose concentration, acidosis and impaired carbohydrate, protein and fat metabolism. Uncontrolled diabetes leads to coma and death.

**diindolylmethane (DIM):** a bio-available indole, a phytonutrient found in cruciferous vegetables which promotes the metabolism of oestrogen to its weaker form.

**dilatation:** to open up passageways, airways or blood vessels enabling an increase in blood or air flow.

**dimethylglycine (DMG):** a methyl donor, important in methylation reactions during detoxification and the synthesis of brain chemicals (neurotransmitters). A supplement commonly used in autism and ADHD to improve concentration and mood.

**disaccharides:** two glucose units: maltose, lactose and sucrose

**docosahexanoic acid (DHA):** A long chain essential fatty acid of the omega 3 series found in fish oils. Important for the brain and the eyes.

**dysbiosis:** an unhealthy balance of bacteria, fungi and/or parasites in the large intestine.

## E

**emulsifier:** usually refers to a compound which increases the solubility of fats in a water environment by breaking the fats into minute globules so that they are dispersed throughout the fluids. Lecithin and bile acids are strong emulsifiers.

**endogenous:** a substance produced by the body.

**endotoxin:** a toxin produced by the body.

## Glossary

**enzyme:** a protein manufactured by living cells that catalyses the conversion of one substance to another via chemical reactions.

**eicosapentanoic acid (EPA):** A long chain essential fatty acid of the omega 3 series found in fish oils.

**exogenous:** a substance that originates from a source outside the body.

**exotoxin:** an environmental toxin; from a source outside the body.

**extracellular:** refers to the environment outside the cell

### F
**fat-soluble:** mixes with fats or organic solvents but not with water.

**free radicals:** molecules which contain highly reactive, negatively charged atoms which will attack and destroy cell membranes and intracellular structures ultimately causing cell death. Formed naturally in the body during metabolism. Usually deactivated by the anti-oxidants. Pollution increases the free radical load on the body.

**functional liver detoxification profile (FLDP):** A laboratory test that indicates the relative activity of the liver detoxification pathways.

### G
**gamma-linolenica acid (GLA):** active form of linoleic acid, converted by the liver from linoleic acid (omega 6 series). A high fat diet combined with nutrient deficiencies inhibits this conversion. Deficiency of GLA leads to cell permeability and eczematous lesions. Evening Primrose Oil is a natural source of this fatty acid.

**glucagon:** a hormone released by the pancreas in response to a falling blood glucose concentration. It stimulates the liver to convert stored glucose (glycogen) to glucose.

**glucocorticoid hormone:** commonly referred to as corticosteroid, a hormone released by the adrenal glands in response to stress or low blood sugar. It stimulates the breakdown of body protein which can be used for energy, sparing glucose for the brain and nervous system. It is important for moderating inflammatory conditions.

**glucogenic acids:** acids formed during the initial metabolism of carbohydrates and specific amino acids which enter the energy cycle via the glucose pathway.

**glucose:** a simple sugar found in carbohydrate rich foods. An important source of energy for the brain and the nervous system.

**glucuronidation:** a conjugation pathway important for the detoxification of bilirubin and oestrogen.

**glutathione:** a tripeptide composed of glycine, glutamic acid and cysteine; important as an antioxidant and as a conjugating agent in the glutathione detoxification pathway.

**glutathione-S-transferase:** an enzyme that transfers toxins to the glutathione conjugating detoxification pathway.

**glycogen:** glucose as stored by the body in the liver and muscles. It is the human form of starch.

**glycination:** the conjugation of compounds with glycine for detoxification, such as in the conversion of bile acids to bile salts.

### H
**hepatic:** pertaining to the liver

**histamine:** a chemical released by mast cells during an allergic reaction leading to hives, asthma and eczema.

**homocysteine:** an intermediate metabolite produced from the incomplete recycling of methionine, usually due to a deficiency of B12, folic acid and/or B6. Elevated levels are a risk factor for heart disease.

**hormones:** complex chemical compounds released from various endocrine glands into the circulation where they target specific tissues stimulating activity.

**hypertension:** high blood pressure.

### I
**indole 3 carbinole (I3C):** a phytonutrient found in cruciferous vegetables that promotes the conversion of oestrogen to its weaker form.

**inflammatory response:** a symptom of both healing and disease, often accompanied by fever. A protective reaction by the body to irritation or injury. An inflammatory response that resolves naturally without the use of medication indicates a high vitality or healing capacity.

**inositol:** a raw ingredient of lecithin, essential for the metabolism of fats. It also inhibits cholesterol synthesis in the liver.

**insulin:** a hormone secreted by the pancreas in response to rising blood glucose levels. It facilitates the uptake of glucose by the cells for energy or storage thereby reducing blood glucose concentration. It is also important in the metabolism of fats, carbohydrates and proteins.

**insulin resistance:** a reduction of insulin receptors at the cell membrane leading to relative insulin resistance and a rise in both blood sugar and insulin.

**intracellular:** refers to the environment within the cell.

## K

**ketogenic acids:** acids created by the initial metabolism of fats and some proteins which enter the energy cycle via the fat pathway.

**kidney filtrate:** formed when blood circulates through the kidney filtration system which separates blood cells and blood proteins from the fluids. Most of the fluids, along with nutrients, are reabsorbed by the kidney while excess nutrients, acids and various waste products, are concentrated and excreted in the urine.

## L

**lactase:** the enzyme which breaks down milk sugar.

**lactose:** a disaccharide composed of glucose and galactose; commonly found in milk (milk sugar).

**leaky gut:** a condition when the gastrointestinal tract becomes permeable to dietary substances which gain access to the systemic circulation and may cause reactions. Dysbiosis or allergic reactions at the gut may be causative factors.

**lecithin:** a phospholipid essential for the metabolism of fats and the elimination of cholesterol. Deficiencies lead to diseases of the nervous system, liver, kidney and heart. Important also for the integrity of the cell membrane.

**linoleic acid:** an essential fatty acid of the omega 6 series found in nuts, seeds, whole grains and unrefined cold-pressed oils, such as sunflower and safflower oils. Heating of these oils destroys the biological value of these fatty acids and they behave as saturated fats. It stimulates the manufacture of lecithin by the liver and is therefore important in the reduction of liver fat in liver cleansing.

**linolenic acid:** an essential fatty acid of the omega 3 series found in oily fish and linseeds. It stimulates the manufacture of lecithin by the liver and is therefore important in reducing liver fat during liver cleansing. It also increases the clotting time of the blood and therefore is protective against heart disease and thrombosis.

**lipid:** a fat.

**lipo:** relating to fat

**lipoprotein:** a compound containing a fatty core of triglycerides and cholesterol surrounded by water-soluble components, lecithin and apoproteins. They are formed by the liver and exported as VLDLs (very low density lipoproteins) and converted to LDLs (low density lipoproteins) by the tissues. The liver also makes HDLs (high density lipoproteins) which are involved in the transport of cholesterol for elimination. HDLs are protective against heart disease, while high LDLs are associated with a greater risk of heart disease.

**lipotrophic agent:** a reducer of fat

**lipotrophic factors:** nutrients required by the liver for the manufacture of apoproteins and lecithin. Lipotrophic agents are simply reducers of liver fat.

**low density lipoprotein (LDLs):** A blood fat which contains more cholesterol than triglyceride. High levels indicate high cholesterol and are a risk factor in heart disease.

## M

**magnesium (Mg):** a major mineral found mainly inside the cell, involved in energy production, nerve impulse transmission, and muscle relaxation; maintains a high potassium environment within the cell and is involved in the secretion and activity of hormones. Necessary for absorption and retention of calcium. Optimum ratio between dietary calcium and magnesium should be no greater than 2:1. Tea, coffee and alcohol cause magnesium losses. RDI: 350mg.

**metabolic acids:** acids produced by the body during metabolism which cannot be eliminated via the lungs. A build up of these acids can accumulate on low carbohydrate, high fat and high protein diets. Elimination is slow (around 7 days) and occurs via the kidneys, which can lead to a cumulative acidic load on the body and a taxing of kidney function. Large amounts of these acids are produced in diabetes mellitus.

**metabolism:** the total of all biochemical reactions in the body. It is the "activity" of the body.

**metallothionein:** a sulphur-containing protein that chelates heavy metals. Zinc is required for its synthesis.

**methionine:** an essential sulphur-containing amino acid which is the parent compound for many detoxification reactions in the liver including methylation, sulphation and glutathionation.

**methylation:** the transfer of a methyl group (CH3) to a substance; important in detoxification pathways and in the synthesis of neurotransmitter chemicals.

**methylcobalamin:** the active form of B12; required by the central nervous system.

**methyltetrahydrofolate (5-MTHF):** the active form of folic acid.

### N

**N-acetyl cysteine (NAC):** the activated form of cysteine; an important antioxidant and chelator of heavy metals. Important in viral infection.

**neurotransmitters:** chemicals released from nerve terminals that are important for the transmission of nerve signals throughout the body via the nervous system and in the brain. Neurotransmitters include serotonin, acetylcholine, adrenaline, noradrenaline and dopamine.

### O

**obligatory loss:** the minimum amount of a nutrient required by the body to function.

**oedema:** fluid retention causing swelling particularly around the ankles, abdomen, hands, fingers and face.

**oestrogen:** a female sex hormone secreted by the ovaries associated with menstruation. Protective against body tissue breakdown. Loss of oestrogen at the menopause partly accounts for the accelerated loss of bone mass (osteoporosis) encountered by some women.

**oestrogen dominance:** a relative oestrogen dominance to progesterone deficiency. This situation is seen in anovulatory cycles and prior to and during the menopause.

**opioids:** short peptides, often derived from the incomplete digestion of milk and gluten (casomorphin and gliadorphin, respectively) that attach to opiate receptors in the brain.

**osteoporosis:** a greater than normal rate of bone loss resulting in decreased bone density and increased risk of bone fracture. Post-menopausal women are particularly vulnerable.

### P

**parathyroid hormone (PTH):** a hormone secreted by the parathyroid glands which maintains blood calcium concentrations when levels fall. It regulates absorption of calcium from the gut, the movement of calcium from the bones and increases the retention of calcium by the kidneys.

**pathogens:** any micro-organism capable of producing disease. (Pathogenic: disease causing).

**phenol:** a chemical found in many fruits and vegetables that may mimic our neurotransmitters and create learning and concentration difficulties, if not detoxified.

**phenol sulfotransferase (PST):** the enzyme responsible for the detoxification of phenols, particularly by the brain.

**phospholipids:** a class of compound within the body containing phosphoric acid, fatty acids and a nitrogenous base. It mixes with both fats and water and is therefore important in the packaging and transport of fats and forms the lipid bi-layer at the cell membrane. Lecithin is the main phospholipid in the body.

**polycystic ovarian syndrome (PCOS):** a condition where many follicular cysts develop in the ovaries. This is usually due to anovulatory cycles where the ovum fails to mature and be released.

**polyunsaturated fatty acids (PUFAs):** these are found in whole grains, nuts and seeds, and the oils of these products. Linoleic and linolenic acid are examples of PUFAs. The extraction and processing of these oils renders them biologically inactive and they behave as saturated fats. Diets high in unrefined PUFAs stimulate the production of lecithin which reduces cholesterol levels in the body.

**potassium (K):** a major mineral and the key mineral within the body cell. Regulates nerve transmission, muscle tone and the energy cycle. RDI 2,500mg - 6,000mg.

**progesterone:** a female sex hormone secreted by the ovarian follicle. Associated with the second phase of the menstrual cycle, development of the placenta and maintenance of pregnancy.

**pyridoxal-5-phosphate (P5P):** an activated form of vitamin B6.

## R

**RDI:** recommended daily intake referring to food nutrients.

## S

**S-adenosylmethionine (SAMe):** the activated form of methionine which donates methyl groups for detoxification, oestrogen metabolism and the synthesis of neurotransmitters. It is a useful supplement for depression and oestrogen dominance with cholestasis, gall stones and/or jaundice.

**salicylate:** a naturally occurring substance found in brightly coloured fruits, vegetables and nuts, and used as a food preservative which may cause adverse reactions in chemically sensitive individuals. Salicylates are chemically related to phenols.

**sodium (Na):** a major mineral governing the fluids outside the cells. Involved in transmission of nerve impulses, fluid balance and the acid/alkaline balance. RDI: 1,000mg-2,000mg

**synthesise:** to manufacture or make.

## T

**thimerosal:** a mercury-containing preservative, commonly used in vaccinations.

**thiol:** a sulphur-containing group found in many compounds that have anti-oxidant properties or involved in detoxification pathways.

**thrombosis:** a blood clot which may occlude a blood vessel reducing blood supply to the area. In the heart this is known as a coronary thrombosis and in the brain, cerebral thrombosis or stroke.

**trimethylglycine (TMG):** commonly known as betaine, a methyl donor and co-factor in the regeneration of homocysteine to methionine.

**toxin:** a poison which damages living cells and may be difficult to eliminate by the body.

**triglycerides:** principle fat found in the blood. Manufactured by the liver and consists of three fatty acids attached to a glycerol nucleus. Fatty acids are transported to tissues as triglycerides to be used for energy or building blocks in cell membranes. Diets high in saturated fat promote triglyceride formation.

**tumour necrosis factor (TNF):** a chemical released by the body during inflammation which causes the shrinkage and death of tumours.

## V

**visceral adipose tissue (VAT):** fats that are deposited in the internal organs.

**volatile acids:** acids produced by the body during metabolism which can be eliminated through the lungs. Carbonic acid is a volatile acid.

## W

**water-soluble:** mixes with water but not with fats or organic solvents.

# Index

## A
**acid-forming foods** 57, 61
**acid/alkaline balance**
    dietary contributions 56
**acidity**
    calcium, precipitation of 40
    degenerative disease 40
    fats and 61
    neutral foods 65
    protein 62
    renal elimination 55, 62
    sodium 40, 62
**acids**
    glucogenic 55
    ketogenic 55
    metabolic 55
    volatile 55
**acrylamides** 210
**ADHD**
    dysbiosis 147
    food sensitivities 141
    potassium status 40
**advanced glycosylation end products** 76, 122, 170
**alcohol**
    blood sugar, effects on 166
    insulin and 166
    oestrogen metabolism 153
**aldehydes** 128, 142
**allergies**
    dysbiosis 186
    food 104, 140
    food, table 128
    inflammation 75
    prostaglandins 180

**alpha lipoic acid** 130
    chelation 145, 149
**Alzheimer's disease** 122
    degenerative disease, and 76
    heavy metals 144
**amines**
    food 127
    food sensitivities, table 128
**animal protein**
    dietary recommendations 197
**antibiotics**
    dysbiosis 186
    liver fat 110
**antioxidants** 184
**apple cider vinegar** 58
**arthritis**
    enteropathic 101
    inflammatory process in 75
**ASD** 146
**Asperger's syndrome** 146
**assessing vitality, chart** 75
**asthma**
    allergy, food 140
    allergy, food table 128
    calcium 48
    eczema link 86, 100
    magnesium 48
**autism** 146
    dysbiosis 147
    food sensitivities 141
    mercury 146
**autoimmune disease**
    chronic inflammation 76
    food sensitivities 142–143

## B
**B12**
    homocysteine metabolism 135
**B6**
    blood sugar control 165
    homocysteine metabolism 135
**beetroot**
    juicing and blood sugar 58
**beta-glucuronidase** 138
**betacarotene**
    food sources 186
**bile**
    contents of 103
    toxin removal 79, 103
**bile acids**
    cojugation of 134
    fibre, role of 115–116
    recycling of, diagram 116
    synthesis from cholesterol 103
**bilirubin clearance**
    Gilbert's syndrome 136
    oestrogens 136, 138
**blood sugar**
    alcohol, effects on 166
    dietary regulation, tips 166
    fibre 166
    hormonal influences 162
**blood sugar, low**
    *See* hypoglycaemia
**bowel flora products** 186
**B vitamins**
    food sources, table 182

## C
**calcium**
    asthma 45, 48
    average food values, table 43, 46

eczema 45
food sources, table 178
magnesium balance 42
magnesium imbalance, symptoms of 49
obligatory loss 44
RDI 42
renal clearance 44
vitamin D 42
**calcium D glucarate** 139
**cancer**
    Gerson Therapy 59
    hormone-sensitive 136
    immune response 79
    inflammation, role of 80
    liver, free radicals 129
    xeno-oestrogens 123
**candida**
    aldehydes 128
    allergy 186
    chronic fatigue syndrome 128
**carbohydrates**
    energy source 65
    insulin, response to 160
    percentage in foods, table 67
**carbonic acid** 54, 55
**casomorphin** 141
**castor oil pack**
    method 85
**celery**
    juicing 58
**chamomile tea enema** 120
**chelation**
    heavy metals 144
    nutrients involved in 144-145
**chemical sensitivities** 127
**child disintegrative disorder** 146
**chlorella** 150
    chelation 145
**cholesterol**
    content in foods, table 113
    conversion to bile acids 111

fibre, role of 116
heart disease 116
insulin resistance 168
precursors for synthesis 111
**Christopher, Dr. J.**
    regenerative diet 59
    three-day cleanse 59
**chromium**
    blood sugar control 167
**chronic fatigue syndrome**
    candida 128
    case study 78
**cilantro, heavy metal removal** 145, 150
**clay**
    diarrhoea 84
**clay pack**
    method and preparation 86
**clostridia** 141
**coeliac disease** 143
**coffee enema** 119
    method 120
    toxic crisis 83
**constipation** 104
    oestrogen dominance 138
**contraceptive pill**
    *See also* oral contraceptives
    bile salt metabolism 111
**cortisone**
    blood sugar metabolism 162
**cruciferous vegetables** 138

**D**

**dairy products**
    dietary recommendations 197
**dehydration**
    causes of 175
**depression** 145
    brain chemicals 145
    iodine deficiency 146
    oestrogen dominance 146
    stress 146
**dermatitis** 104
    inflammation 75

**detoxification**
    *See* liver detoxification
**detoxification crisis**
    management of 83, 89
    symptoms of 89
**DHA**
    *See* docosahexanoic acid
**diabetes**
    complications of 76, 170
    exercise 171
    fructose 171
    heart disease 170
    inflammation 75
    insulin resistance, diagram 169
**diarrhoea**
    clay, use of 84
**dietary recommendations** 197-200
**digestive enzymes** 142
**dimethylglycine (DMG)** 135
**disease crisis**
    management of 86
    symptoms of 80
**DMSA**
    chelation 144, 145
**docosahexanoic acid (DHA)** 153
    brain signalling 153, 180
    food sources 180
**dysbiosis**
    ADHD, autism 141, 147
    antibiotics 186
    herbs for 186
    immune suppression 186
    iodine deficiency 141
    phenols 141

**E**

**eczema** 104
    allergy, food 140
    allergy, food table 128
    asthma, link 86, 100
**eggs**
    dietary recommendations 197

**eicosapentanoic acid (EPA)** 153
    food sources 180
**eliminative channels** 96
    kidneys, symptoms in 102
    liver, symptoms of congestion 103
    lymphatic system, symptoms in 96
    mucous membranes, symptoms 101
    skin, symptoms in 100
**endometriosis** 136
**enemas**
    chamomile tea 120
    coffee 119
    herbal 120
**energy cycle**
    nutrients required 55
**enteropathic arthritis** 101
**EPA**
    See eicosapentanoic acid
**essential fatty acids**
    See also EPA, DHA
    hydration 180
    inflammation, role in 180
**evening primrose oil** 153, 180
**extra-cellular matrix**
    composition of 175

**F**

**fasting**
    keto-acid production 60
**fat intolerance**
    liver detoxification 134
**fats**
    acidity 61
    percentage in foods, table 67
**fats and oils**
    dietary recommendations 200
**fever**
    management of 84, 90
**fibre**
    blood sugar control 162, 166
**fibre, insoluble**
    nutrient deficiencies 116

**fibre, soluble**
    bile acids 116
    cholesterol, reduction of, diagram 117
    foods 115
    oestrogen clearance 138
    toxin removal 116
**fibrocystic breast disease** 136
    iodine deficiency 138
**fibroids** 136
**fibromyalgia** 142
**flaxseed oil** 153, 180
    dietary recommendations 200
**folinic acid**
    oestrogen metabolism 139
**follicle stimulating hormone** 137
**food allergies** 104
    See also food sensitivities
    allergic reactions 128
    dairy 142
    Phase 1 liver detoxification 127–128
    Phase 2 liver detoxification 140
    reactions, table 128
    wheat 142
**food cravings**
    blood sugar control 158
**food intolerances** 104
**food sensitivities**
    ADHD, autism 141
    allergic reactions 128, 140
    amines, table 128
    phase 2 liver detoxification 140
    phenols and salicylates 141
**food tables**
    B vitamins, food sources 182
    calcium, food sources 178
    calcium and magnesium, average values 43
    calcium and magnesium, average values per portion 46
    cholesterol and lipotrophic nutrients 113

    CHOs, fats and proteins, percentage in foods 67
    magnesium, food sources 178
    selenium, food sources 184
    sodium values in seasoning and snacks 36
    vitamin C, food sources 185
    vitamin E, food sources 185
**free radicals**
    antioxidants 184
    chronic disease 75
    liver detoxification 130
**fructose**
    blood sugar 166
    diabetes 143, 171
**fruits**
    dietary recommendations 200
**functional liver detoxification (FLDP)**
    profile 132
**fungal overgrowth**
    See dysbiosis

**G**

**gall stones**
    case study 118
    cholesterol metabolism 106
    glycination pathway 134
    oestrogen metabolism 134
**gamma-linolenic acid** 153
    food sources 180
**gelatin, hydration** 176
**genetic variance**
    liver detoxification 124, 133
**Gerson, Dr. Max** 38
    inflammation, role in cancer 80
**Gerson Therapy** 59
    coffee enema 119
**GLA**
    See gamma-linolenic acid
**glandular fever** 97, 106
    case study 99
**gliadorphin** 141
**globe artichoke** 130

**glucogenic acids** 55
**glucuronidation**
    oestrogen clearance 136, 138
**glutamine**
    colonocytes, fuel for 142
**glutathione**
    free radicals 130
**glutathione-S-transferase**
    coffee enema 119, 130
    free radicals 130
    herbal support for 130
**gluten intolerance** 141, 143
**glycogen**
    hepatic synthesis 160
**glycoproteins, hydration** 176
**glycosaminoglycans**
    food sources 176
    hydration 175
**gout** 56
**grains**
    dietary recommendations 199
    preparation of 198
**green juice, recipe** 58
**green tea** 130
**gruel, in detoxification** 83

**H**

**healing crisis**
    management of 84, 89
    suppression of 80
    symptoms of 80, 84, 89
**heart disease**
    cholesterol and 116
    diabetes 170
    homocysteine 135
    inflammation 75
    liver congestion 105
    magnesium 48
**heavy metals**
    ADHD, ASD 144
    cancer 144
    chelation 144
    chronic degenerative disease 144

    depression 144
    detoxification 144
    environmental exposure 123
    epilepsy 144
    iodine deficiency 144, 149
    selenium, in detoxification 145
    vaccination 147
**hepatitis** 106
**histamine, allergy** 140
**homocysteine** 135
**honey**
    dietary recommendations 201
**hydration** 175
    glycosaminoglycans 177
    water intake 176
**hyperactivity**
    *See* ADHD
**hyperglycaemia**
    *See* diabetes
**hypoglycaemia**
    ageing, effects on 165
    alcohol, effects on 166
    case study 163
    magnesium, role in 162
    regulation by liver 105, 160
    stimulants, effects on 162
    symptoms of 158, 159

**I**

**immune response, healing reaction** 96
**immune tolerance** 140
**indole 3 carbinole** 138
**infertility**
    liver congestion 105
    oestrogen dominance 136
    xeno-oestrogens 123
**inflammation**
    chronic disease 75, 76
    cycle of, diagram 77
    healing response 79
    scar tissue formation 77, 122
**inositol**
    cholesterol, reduction of 116

**insulin**
    alcohol, effect on 166
    antagonism by hormones 162
    blood sugar control 160
    glycogen synthesis, and 160
**insulin-dependent diabetes (IDDM)** 170
**insulin resistance**
    cholesterol synthesis 168
    depression 146
    iodine deficiency 169
**iodine deficiency**
    breast cancer, risks 138
    depression 146
    dysbiosis 141
    heavy metals 144, 149
    insulin resistance 169
**irritable bowel syndrome** 142
    food sensitivities 141

**J**

**jaundice** 103

**K**

**ketogenic acids** 55
**kidneys**
    acidity, removal of 102
    calcium, control of 44
    pH, control of 102

**L**

**leaky gut** 142
**lecithin** 181
    content in foods 113
    structure of 109
    synthesis of 110
**legumes**
    dietary recommendations 198
    preparation of 198
**lemon barley, recipe** 117
**lemons, juicing** 58
**linoleic acid**
    cholesterol metabolism 111
    food values, table 114
**lipoic acid**
    *See* alpha lipoic acid

lipoproteins
    packaging by the liver  108
liver congestion
    hormonal imbalance  105
    symptoms of  103-106
liver detoxification
    bilirubin  136
    chemical sensitivities  127
    food sensitivities  127
    genetic variance  124, 133
    herbs, support for  130
    oestrogen clearance  134, 136, 138
    phase 1, nutrients required, table  131
    phase 1, overactive  129
    phase 1, underactive  127
    phase 2, nutrients required  133
    phase 2, nutrients required, diagram  135
    phase 2, nutrients required, table  152
    phase 2 pathways  132
    sulphation pathway, diagram  144
    two phases of  126
low blood sugar
    *See* hypoglycaemia
low density lipoproteins (LDLs)
    cholesterol  116
Lugol's solution  149
luteinizing hormone  137
lymphatic system  96-98
    congestion, symptoms of  97
    toxins, removal of  79

## M

magnesium
    asthma  45, 48
    average food values, table  43, 46
    blood sugar control  162
    calcium balance  42-44
    calcium imbalance, symptoms of  49
    deficiency, refined grains  43
    deficiency, symptoms of  48
    depleting factors  44
    eczema  45
    energy  47, 162, 165
    food cravings  47
    food sources, table  178
    heart disease  48
    high blood pressure  45
    muscle cramps  47
    nerve impulse  47
    RDI  32
    sodium/potassium pump  47
mercury
    hair analysis  147
    removal, tips on  149
    vaccination  147
metabolic acids  39
    renal elimination  55, 56
methionine  133
methionine-homocysteine pathway
    nutrients required, diagram  135
methylcobalamin  151
migraine, hormonal  136
milk protein allergy  142
minerals
    competitive inhibition  182
    elemental weight in supplements  182-183
mono-amine oxidase inhibitors (MOAIs)  127
mono-amine oxidases (MAOs)  127
multiple chemical sensitivities  128
multiple sclerosis
    heavy metals  144

## N

n-acetylcysteine (NAC)  130
    chelation  145, 149
neutral foods
    acidity  65
non-insulin-dependent diabetes (NIDDM)
    onset of, diagram  169

## O

obligatory loss
    calcium  44
    sodium  35
oestrogen dominance  136-139
    case study  118
    causes of  137
    symptoms of  136-139
oestrogen metabolism
    bilirubin clearance  138
    fibre, role in  138
    folinic acid  139
    gall stones  134
    glucuronidation  134, 136
    liver detoxification  138-139
    methylation  134, 138
    phase 1 liver detoxification  138
    phase 2 liver detoxification  138
    s-adenosyl methionine  134
oestrogens, environmental  123
    infertility, effects on  123
omega 3 series  153
    prostaglandins  180
omega 6 series  153
    prostaglandins  180
oral contraceptives
    *See also* contraceptive pill
    bile salt metabolism, inhibition of  111, 115, 118
    ovulation, inhibition of  137

## P

pain
    management of  84-86, 90
parathyroid hormone
    calcium metabolism  44-45
pathological detoxifier  129
pervasive developmental disorder  146
Phase 1 liver detoxification
    nutrients required, table  131
phase 2 liver detoxification
    nutrients required, diagram  135

phenols
    ADHD, autism  141
    brain signal inhibition  141
    depression  141
    detoxification of  141
    digestion of  141
    dysbiosis  141
    food sensitivities  141
phenol sulphotransferase  141
    ADHD, autism  147
phosphatidyl choline
    structure of  109
phytic acid
    neutralisation of  198
poly-cystic ovarian syndrome (PCOS)
    iodine  138
potassium
    average values, processed foods  37
    RDI  36
    sodium exchange for  38, 39
    sodium ratio  32
pre-menstrual syndrome
    liver congestion  105
prebiotics  143, 186
pregnancy
    detoxification during, case study  66
prostaglandins
    allergy, inflammation  180
prostatic hypertrophy, role of oestrogens  138
protein
    acidity  62, 63
    average values in foods, table  61
    combining second-class  63
    percentage in foods, table  67
    requirements  61, 63
    stress  63
psoriasis  104
    arthritic  101
    inflammation  75

R
recipes
    avocado & kiwi fruit salsa  244
    barley with dried fruit compote  219
    bean & nut roast  249
    bean goulash  248
    bean salad with tuna  229
    beetroot salad  233
    bircher muesli  218
    broad bean soup with mint  222
    brown rice salad, nuts & vegetables  233
    brown rice salad, parsley & pine nuts  230
    cabbage & red capsicum  263
    cashews & zucchini with buckwheat  229
    cassoulet  253
    chicken stock  239
    chickpea burgers  249
    chickpea flour pancakes  228
    coleslaw with savoury tofu dressing  233
    cooked salad  234
    curried chickpeas  250
    curried tofu  251
    dahl soup  222
    eggplant dip  243
    eggplant lasagne  262
    eggplant omelette  224
    fava bean dip  240
    fish with roasted vegetables  253
    fish with tandoori marinade  255
    fresh fruit salad with yoghurt  219
    fruit scones  266
    gazpachio  223
    granola  219
    granola biscuits  266
    gravy  239
    guacamole  243
    hazelnut zucchini loaf  261
    honey cheesecake  266
    hummus  228
    Indian curry paste  245
    Indian dosas  252
    laksa  256
    lentil burgers  248
    lentil curry  250
    maize bread  266
    Mexican chilli with corn tortillas  251
    minestrone soup  223
    muesli  218
    nut moussaka  263
    paella  254
    pasta with creamy lentil sauce  250
    pasta with tuna & tomato sauce  254
    pilau rice  262
    porridge  218
    potato salad  234
    raita  244
    ratatouille  261
    red cabbage & apple  262
    salad nicoise  234
    savoury tofu dressing  235
    seviche with Mediterranean salsa  255
    soaked muesli with fresh fruit  218
    Spanish omelette  224
    spicy eggplant  243
    spicy Moroccan lentils  227
    spicy mushroom sauce  238
    spinach & red capsicum salad  233
    sun-dried tomato & chilli pesto  240
    sun-dried tomato, lemon & garlic pesto  240
    tahini dip  243
    Thai-style yellow curry with fish  258
    Thai chicken green curry  257
    Thai fish red curry  257
    Thai fish salad  256
    Thai green curry paste  245
    Thai red curry paste  245
    tofu garlic dip  240
    tomato & coriander salsa  244
    tomato & red capsicum sauce  238
    tomato sauce  238
    tuna risotto  256
    vegetable stock  239
    vinaigrette  235

wild rice salad with orange & mint 230
yoghurt fruit salad dressing 219
**Rett's disorder** 146

## S
**s-adenosyl methionine (SAMe)**
    oestrogen metabolism 134
**salicylates**
    food sensitivities 141
**schizandra** 130
    liver detoxification 130
**selenium** 184
    food sources 184
    glutathione 145
    heavy metal detoxification 145, 150
**serotonin**
    depression 145
**short chain fatty acids (SCFAs)**
    colonocytes, fuel for 142
**sodium**
    acidity 40, 62
    average values, processed foods 37
    elimination, renal 38
    extracellular/intracellular ratio 38
    obligatory loss 35
    potassium exchange for 36, 38, 39
    potassium ratio 32
    RDI 35
    sweat losses 35
**sodium/potassium pump** 38
    magnesium 47
**soy products**
    dietary recommendations 199
    phytosterols 200
    thyroid function 200
**stimulants**
    blood sugar, effects on 162
**St Mary's thistle** 130
    liver detoxification 130
**stress**
    depression 146
    insulin resistance 168

protein breakdown 63
**sulphation pathway**
    liver detoxification, diagram 144
**sunflower seed oil**
    dietary recommendations 200
**syndrome X**
    *See* metabolic syndrome

## T
**TCM, liver disharmony** 125
**thimerosal, vaccination**
    autism, incidence of 147
**thyroid function**
    soy products and 200
**tofu**
    phytates 200
**tonsillitis** 103
**toxic crisis**
    coffee enema 83
    management of 83, 89
    symptoms of 83, 89
**toxins**
    breast milk 101
    cellular elimination 56
    dioxins, PCBs 123
    endogenous 39
    environmental 123
    foetal exposure 101
    xeno-oestrogens 123
**trans fats, dehydration** 180
**trimethylglycine (TMG)** 135
**turmeric** 130
    liver detoxification 130

## V
**vaccination** 73
    autism, incidence of 147
    mercury toxicity 147
**vegetable juices**
    ingredients for 58
**vegetables**
    detoxification, amounts required 57
    dietary recommendations 197-198

energy values 57
protein value 63
**vitality**
    chronic disease 75
    drug medication 74
    infectious illness 73
    measuring 72, 75
    stress, effects of, diagram 98
    suppression of 74
**vitality questionnaire** 193
**vitamins**
    B
        food sources, table 182
    B6
        blood sugar control 165
    C
        RDI 185
    D
        calcium absorption 42
        food sources, table 179
        RDI 179
    E
        food sources 185
        RDI 185
**volatile acids** 55

## W
**water frying** 200, 210
**water intake**
    hydration 176
**weight loss**
    muscle bulk 162
**wheat protein allergy** 142

## X
**xeno-oestrogens**
    *See* oestrogens, environmental

## Z
**zinc**
    blood sugar control 167
    deficiencies 183
    vegetarianism, and 183

Made in the USA
Charleston, SC
08 August 2014